ROBOTIC SURGERY IN OTOLARYNGOLOGY HEAD AND NECK SURGERY

***System requirements*:**

- **Operating System—Windows Vista or above**
- **Web Browser—Google Chrome, Mozilla Firefox, Internet Explorer 9 and above**
- **Essential plugins—Java & Flash player**
    - Facing problems in viewing content—it may be your system does not have Java enabled.
    - If Videos do not show up—it may be the system requires Flash player or need to manage Flash setting. To learn more about Flash setting click on the link in the help section.
    - You can test Java and Flash by using the links from the help section of the CD/DVD.

Accompanying CD/DVD Rom is playable only in Computer and not in DVD player.

CD/DVD has Autorun function—it may take few seconds to load on your computer. If it does not works for you then follow the steps below to access the contents manually:

- Click on My Computer
- Select the CD/DVD drive and click open/explore—this will show list of files in the CD/DVD
- Find and double click file—"launch.html"

For more information about troubleshoot of Autorun click on:
http://support.microsoft.com/kb/330135.

ROBOTIC SURGERY IN OTOLARYNGOLOGY HEAD AND NECK SURGERY

Editor

Nilesh R Vasan MD FRACS
Associate Professor
Jesus E Medina Chair in Otolaryngology
Department of Otolaryngology—Head and Neck Surgery
The University of Oklahoma
Health Sciences Center
Oklahoma City, Oklahoma, USA

Foreword

Jesus E Medina

JAYPEE *The Health Sciences Publisher*
New Delhi | London | Panama | Philadelphia

Jaypee Brothers Medical Publishers (P) Ltd

Headquarters
Jaypee Brothers Medical Publishers (P) Ltd.
4838/24, Ansari Road, Daryaganj
New Delhi 110 002, India
Phone: +91-11-43574357
Fax: +91-11-43574314
E-mail: jaypee@jaypeebrothers.com

Overseas Offices
J.P. Medical Ltd.
83, Victoria Street, London
SW1H 0HW (UK)
Phone: +44-20 3170 8910
Fax: +44(0)20 3008 6180
E-mail: info@jpmedpub.com

Jaypee-Highlights Medical Publishers Inc.
City of Knowledge, Bld. 237, Clayton
Panama City, Panama
Phone: +1 507-301-0496
Fax: +1 507-301-0499
E-mail: cservice@jphmedical.com

Jaypee Medical Inc.
The Bourse
111 South Independence Mall East
Suite 835
Philadelphia, PA 19106, USA
Phone: +1 267-519-9789
E-mail: jpmed.us@gmail.com

Jaypee Brothers Medical Publishers (P) Ltd.
17/1-B, Babar Road, Block-B, Shaymali
Mohammadpur, Dhaka-1207
Bangladesh
Mobile: +08801912003485
E-mail: jaypeedhaka@gmail.com

Jaypee Brothers Medical Publishers (P) Ltd.
Bhotahity, Kathmandu, Nepal
Phone: +977-9741283608
E-mail: kathmandu@jaypeebrothers.com

Website: www.jaypeebrothers.com
Website: www.jaypeedigital.com

Inquiries for bulk sales may be solicited at: jaypee@jaypeebrothers.com

Robotic Surgery in Otolaryngology—Head and Neck Surgery

First Edition: 2016

ISBN: 978-93-5152-901-9

Printed at Ajanta Offset & Packagings Ltd., New Delhi

Dedicated to

My wife Dimple and sons Dylan and Krish

Contributors

Eun Chang Choi MD PhD
Professor and Chairman
Department of Otorhinolaryngology
Yonsei University, College of Medicine
Director
Yonsei Head and Neck Cancer Center
Severance Hospital
Yonsei University Health System
Seoul, South Korea

Woong Youn Chung MD PhD
Professor
Chief, Endocrine Surgery Division
Department of Surgery
Yonsei University, College of Medicine
Seoul, South Korea

Julia A Crawford MBBS FRACS
Advanced Head and
Neck Surgical Fellow
Florida Hospital Celebration Health
Florida, USA

William S Duke MD
Assistant Professor
Department of Otolaryngology
Associate Surgical Director
GRU Thyroid and Parathyroid Center
Georgia Regents University
Augusta, Georgia, USA

Umamaheswar Duvvuri MD PhD
Assistant Professor
Director of Head and
Neck Robotic Surgery
University of Pittsburgh
VA Pittsburgh Health System
Pittsburgh, Pennsylvania, USA

Peter T Dziegielewski MD FRCSC
Assistant Professor
Head and Neck Oncologic and
Microvascular Reconstructive Surgery
Department of Otolaryngology
University of Florida
Florida, USA

Eric M Genden MD FACS
The Isadore Friesner Professor and
Chairman of Otolaryngology—
Head and Neck Surgery
Professor of Immunology
Professor of Neurosurgery
The Icahn School of
Medicine at Mount Sinai
New York, USA

Tamer Abdel-Halim Ghanem MD PhD
Henry Ford Health System
Detroit, Michigan, USA

Ehab Hanna MD FACS
Professor and Vice Chairman
Director of Skull Base Surgery
Department of Head and Neck Surgery
Medical Director Head and Neck Center
University of Texas
MD Anderson Cancer Center
Houston, Texas, USA

Emad Kandil MD FACS FACE
Edward G Schlieder
Chair in Surgical Oncology
Chief, Endocrine Surgery Section
Department of Surgery
Tulane University School of Medicine
New Orleans, Louisiana, USA

Yoon Woo Koh MD PhD
Professor
Department of Otorhinolaryngology
Yonsei Head and Neck Cancer Center
Yonsei University, College of Medicine
Seoul, South Korea

Michael E Kupferman MD
Associate Professor
Department of Head and Neck Surgery
MD Anderson Cancer Center
Houston, Texas, USA

Jandee Lee MD PhD
Department of Surgery
Yonsei University, College of Medicine
Seoul, South Korea

J Scott Magnuson MD FACS
Chief Medical Officer
Florida Hospital Celebration Health
Professor of Otolaryngology—
Head and Neck Surgery
University of Central Florida
College of Medicine
Medical Director Head and Neck Surgery
Celebration Health
Director, Robotic Head and Neck
Surgery
Florida Hospital
Nicholson Center for Robotic Surgery
Florida Hospital Nicholson Center
Global Faculty Board Member
Florida, USA

Vikas Mehta MD MPH FACS
Assistant Professor
Otolaryngology—
Head and Neck Surgery
Director of Robotic—
Head and Neck Surgery
LSU Health Shreveport
Department of Otolaryngology
Shreveport, Louisiana, USA

Anya Joyce Miller MD
Henry Ford Health System
Detroit, Michigan, USA

Salah E Mohamed MD
Division of Endocrine and
Oncologic Surgery
Department of Surgery
Tulane University
School of Medicine
New Orleans, Louisiana USA

Enver Ozer MD
Associate Professor
Department of Otolaryngology—
Head and Neck Surgery
Wexner Medical Center at
The Ohio State University
Columbus, Ohio, USA

Eitan Prisman MD FRCSC
Assistant Professor
Vancouver Hospital and Health Sciences Centre
Vancouver, BC Canada

Chelsey J Smith MD
Head and Neck Fellow
Department of Otolaryngology—Head and Neck Surgery
The University of Oklahoma
Health Sciences Center
Oklahoma City, Oklahoma, USA

David J Terris MD FACS
Surgical Director
GRU Thyroid and Parathyroid Center
Georgia Regents University
Augusta, Georgia, USA

Betty S Tsai Do MD
Assistant Professor
Otology/Neurotology
Department of Otorhinolaryngology
The University of Oklahoma
Health Sciences Center
Oklahoma City, Oklahoma, USA

Raymond K Tsang MBChB FRCSEd(ORL) FHKCORL FHKAM (Otorhinolaryngology)
Clinical Assistant Professor
Department of Surgery
University of Hong Kong
Queen Mary Hospital, Hong Kong, China

Nilesh R Vasan MD FRACS
Associate Professor
Jesus E Medina Chair in Otolaryngology
Department of Otolaryngology—Head and Neck Surgery
The University of Oklahoma
Health Sciences Center
Oklahoma City, Oklahoma, USA

William I Wei MS FRCS FRCSEd FRACS(Hon)
Director
Li Shu Pui ENT
Head and Neck Surgery Centre
Hong Kong Sanatorium and Hospital
Hong Kong, China

Hilliary N White MD FACS
Head and Neck Surgery Center of Florida
Florida Hospital Celebration Health
Associate Professor of Otolaryngology—Head and Neck Surgery
University of Central Florida
College of Medicine
Florida, USA

Foreword

The circle is now complete. The student has surpassed his mentor.

For an academician it is immensely gratifying to witness the gradual transformation of a student, learner into a master of his or her own trade. Nilesh Vasan, our Fellow in training a few years ago had the courage, discipline and creative hard work to gradually become an expert in a new and promising area of our discipline: *Robotic Surgery in Otolaryngology—Head and Neck Surgery*.

Commendably, Dr Vasan has channeled his latest efforts towards the production of a timely textbook in which he, and other respected clinicians, share what they have learned as they dedicated themselves to advancing robotic surgery in our specialty. They have collectively succeeded in preparing a valuable source in which trainees and practitioners of head and neck surgery will find excellent descriptions of anatomy from a pertinent perspective, innovative surgical instruments and techniques that are described with the subtle nuances that often can be only offered by someone who has taken part in their development. The book is generously illustrated throughout with color drawings of uniform style and high quality; they add considerably to the clarity of the descriptions.

The editor and all the contributing authors are to be praised for crafting a book that I am sure will be a welcomed addition to many personal and institutional libraries.

Jesus E Medina MD FACS
Professor
Department of Otolaryngology—
Head and Neck Surgery
Oklahoma City, Oklahoma USA

Preface

We now live in a time where it is possible to operate on our patients "removed" from the surgical table. Indeed what was previously depicted in science fiction is now a science fact.

Since the FDA approved transoral robotic surgery in late 2009, many Otolaryngologists—head and neck surgeons have taken the challenge to further their training and become credentialed in the use of the "da Vinci robotic surgical system".

The da Vinci robot is particularly well-suited for our patients; it enables us to operate in areas previously hard to access such as the base of tongue. Over the last few years, operations using the robot have been developed and taught by our colleagues who are at the forefront of this new technology thereby becoming the "pioneers" for robotic surgery. We are fortunate that these leaders are contributing authors for *Robotic Surgery in Otolaryngology—Head and Neck Surgery*.

Since robotics in Otolaryngology is still in its infancy, the operations that have been described in this book will almost certainly undergo significant change. Within short order, I would expect this book to become outdated and in fact this is what we should all want! Continued refinements in performing these operations, development of assistive tools and modifications to the da Vinci surgical system itself such as the new da Vinci XI system will, I am sure, make the current robotic system resemble a hammer in the not so distant future.

Robotic Surgery in Otolaryngology—Head and Neck Surgery has been structured so robotic head and neck procedures can be described and shown in a clear and concise manner with the use of photographs, diagrams and video; our hope is that others will take this information and further the field. This book has been divided into four sections where the robot is currently used. A section entitled "Robotic Procedures in Evolution" which describes robotic procedures that are currently in the process of study is included with the real possibility that they may one day become commonplace.

Nilesh R Vasan MD FRACS

Acknowledgments

It is an odd task to thank all the people who have in some way helped make this book possible because there are so many, beginning with my parents and teachers in New Zealand who pointed me in the right direction to those individuals that have encouraged and supported me during my adventures in the United States.

For *Robotic Surgery in Otolaryngology—Head and Neck Surgery*, I must thank my mentor and good friend Jesus E Medina MD FACS In addition to teaching me all his tricks during my Fellowship with him, he instilled and continues to so instill in me the importance of caring for our patients using the best available evidence and adopting innovation in medicine, when the evidence suggests that it is time to do so. It was back in 2009, after the FDA approved transoral robotic surgery, that he cornered me and gave me an Intuitive Surgical brochure saying "you should get into this".

I also wish to thank all the contributors who have taken time from their busy schedules to commit to this book. These individuals are leaders within our field that not only perform robotic surgery for otolaryngology—head and neck conditions but also assess, innovate, modify and publish their results so the rest of us can learn from them.

Finally, I must thank our patients who readily place their trust and ultimately their lives in our hands. They accept our recommendations and are often willing to undergo innovative new treatments in the hope of a cure for their own conditions and for the future care of others. They are truly the bravest people I know!

Finally, I would also like to thank Shri Jitendar P Vij (Group Chairman), Mr Ankit Vij (Group President), Ms Chetna Malhotra Vohra (Associate Director) and Ms Angima Shree (Development Editor) of M/S Jaypee Brothers Medical Publishers (P) Ltd., New Delhi, India.

Contents

Section 1: Transoral Robotic Surgery (TORS)

Section 2: Thyroid

Section 3: Head and Neck Reconstruction

Section 4: Robotic Procedures in Evolution

Video Legends

Video 1.1: Right transoral robotic radical tonsillectomy.

Video 2.1: TORS for base of tongue cancer.

Video 3.1: Right hypopharyngeal transoral robotic surgery.

Video 5.1: TORS-Lingual tonsillectomy and sleep nasoendoscopy.

Video 6.1: Robotic total thyroidectomy/central node dissection via right axillary approach.

Video 8.1: Robotic Thyroidectomy—Facelift Approach.

Video 9.1: Transoral robotic surgery free flap.

Video 12.1: Robotic-Assisted Surgery for recurrent Nasopharyngeal cancer.

Section 1

Transoral Robotic Surgery (TORS)

Chapter Outline

- Transoral Robotic Surgery for Tonsil Cancer
- Transoral Robotic Surgery for Base of Tongue Tumors
- Transoral Robotic Surgery—Hypopharynx
- Transoral Robotic Supraglottic Laryngectomy (TORS-SGL)
- Transoral Robotic Surgery for Obstructive Sleep Apnea

Chapter 1 Transoral Robotic Surgery for Tonsil Cancer

Julia A Crawford, Hilliary N White, J Scott Magnuson

INTRODUCTION

Unlike the decreasing incidence of laryngeal, oral and hypopharyngeal squamous cell carcinoma (SCC), the incidence of oropharyngeal squamous cell carcinoma (OPSCC) has shown a marked increase over the past decade.[1-3] Corresponding to this change in incidence has been the change in the overall patient demographic from that of an older population with a strong tobacco and alcohol history to that of a younger population with little or no history of either tobacco or alcohol use.

This increasing incidence is related to infection with the human papilloma virus (HPV) subtype 16 and 18 with up to 84% of HPV-associated head and neck cancers positive for HPV-16.[4-6] This is presumed to be due to societal changes in lifestyle and sexual behaviors that may predispose to infection in the oropharynx. The importance of this is related to the corresponding change in survival patterns. Compared with the traditional smoking-associated head and neck squamous cell carcinoma (SCC), HPV-related oropharyngeal carcinoma has a more favorable natural history and seems to be more responsive to treatment, irrespective of the treatment regime that is utilized.[3-4,7] Consequently, patients with HPV-positive malignancies tend to have better long-term survival than those with HPV-negative head and neck SCC and are more likely to experience chronic therapy-induced morbidity.[8] Thus, long-term quality of life considerations are even more relevant to the multidisciplinary team coordinating the care of these patients.[9]

The review of oropharyngeal carcinoma treatment by Parsons et al. (2002) reported on 6,400 patients with OPSCC treated with surgery, surgery plus radiotherapy or primary radiotherapy at North American academic medical institutions.[10] Despite a comparable cumulative 5-year survival between treatment groups, the radiotherapy alone treatment arm had a significantly decreased risk of severe complications.[11] This led the authors to recommend non-operative over operative management of these cancers regardless of stage. However, the rise of minimally invasive surgery adapted to suit the oropharynx has recently started to challenge this prevailing treatment strategy because of decreased morbidity associated with this form of treatment.[10,12-15]

RATIONALE FOR PROCEDURE

The issue with approaching the oropharynx surgically has always been one of access. The morbidity of this type of surgery was related to the severe disruption to the speech and swallowing musculature. Results of this type of dramatic surgery affected patients' quality of life due to disfigurement and the impact on their ability to participate in the social necessities of eating, drinking and speaking. In the context of purely transoral approaches for tonsillar carcinoma, this restricted surgical access limited the indications for transoral resections of malignant neoplasms to those confined to the tonsillar fossa without significant extension to the surrounding areas.[16] The aim of minimally invasive surgery is to reduce this morbidity without compromising oncologic outcomes.[17,18]

Reports of minimally invasive surgery for oropharyngeal carcinoma have burgeoned in recent years driven by a desire to offer a less morbid alternative to chemoradiation.[9] The potential for this has become increasingly important due to the change in epidemiology of oropharyngeal carcinoma with patients with HPV-related SCC having a better long-term survival than those with HPV-unrelated head and neck SCC. Furthermore, any new treatment paradigm that is aimed at reducing morbidity must do so without compromising local and regional tumor control rates.[8]

These minimally invasive approaches have included transoral laser microsurgery and, in more recent years, transoral robotic surgery (TORS).[19-28] In contrast to traditional open surgical resection, these endoscopic procedures provide excellent oncologic outcomes while preserving speech and swallowing function.[25,26] With appropriate adjuvant therapy, TORS achieves equivalent or superior oncologic results when compared to other surgical and nonsurgical treatments while also achieving excellent functional outcomes.[27] Furthermore, the key to preserving function of the oropharynx during cancer treatment is to minimize damage to the surrounding musculature and motor and sensory nerves of the pharynx and it is in this function that the role of TORS comes to the fore.[28]

APPLIED ANATOMY-RADICAL TONSILLECTOMY

The pharynx extends from the base of skull to the lower border of the cricoid cartilage and is divided into nasal, oral and laryngeal segments. The area of importance for TORS surgery is the oropharynx that extends from the soft palate to the epiglottis. The main sites of resection include the palatine tonsil and the pharyngeal base of tongue. When undertaking a TORS radical tonsillectomy, the anatomy is effectively made up of a box with superior, inferior, lateral and medial boundaries. The transoral approach to these anatomical boundaries is unique when compared to open surgery.

The superior border of the resection is dependent on the extent of tumor involvement of the soft palate. In beginning this part of the resection, the surgeon will dissect through the superior pharyngeal constrictors, supratonsillar space and muscles of the soft palate through to the posterior free edge of the palate. When moving on to address the lateral border, an incision is made through the mucosa of the retromolar trigone and subsequently through the superior pharyngeal constrictors to encounter the parapharyngeal space.

The superior pharyngeal constrictor muscle is separated from the underlying buccopharyngeal fascia by loose areolar tissue. Deep to this buccopharyngeal fascia lies the medial pterygoid superiorly and parapharyngeal space more inferiorly. The internal carotid artery is protected in the region of the parapharyngeal space only by a layer of fat and pulsations can often be appreciated in this region. The surgeon should avoid dissecting lateral to the pharyngeal fat pad so as not to encounter the internal carotid artery and so that this fat provides protection to the carotid arterial system postoperatively.[29]

The lateral and inferior borders merge in the region of the stylopharyngeus and styloglossus. The stylopharyngeus muscle spans from the base of the styloid process lateral to the superior constrictor before passing between the superior and middle constrictor muscles to attach onto the posterior border of the thyroid cartilage and the palatopharyngeus muscle. The styloglossus muscle is positioned more superficially and laterally to the stylopharyngeus and arises from the inferior and lateral edge of the styloid process broadening out as it descends to insert into the lateral aspect of the tongue. Following identification of these muscles, the surgeon will typically encounter the glossopharyngeal nerve.

The inferior border is defined by the tongue base and is largely composed of lymphoid tissue. The degree of anatomy encountered will depend on the extent of the tumor. The most important structure to be aware of in this area is the lingual artery that lies on the medial border of the hyoglossus muscle. The final and medial border of the box is the posterior pharyngeal mucosa and musculature merging with the superior border at the soft palate.

INDICATIONS AND CONTRAINDICATIONS

The introduction of TORS to the treatment armamentarium for oropharyngeal carcinoma has significantly widened the scope for surgery as the primary treatment modality. Since Food and Drug Administration (FDA) approval in 2009, multiple studies have shown favorable outcomes using TORS for the treatment of early, late and recurrent stage oropharyngeal malignancies.[24-28]

As such, the primary indication for TORS is any biopsy proven SCC of the oropharynx where there is adequate intraoral access. Currently, the FDA has approved TORS for T1 and T2 stage tumors only. The contraindications for TORS can be broken down into tumor- and nontumor-related reasons (Table 1.1).

If the tumor has a large soft palate component and resection would result in significant long-standing velopharyngeal insufficiency then other treatment options should be considered. A locally advanced tumor involving the pterygoid muscles, bone, extrinsic muscles of the tongue, prevertebral muscles or the carotid on imaging should not be approached operatively. Involvement of these structures is likely if the tumor is fixed on palpation. Similarly, in these circumstances the patient will have significant trismus that impairs trans-oral access. Patients who have advanced or unresectable neck disease are unlikely to benefit from surgical resection as they will require postoperative chemoradiotherapy.

Table1.1: Surgical indications and contraindications for TORS Radical Tonsillectomy

Indications	
• Biopsy proven squamous cell carcinoma of the oropharynx • T1, T2 stage tumors (FDA)	
Relative contraindications	
• Anatomical limitations to intraoral access • Anatomical limitations to neck extension • Aberrant carotid artery anatomy • Medical contraindications to transoral surgery in which an open wound heals by secondary intention • Resultant defect postresection that limits patients speech and/or swallowing • Likely treatment requiring chemoradiotherapy	
Absolute contraindications	
Tumor-related	*Nontumor-related*
• Stage IVC disease • Pharyngeal involvement requiring resection of >50% of the posterior pharyngeal wall • T4a disease with mandibular or hard palate invasion, medial pterygoid involvement with resultant trismus or deep involvement of the tongue base to the level of the genioglossus • Radiological evidence of carotid artery involvement • Fixation on palpation with radiological evidence of invasion lateral to the constrictors or posterior into the prevertebral fascia • Unresectable neck disease	• Medical contraindications for either general anesthesia or surgery

Nontumor-related factors include significant medical comorbidities that increase anesthesia risk or increase postsurgical risk. The need for anticoagulation may also affect the decision to pursue a surgical route. Patients who have difficult intraoral access or limited neck extension may not be surgical candidates.

PREOPERATIVE ASSESSMENT

The National Comprehensive Cancer Network includes the following in their 2013 guidelines for the initial evaluation and work-up of OPSCC: history and physical, biopsy, tumor HPV testing, chest imaging, computed tomography (CT) with contrast and/or magnetic resonance imaging of both the primary site and neck, consideration of positron emission tomography CT for stage III-IV disease, dental evaluation as indicated and examination under anesthesia as clinically indicated. Furthermore, multidisciplinary consultation should be arranged as indicated.[30]

For TORS, there are specific considerations that affect the feasibility of robotic surgical intervention. These relate to the contraindications stated previously. First a physical examination is performed to assess limitations to access and tumor resectability. A mild degree of trismus could indicate extension beyond the constrictor muscles into the pterygoid musculature. Additionally, on palpation, the tumor should not be fixed to the lateral tissues.

Radiographic imaging will aid in determining the degree of infiltration of the tumor into the parapharyngeal space and lateral neck. This helps the evaluation of surrounding structures such as the pterygoid muscles and carotid artery. Finally, staging endoscopy under a general anesthetic confirms tumor resectability by evaluating the intraoral accessibility of the tumor and the full extent of the tumor.

INSTRUMENTATION

General Surgical Instruments

The necessary general surgical instruments include a headlight, Yankauer suction, a suction electrocautery device, long forceps and a Hurd retractor, tonsil dissector and pillar retractor.

Access Instruments

Two commonly used mouth gags include the Davis-Meyer gag (Karl Storz America) and the Feyh-Kastenbauer-Weinstein-O'Malley retractor (Gyrus ACMI, Germany). Each system includes multiple tongue blades of different lengths and shapes that are typically sufficient for the procedure. The retractor system is suspended upon a stationary table or a suspension arm that is fixed to the side of the surgical bed.

Robotic Instrumentation

The surgery is performed with the da Vinci Surgical System manufactured by Intuitive Surgical, Sunnyvale California. The robotic instrumentation includes a high definition camera and the articulated instruments arms. The two high definition cameras that are used during TORS surgery include a 0° and 30° camera. For radical tonsillectomy, the 0° camera is used, while for base of tongue surgery the 30° camera allows better visualization. Both the 12 mm and the 8 mm diameter scopes have excellent optics and allow for adequate working space in

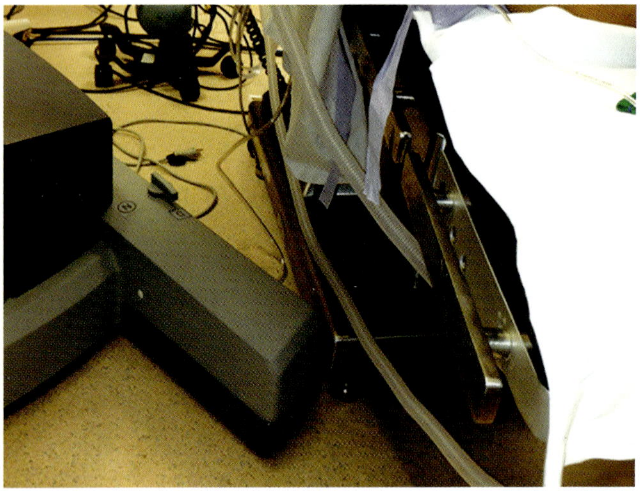

Fig. 1.1: The surgical robot base forms a 30° angle with the operating table to achieve optimal deployment of the robotic arms.

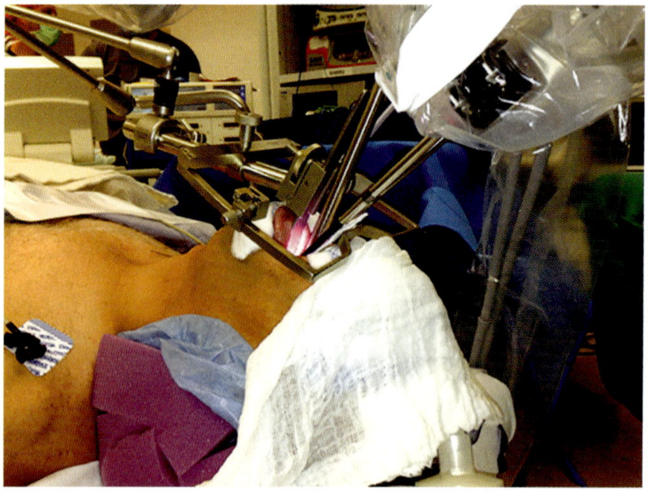

Fig. 1.2: The patient in suspension with the robotic arms docked.

the mouth. They provide magnification up to 10×, resulting in a clear three-dimensional image.

In addition to the camera in the working space, two additional instruments are used. These 5 mm articulated EndoWrist instruments include a grasping instrument and a cautery instrument. A compatible laser fiber can be used in place of the cautery instrument.

OPERATIVE SETUP

The patient is positioned supine and intubated with a nasotracheal tube, preferable through the nares opposite to the tumor. The patient's head is then turned 180° from the anesthesia cart. A stitch is placed in the anterior portion of the tongue to assist in retraction and positioning of the tongue. The mouth gag is placed to provide adequate exposure of the primary tumor using a surgical headlight for visualization. At this point the surgical table is lowered to the lowest position possible. The robotic patient side cart is then wheeled to the bedside towards the patient's head such that the base of the robot is approximately at a 30° angle with the base of the surgical table (Fig. 1.1). The robotic base may be on the patient's left or right side depending on the room setup.

The three robotic arms are aimed towards the patient's mouth and positioned in a triangular format (Fig. 1.2). The camera is placed in the center arm and the grasping instrument and cutting instrument are placed in the side arms. The grasping instrument should be placed on the contralateral side to the tumor. The instruments are inserted into the patient's mouth so that the apexes of the instruments meet at the area surrounding the tumor. Care should be taken to ensure that the instruments themselves will not clash, that their movement will not be obstructed by intraoral structures and that they safely move within the patient's oral cavity.

OPERATIVE TECHNIQUE

Transoral robotic surgery procedures are designed around the philosophy of en bloc resection. For radical tonsillectomy, the borders of resection include the soft palate superiorly, the pterygoid muscles and mandible laterally, the base of tongue inferiorly, the posterior pharyngeal wall medially and the constrictor muscles and parapharyngeal fat as the deep margin.

The initial incision is made along the soft palate through the superior constrictor muscles until the parapharyngeal fat is identified (Fig. 1.3). Next, the incision is carried laterally down to the tongue base following the medial pterygoid muscle (Fig. 1.4). At this point, the lingual nerve may be identified and care must be taken to avoid injury. Blunt dissection in the parapharyngeal fat using the cautery tip is helpful to identify blood vessels. Vessels that are encountered may be managed with hemoclips or electrocautery (🎥 1.1).

Next, the inferior margin is incised along the base of tongue (Fig. 1.5). This allows medial rotation of the tumor. The stylopharyngeus and styloglossus muscles are divided to complete the resection of the deep margin (Fig. 1.6). Finally, the medial margin is incised along the posterior pharyngeal wall (Fig. 1.7). Keeping close attention

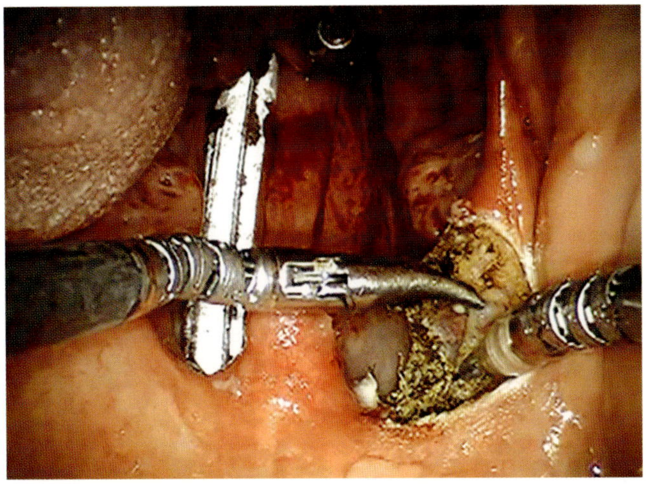

Fig. 1.3: Superior border through soft palate and superior constrictors.

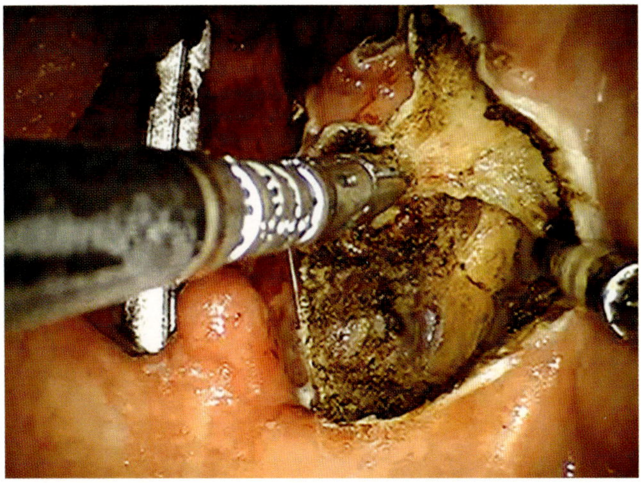

Fig. 1.4: Lateral border showing parapharyngeal fat and medial pterygoid.

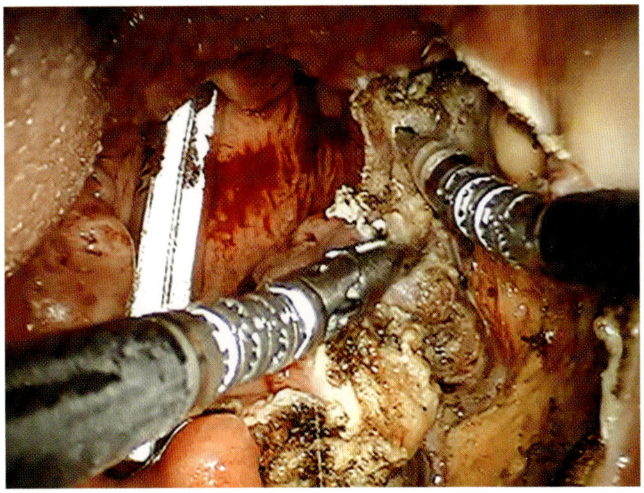

Fig. 1.5: Inferior border through lingual tonsil. The submandibular gland is also seen.

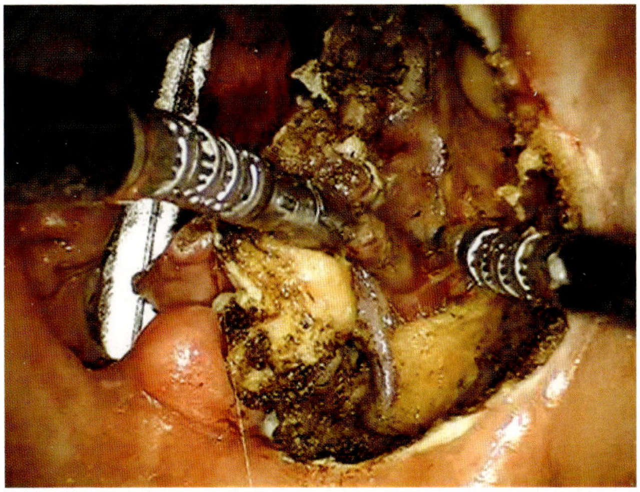

Fig. 1.6: The cut end of styloglossus is held in the Maryland forceps.

to the correct anatomical configuration of the resected specimen, the tumor is removed by the assistant and the margins are appropriately marked by the primary surgeon (1.1).

Final inspection of the surgical bed is performed to ensure adequate hemostasis. Throughout the resection, the bedside assistant is helpful by providing additional traction, suction, placement of hemoclips and cautery.

The robot is then removed from the patient's bedside and the patient is taken out of suspension. For large resections, a nasogastric feeding tube is placed under direct visualization and secured to the nasal septum with a suture. The patient's bed is then rotated back to the anesthesia service where the patient is awakened and extubated.

EARLY POSTOPERATIVE CONSIDERATIONS

The most serious postoperative issues relate to tongue-base swelling, hemorrhage and airway compromise. Procedures lasting < 40 minutes typically cause little tongue-base swelling. Perioperative intravenous steroids also help limit swelling. Immediate postoperative hemorrhage may occur as a result of the release of occlusive pressure from the mouth-gag. This typically requires immediate return to the operative room for control of hemorrhage.

Airway compromise can occur as a result of tongue edema, postoperative hemorrhage or both. White et al. (2013) demonstrated the safety of immediate extubation

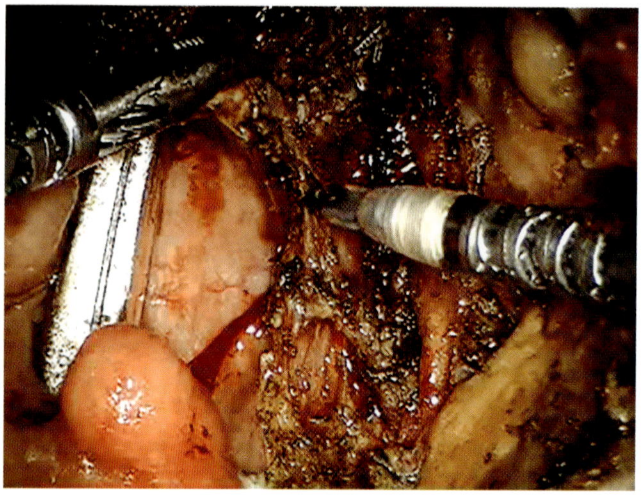

Fig. 1.7: The specimen is freed by cutting through the medial border of posterior pharyngeal wall mucosa and muscle.

and low incidence of serious postoperative complication allowing for hospital discharge on the first postoperative day.[31] On the day after surgery, prior to discharge, a speech pathologist assesses the patient for swallowing safety and determines the extent of immediate safe postoperative oral intake.

MANAGEMENT OF THE NECK

The staging and prognosis of oropharyngeal SCC is intimately tied to the status of the cervical lymph nodes. Between 66% and 76% of patients with tonsillar OPSCC will present with clinically positive nodal disease, most commonly in the jugulodigastric nodal group.[32] Due to the high risk of occult nodal disease, most clinicians recommend treating the neck for these primary tumors particularly as the instance of occult metastases in a clinically node-negative neck in OPSCC has been reported to be greater than 30% in some series.[33-34] The benefit of surgical management of the neck lies in its ability to provide important staging and prognostic information. Pathology of neck specimens provides information regarding size of metastases, number of involved nodes, presence of extracapsular spread, additional tumor deposits and micro metastases.

Neck dissection may be offered to patients as a staged or concurrent procedure. It is helpful to perform the neck dissection prior to the TORS operation so that major branches of the external carotid artery may be ligated. This may reduce the risk of serious intraoperative and postoperative hemorrhage during the TORS component of the patient's management.

MANAGEMENT OF COMPLICATIONS

Complications arising from TORS surgery may occur intraoperatively or postoperatively. Arterial bleeding during the procedure can be managed with either electrocautery or hemoclips. While rare, postoperative arterial bleeding may require operative management. Additionally, pharyngeal edema may occur within the first 24 hours following surgery. The development of edema can be reduced by limiting the length of time a patient is held in suspension and the administration of intravenous steroids. Observation in a high-acuity ward with specialty-trained nurses is recommended. Continuous pulse oximetry may be warranted particularly in patients with a history of obstructive sleep apnea.

Patients may also be at risk of developing aspiration pneumonia postoperatively depending on the extent of resection. It may be helpful to perform a preoperative swallow evaluation to aid in any early identification of swallowing deficits. Insertion of a nasogastric tube and assessment of swallowing function by a specialized Head and Neck trained speech therapist prior to commencing a diet postoperatively may also decrease this risk.

Long-term complications include velopharyngeal incompetence with rhinolalia and/or nasopharyngeal regurgitation of liquids. This will often be transient. However, if at the time of surgery there is a large soft tissue defect, a pharyngoplasty or pedicled buccal fat pad flap can be used to minimize the risk. The rates of tracheostomy or PEG (percutaneous gastrostomy tube)dependence postradical tonsillectomy are most commonly related to the adjuvant therapy that the patient receives and does not need to be addressed here.[26]

FOLLOW-UP

The patient is typically discharged 1 day after surgery and returns at 1 week for a further speech and nutrition assessment. Additionally, the pathology is reviewed and a determination for adjuvant therapy is made if this is indicated.

The patient then returns for routine follow-up for cancer surveillance and follow-up speech assessment as needed.

RESULTS

The evidence for TORS as a viable alternative to chemoradiation as the primary treatment for oropharyngeal carcinoma is quickly gaining a substantial base. Preliminary data related to local control, disease-specific survival and overall survival using TORS as first-line therapy is encouraging thus far.[25-28]

Feasibility

The data from a recent multicenter study published in Laryngoscope was able to document the feasibility, safety and adequacy of surgical margins of TORS for the diagnosis and treatment of selected oropharyngeal tumors. In terms of feasibility, 98.9% of the intent-to-treat population underwent successful TORS without any need to convert to open surgery compared to a 5.9% conversion in nonrobotic surgery. The overall incidence of positive tumor margins was 4.3% that compares favorably with nonrobotic transoral surgical resection.[25]

White et al. (2013) published on the learning curve for TORS. A single tertiary care academic institution's experience with TORS for head and neck tumors over a 4-year period was analyzed and the treatment trends and clinical outcomes were reported on. They demonstrated a significant decrease in operative time, length of intubation and length of stay as TORS experience increased. There was no significant difference over time in the number of cases that could not be performed robotically, the positive margin status or the number of tracheostomies and feeding tubes required.[31]

Oncologic Outcomes

The local control rates have, to this point, been consistently favorable for early stage oropharyngeal carcinoma. Combined results from two tertiary referral centers published by White et al. (2010) at 2 years follow-up showed a local control rate of 86.5%.[13] Similarly, the control rate published by Weinstein et al. (2012) was 97% with a mean follow-up of 2.7 years while the 2-year recurrence-free survival reported by Moore et al. was 92.4%.[25,27-28]

Functional Outcomes

Due to the minimally invasive nature of TORS, the functional outcomes of patients undergoing these procedures have been favorable. Weinstein et al. (2012) published a 5% PEG dependence, which can be used as a surrogate indicator for preservation of swallowing function, in patients treated primarily with TORS. This was significantly lower than those treated with other available surgical and nonsurgical therapy.[35]

Sinclair et al. (2011) published on patient-perceived objective functional outcomes following TORS by administering the M. D. Anderson Dysphagia Inventory pre- and post-operatively. Following TORS for T1 and T2 oropharyngeal SCC, approximately one-third of patients experienced a sustained decrease in perceived swallowing function. However, ongoing improvement continued over time even after 12 months. White et al.'s (2010) analysis of functional outcomes of 89 patients from two tertiary referral centers showed no gastrostomy dependent patients at last follow-up.[13] Moore et al. (2012) followed 66 TORS patients, 97% of whom had returned to oral diet within 3 weeks of surgery with a long-term gastrostomy tube rate of 4.5%.[27]

FUTURE DIRECTIONS

The management of patients with OPSCC continues to evolve with both advances in therapeutic regimens and evolution of our understanding of the underlying pathophysiology of the disease process. Currently, the oncological outcomes in patients with HPV-positive OPSCC remain similar regardless of treatment and thus an appreciation of the functional outcomes represents a significant and fundamental consideration when formulating management recommendations.

While there is a paucity of long-term follow-up for TORS patients, the available data is promising in terms of both oncological and functional outcomes when compared to the best available treatment. Several trials comparing chemoradiotherapy to primary surgery are currently underway and hopefully the analysis of outcomes from these studies will allow for greater evidence basis for current treatment paradigms.

The utility of TORS as part of surgical salvage for recurrent or residual tumors is also promising. Surgical salvage may be the only viable treatment option for recurrent tumors of the oropharynx in the setting of previous radiotherapy. A recent study by White et al. (2013) demonstrated that TORS offers an alternative surgical approach to recurrent tumors of the oropharynx with acceptable oncological outcomes and better functional outcomes than traditional open surgical approaches.[15]

Another application for TORS may lie in the treatment of the unknown head and neck primary tumor. Patel et al. (2013) published a multi-institutional case-series investigating patients with an unknown head and neck primary who underwent TORS to help identify the primary tumor site. Forty-seven patients with an unknown primary following examination and radiological investigation underwent a TORS resection of the tonsil and base of tongue on the affected side. In 72% of cases, a primary site was identified. In cases with only a single metastatic node without extracapsular extension, a complete resection with clear margins would allow for single-modality therapy and/or a reduction in the overall radiation dose.[36] A prospective trial with a standardized preoperative workup and surgical treatment with TORS is warranted to further investigate this as a treatment option; however, the early results are promising.

Emerging evidence suggests that effective primary surgical management of these malignancies may also provide an opportunity for deintensification of adjuvant treatments, namely a decreased dose of radiotherapy, which may result in improvements in patient's post-treatment quality of life, without compromising oncological outcomes.[9]

CONCLUSION

The introduction of TORS for OPSCC is an exciting evolution in the treatment for these increasingly younger patients. While larger prospective trials and longer follow-up times are required, early results suggest that TORS holds promise and that this type of surgery is yet another option for our patients.

VIDEO LEGEND

Video 1.1: Right transoral robotic radical tonsillectomy.

REFERENCES

1. Chaturvedi AK, Engels EA, Anderson WF, et al. Incidence trends for human papillomavirus-related and -unrelated oral squamous cell carcinomas in the United States. J Clin Oncol. 2008;26:612-9.
2. Ryerson Am, Peters ES, Coughlin SS, et al. Burden of potentially human papillomavirus-associated cancers of the oropharynx and oral cavity in the US, 1998-2003. Cancer. 2008; 113:2901-9.
3. Genden E. The role for surgical management of HPV-related oropharyngeal carcinoma. Head Neck Pathol. 2012; 6:S98-S103.
4. Cohan DM, Popat S, Kaplan SE, et al. Oropharyngeal cancer: current understanding and management. Curr Opin Otolaryngol Head Neck Surg. 2009;17:88-94.
5. Kreimer AR, Clifford GM, Boyle P, et al. Human papillomavirus types in head and neck squamous cell carcinoma worldwide: a systematic review. Cancer. 2005;14:467-75.
6. Hobbs CG, Sterne JA, Bailey M, et al. Human papillomavirus and head and neck cancer: a systematic review and meta-analysis. Clin Otolaryngol. 2006;31:259-66.
7. Shah KV, Westra WH. Genital HPVs in the aerodigestive tract: etiologic association with a subset of oropharyngeal/tonsillar cancers and with recurrent respiratory papillomatosis. Dis Markers. 2007;23:235-45.
8. Ang KK, Surgis EM. Human papillomavirus as a marker of the natural history and response to therapy of head and neck squamous cell carcinoma. Semin Radiat Oncol. 2012;22(2):128-42.
9. Dowthwaite SA, Franklin JH, Plama DA, et al. The role of transoral robotic surgery in the management of oropharyngeal cancer: a review of the literature. ISRN Oncol. 2012;945162:1-14.
10. Moore EJ, Hinni ML. Critical review: transoral laser microsurgery and robotic-assisted surgery for oropharynx cancer including human papillomavirus-related cancer. Int J Radiat Oncol Biol Phys. 2013;85(5):1163-7.
11. Parsons JT, Mendenhall W, Stringer SP, et al. Squamous cell carcinoma of the oropharynx: surgery, radiation therapy, or both. Cancer. 2002;94:2967-80.
12. Boudreaux BA, Rosenthal EL, Magnuson JS, et al. Robot-assisted surgery for upper aerodigestive tract neoplasms. Arch Otolaryngol Head Neck Surg. 2009;135(4):397-401.
13. White HN, Moore EJ, Rosenthal EL, et al. Transoral robotic-assisted surgery for head and neck squamous cell carcinoma: One- and 2-year survival analysis. Arch Otolaryngol Head Neck Surg. 2010;136(12):1248-52.
14. Iseli TA, Kulbersh BD, Iseli CE, et al. Functional outcomes after transoral robotic surgery for head and neck cancer. Otolaryngol Head Neck Surg. 2009;141:166-71.
15. White HN, Ford S, Bush B, et al. Salvage surgery for recurrent cancers of the oropharynx: comparing TORS with standard open surgical approaches. JAMA Otolaryngol Head Neck Surg. 2013;139(8):773-8.
16. Weinstein FS, O'Malley BW, Jr, Snyder W, et al. Transoral robotic surgery: radical tonsillectomy. Arch Otolaryngol Head Neck Surg. 2007;133(12):1220-6.
17. Li RJ, Richmon JD. Transoral endoscopic surgery: new surgical techniques for oropharyngeal cancer. Otolaryngol Clin North Am. 2012:45:823-44.
18. Moore EJ, Henstrom DK, Olsen KD, et al. Transoral resection of tonsillar squamous cell carcinoma. Laryngoscope. 2009;119:508-15.
19. Steiner W, Fierek O, Ambrosch P, et al. Transoral laser microsurgery for squamous cell carcinoma of the base of tongue. Arch Otolaryngol Head Neck Surg. 2003;129:36-43.
20. Grant DG, Salassa JR, Hinni ML, et al. Carcinoma of the tongue base treated by transoral laser microsurgery, part one: untreated tumors, a prospective analysis of oncologic and functional outcomes. Laryngoscope. 2006;116: 2150-5.
21. Haughey BH, Hinni ML, Salassa JR, et al. Transoral laser microsurgery as primary treatment for advanced-stage oropharyngeal cancer: a United States multicenter study. Head Neck Surg. 2011;33:1683-94.

22. Grant DG, Hinni ML, Salassa JR, et al. Oropharyngeal cancer: a case for single modality treatment with transoral laser microsurgery. Arch Otolaryngol Head Neck Surg. 2009; 135:1225-30.
23. Hockstein NG, Nolan M, O'Malley BW. Robotic microlaryngeal surgery: a technical feasibility study using the da Vinci surgical robot and an airway mannequin. Laryngoscope. 2005;115:780-5.
24. O'Malley BW, Jr, Weinstein GS, Snyder W, et al. Transoral robotic surgery (TORS) for base of tongue neoplasms. Laryngoscope. 2006;116:1465-72.
25. Weinstein GS, O'Malley BW, Jr, Magnuson JS, et al. Transoral robotic surgery: a multicenter study to assess feasibility, safety and surgical margins. Laryngoscope. 2012;122:1701-7.
26. Sinclair CF, McColloch NL, Carroll WR, et al. Patient-perceived and objective functional outcomes following transoral robotic surgery for early oropharyngeal carcinoma. Arch Otolaryngol Head Neck Surg. 2011;137(11):1112-6.
27. Moore EJ, Olsen SM, Laborde RR, et al. Long-term functional and oncologic results of transoral robotic surgery for oropharyngeal squamous cell carcinoma. Mayo Clin Proc. 2012;87(3):219-25.
28. Moore EJ, Olsen KD, Kasperbauer JL. Transoral robotic surgery for oropharyngeal squamous cell carcinoma: a prospective study of feasibility and functional outcomes. Laryngoscope. 2009;119:2156-64.
29. Kokot N, O'Malley BW, Weinstein G. Transoral anatomy in the context of TORS. In: Weinstein GS, O'Malley BW (Eds). Transoral Robotic Surgery (TORS). San Diego: Plural Publishing Inc; 2012. pp. 59-84.
30. National Comprehensive Cancer Network. Head and Neck Cancer (Version 1.2014). http://www.nccn.org/professionals/physician_gls/pdf/head-and-neck.pdf. Accessed March 30, 2014.
31. White HN, Frederich J, Zimmerman T, et al. Learning curve for transoral robotic surgery: a 4-year analysis. JAMA Otolaryngol Head Neck Surg. 2013;139(6):564-7.
32. Osborne RF, Brown JJ. Carcinoma of the oral pharynx: an analysis of subsite treatment heterogeneity. Surg Oncol Clin North Am. 2004;13(1):71-80.
33. Pitman KT, Johnson JT, Myers EN. Effectiveness of selective neck dissection for management of the clinically node negative neck. Arch Otolaryngol Head Neck Surg. 1997;123(9):917-22.
34. Van Abel KM, Moore EJ. Focus issue: neck dissection for oropharyngeal squamous cell carcinoma. ISRN Surg. 2012; 2012:547017.
35. Machtay M, Moughan J, Trotti A, et al. Factors associated with severe late toxicity after concurrent chemoradiation for locally advanced head and neck cancer: an RTOG analysis. J Clin Oncol. 2008;26:3582-9.
36. Patel, et al. Robotic surgery for primary head and neck squamous cell carcinoma of unknown site. JAMA Otolaryngol Head Neck Surg. 2013;139(11):1203-11.

Chapter 2 Transoral Robotic Surgery for Base of Tongue Tumors

Umamaheswar Duvvuri, Vikas Mehta

INTRODUCTION

Neoplasms of the base of tongue (BOT) present a therapeutic challenge for treating physicians. This anatomic region contains structures that are critical to speech and swallowing functions. One of the most common tumors arising in this location is malignant squamous cell carcinoma (SCC). However, the differential diagnosis is quite broad and includes lymphoma, granular cell tumors, salivary gland tumors (both benign and malignant), rhabdomyosarcoma and metastatic disease. In addition, benign processes such as ectopic lingual thyroid must be considered. Surgery as a primary modality is a very effective treatment for many of these benign and malignant processes. However, transcervical approaches to the oropharynx often require the placement of tracheostomy and gastrostomy tubes. Furthermore, these patients frequently undergo adjuvant chemoradiotherapy for advanced nodal disease or close surgical margins. For this reason, during the past two decades, surgical treatment of BOT carcinoma has been gradually supplanted by nonoperative therapy; to the extent that many surgeons are unfamiliar with the technique of surgical approaches to the BOT. This is unfortunate as many patients in the primary and salvage treatment setting would benefit from a well-executed resection of their BOT tumor.

Surgical access to this region is difficult, and the choice of approach is dictated by the size and exact location of the lesion. The treating surgeon must be cognizant of the full spectrum of techniques available to access the BOT, while recognizing the impact of each procedure on cosmesis and function. Many BOT tumors can be accessed transorally, so the surgeon needs to be adept at transoral approaches to this anatomic region. For the purposes of this chapter, we will focus on surgical excision of SCC of the BOT.

Rationale for Procedure

The primary advantage of transoral robotic surgery (TORS) over a nonsurgical approach is immediate confirmation of complete extirpation of the primary tumor. Secondary benefits include the ability to more accurately stage the extent of tumor and the opportunity to individualize/deescalate adjuvant treatment strategies. The advantages of the transoral approach over open approaches are the minimal invasiveness of the procedure, the ability to keep the pharyngeal musculature and neural innervation intact, decreased tracheostomy tube and gastrostomy tube dependence postoperatively, the ability to keep the mandible intact and the shorter postoperative recovery time.

The modality used to manage patients with BOT cancer depends on histopathologic diagnosis and lesion size. Both surgical and nonsurgical interventions, such as radiation therapy and chemotherapy, can be considered. The choice to operate upon a patient with a BOT tumor or to treat with chemoradiotherapy is a complicated one. The decision involves many individual patients and treating physician factors. In general, the ability to achieve completely clear surgical margins is one of the primary issues that influence survival. We feel that the ability to achieve clear surgical margins and leave the patient with 50% of the BOT, and at least one intact hypoglossal nerve and lingual artery, is critical in proceeding with TORS. These patients can achieve very good functional swallowing and speech in the post-treatment period with careful follow up and speech and swallowing therapy. If the resection is likely to leave a larger defect, then we typically recommend nonoperative therapy. The controversial and difficult portion of the treatment algorithm comes into play in deeply invasive and bulky tumors on one side of the tongue that falls between these categories. The nodal stage of the patient must also be taken into account. We feel that patients with N2c and N3 diseases will most likely require adjuvant therapy and these patients are best treated with definitive chemoradiotherapy.

Applied Anatomy

The BOT is delineated anteriorly by the circumvallate papillae, laterally by the glossotonsillar sulci and inferiorly by the circumvallate papillae. Squamous cell carcinoma of the BOT often extends to involve the lingual tonsils and potentially the intrinsic tongue musculature. It is important to remember that lingual tonsil tissue, unlike the palatine tonsils, is not encapsulated. Therefore, there is no clear anatomic plane that separates the lingual tonsil tissue from the underlying tongue musculature.

The critical neurovascular structures that are frequently encountered during BOT surgery include the lingual artery, lingual branch of the glossopharyngeal nerve and, rarely, the hypoglossal nerve. The dorsal branch of the lingual artery is encountered at the lateral BOT, in the region of the glossotonsillar sulcus.

HISTORY

The classic history for patients with SCC of the tongue is that of a heavy smoker and/or drinker: a pack-a-day or more for over 10 years with varying degrees of alcohol intake. However, in the recent past, the history has shifted to include a larger number of patients who report being never smokers, or who have stopped smoking in the distant past and have a minimal history for alcohol intake. These patients have a tumor that is related to the human papillomavirus (HPV), an etiologic factor contributing to the development of their cancer. Thus, it is important to take a thorough history of all patients with an emphasis on alcohol and tobacco consumption. It is also important to question whether these patients have engaged in high-risk sexual behaviors, as this may also contribute to the diagnosis of a HPV-related malignancy. Female patients should be questioned about their gynecological history and specifically a history of abnormal Pap smear. It is also important to ascertain whether these patients have complaints of hoarseness, dysphagia, odynophagia or otalgia, all of which may better delineate the primary tumor.

PHYSICAL EXAMINATION

A thorough examination of the head and neck is warranted in all patients who present with SCC of the BOT. An examination of the oral cavity and oropharynx should be performed, ideally with indirect mirror-laryngoscopy to examine the BOT and tonsillar fossae. Bimanual palpation of the BOT and tonsillar fossae is also required. The physical examination should include palpation of the neck to determine whether there are metastatic lymph nodes. These nodes should be assessed to determine if they are fixed to underlying structures or if they are freely mobile. Palpation should also include examination of the thyroid and tracheal regions as well as the nodal lymphatic basins of levels I through VI.

All patients undergo flexible nasolaryngoscopy as this provides a better view of the BOT, tonsil fossae and supraglottic structures. It is important to evaluate the extent of tumor and determine which structures may need to be resected to ensure adequate surgical margins.

Indications

When considering a TORS approach to the BOT, the surgeon must carefully and completely assess the size and local extension of the tumor, as well as adequate surgical access and the ability to achieve clear surgical margins. The TORS approach is ideal for T1 and T2 malignant tumors, exophytic T3 malignant disease or benign tumors with limited extension into surrounding tissues. Patients should be counseled regarding all options to treat their cancers including open surgical approaches.

Contraindications

Contraindications to the TORS approach include: (1) deep tumor invasion into the adjacent parapharyngeal space with tumor fixation, (2) any concern for involvement of major vascular structures such as the carotid or jugular system on physical exam or imaging, (3) bony invasion into the mandible or skull base or (4) clinically significant trismus indicating tumor involvement of the pterygoid musculature, and the potential for decreased surgical access. Tumors that extend deep to the extrinsic tongue musculature (particularly the genioglossus and hyoglossus muscles) can be difficult to extirpate transorally and put the ipsilateral lingual artery, hypoglossal nerve and carotid artery at risk. A careful assessment of clinical and radiographic data must be undertaken preoperatively in order to assess the relationship of the tumor to the genioglossus and hyoid bone. Involvement of, or extension beyond, these structures is a relative contraindication to transoral resection, as it places the lingual artery, hypoglossal nerve and the external carotid artery at significant risk during resection.

Preoperative Workup

Radiographic Imaging

Radiographic workup most commonly involves computed tomography (CT), magnetic resonance imaging (MRI) and positron emission tomography (PET) with CT (PET/CT). Computed tomography scan with intravenous contrast can be acquired rapidly and can provide information regarding primary tumor extension, bony erosion of the mandibular cortex and information regarding cervical metastasis. MRI can be an important adjunct for the evaluation of BOT lesions since it gives more detailed soft tissue information and can demonstrate submucosal tumor extension, thus helping to define whether transoral resection is feasible. The most critical tumor factors to determine on imaging are extent of tumor, the amount of functional BOT involved, the anterior extent of the tumor into the root of tongue and genioglossus muscle, the lateral extent of the tumor into the hyoglossus muscle, hyoid bone, and pharynx and the involvement of critical neck structures such as the internal and external carotid artery. These scans are also critical in assessing the status of the neck lymph nodes. Finally, PET/CT scans can be used to help define extent of primary disease, as well as the presence of locoregional or distant metastases.

Endoscopy

Planning for a TORS resection can be facilitated by an operative examination under anesthesia. We recommend this approach, especially for surgeons who are beginning a TORS program and who do not have extensive experience with other transoral resection methods [such as transoral laser microsurgery (TLM)]. The operative exam under anesthesia does introduce additional expense, anesthesia and patient time. However, these factors are balanced by the advantage gained in mapping the tumor extent and knowing that the tumor can be exposed adequately for ultimate TORS resection. In select cases, this assessment in the operating theatre can be used to perform the lymphadenectomy portion of the procedure and major arteries can be ligated in an elective fashion.

Robotic Approach to the BOT

For patients who meet the preoperative criteria discussed above, a TORS approach to a BOT SCC can be considered as a primary oncologic treatment modality. The overall goal of the robotic BOT resection is to achieve en bloc resection of the primary tumor with adequate surgical margins. Below, we provide a description detailing the intraoperative use of the Da Vinci robotic surgical system (Intuitive Surgical, Sunnyvale, CA) for transoral BOT SCC excision.

Instrumentation

- Operative headlight
- Tooth guard
- Crow Davis, Dingman or FK retractor (Gyrus, Olympus) with various size flat tongue retractor blades
- DaVinci Robotic System, Intuitive Surgical, Sunnyvale, CA
- 5 mm spatula tip monopolar cautery, Intuitive Surgical, Sunnyvale, CA
- 5 mm Maryland dissector, Intuitive Surgical, Sunnyvale, CA
- 2-0 silk suture.

Operative Setup

The operating room set up is shown in Figure 2.1 and is similar to other TORS procedures as described in this book.

Operative Technique

The procedure is performed in the operating room with the patient orally or nasally intubated with an endotracheal tube. The intubation method is based on surgeon preference with no distinct advantage provided with nasal intubation. The teeth are protected by molded thermoplastic splints, which protect both the maxillary and mandibular teeth. Every operation is initiated with an exam under anesthesia, including a direct laryngoscopy and manual palpation of the oropharynx. The tongue is retracted with a suture to improve access. The oral retractor, either a Crowe-Davis, Dingman (Fig. 2.2) or Feyh-Kastenbauer Retractor depending on availability and surgeon preference, is then placed and suspended. At this time, the tumor is palpated to assess the surgical margins. The manual palpation is essential for determining surgical margins and correlating these boundaries with anatomical landmarks such as the lateral pharyngeal walls, hyoid bone etc. Transoral approaches to the BOT are dependent on tumor exposure. The tip of the retractor should be positioned so that the anterior extent of the anticipated tumor cut, taking into account an adequate oncologic margin, is exposed. If possible, exposure should also allow visualization of the inferior aspect of the tumor. If the anatomy does not permit complete exposure of the tumor with the anterior positioning of the retractor, the surgeon must be very careful to clear the margins that can be visualized before advancing and re-exposing the tumor. The dissection must be carefully performed to avoid transecting the tumor

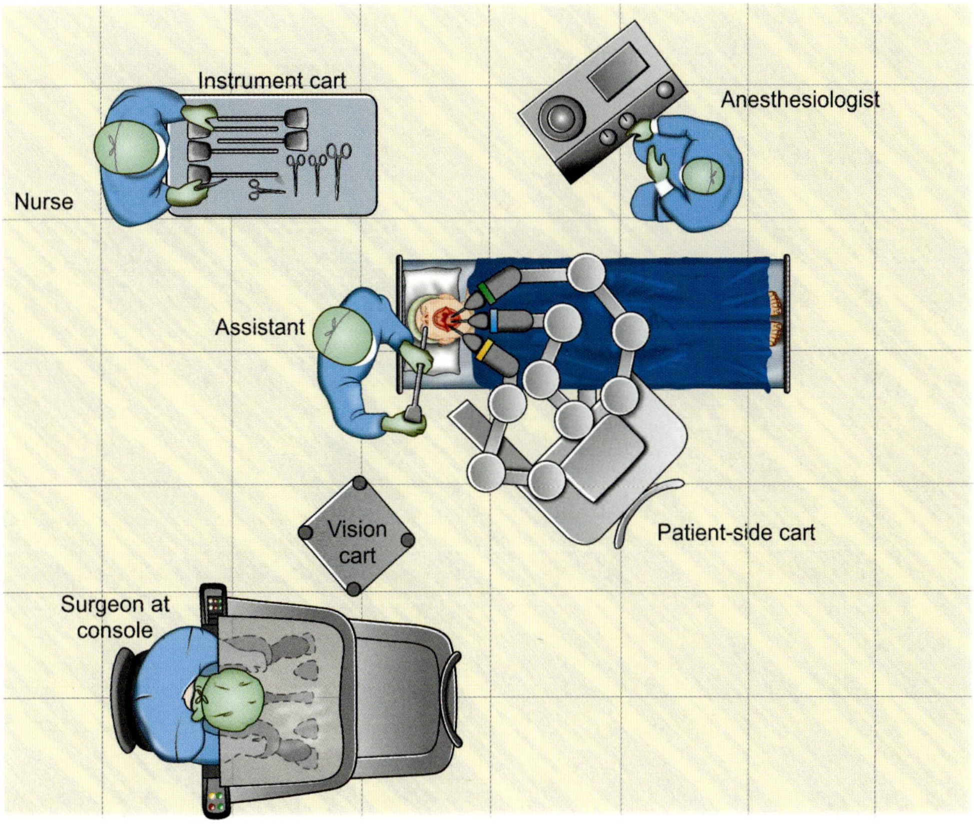

Fig. 2.1: Operating theatre layout for TORS of the base of tongue.

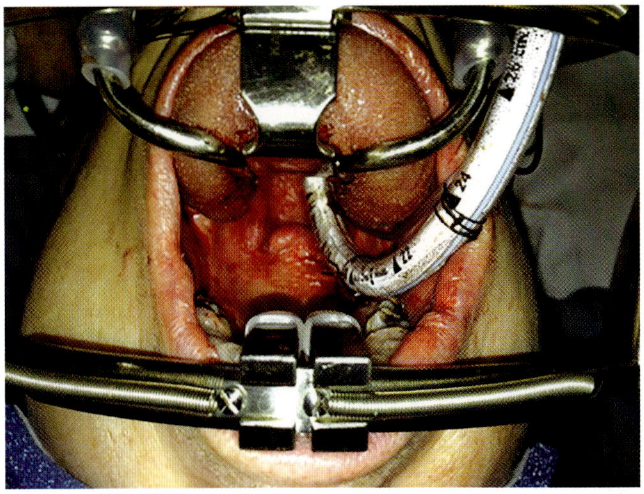

Fig. 2.2: The exposure of the oropharynx is obtained using a Dingman mouth retractor with a flat blade. The endotracheal tube is sutured to one side. The lateral pharyngeal walls and the circumvallate papillae are exposed.

or obtaining positive margins, especially in the deep tongue musculature. Once exposure is achieved, the surgical robot is docked and the working space is optimized (Fig. 2.3).

After positioning the robotic system, the first incision is made horizontally above the anterior border of the tumor, which allows the tumor to "drop" into the surgical field with subsequent cuts (🎥 2.1). Many lateral BOT tumors invade into the tonsillar fossa, thus requiring excision of the tonsil and superior pharyngeal constrictor muscle. The next cut is made vertically along the midline to the vallecula as dictated by the tumor. This cut allows the surgeon to assess the depth of the tumor, and can be

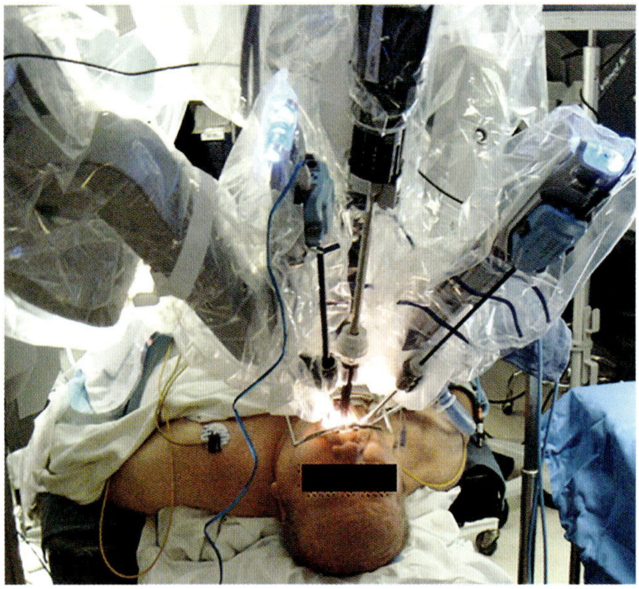

Fig. 2.3: Depiction of the placement of robotic instruments in the transoral robotic surgery approach for base of tongue resection. The patient's mouth is retracted using a Dingman retractor with a flat blade. The da Vinci robot is then docked with instruments in the patient's mouth.

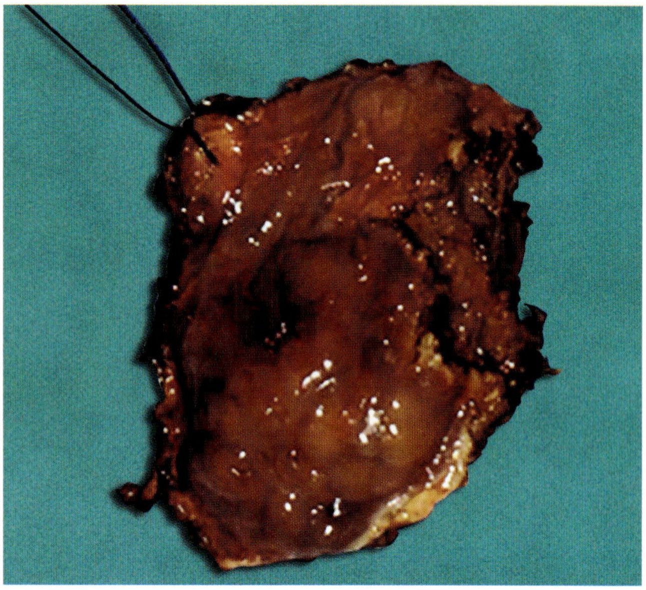

Fig. 2.4: A typical resection specimen is shown. The entire extent of the right base of the tongue is resected from the midline at the circumvallate papillae (marked by suture) to the valleculae (the inferior limit).

made in a generous fashion since there are no major arterial vessels in the midline of the tongue. The cut should ensure that a cuff of normal soft tissue is removed along with the tumor specimen to provide an adequate pathologic margin of resection depending on tumor histology. The surgeon can also grasp this cuff of tissue to provide countertraction throughout the remainder of the procedure. Importantly, since the da Vinci system lacks haptic feedback, the surgeon can frequently leave the surgeon's console and palpate the tumor bed to reassess the margins as the dissection is being performed. Attention is then turned to the lateral cut that is made deep through the constrictor muscles and incorporates the ipsilateral palatine tonsil (2.1). It should be noted that the lingual artery enters the BOT laterally, and there is the possibility of encountering vigorous bleeding if these lateral cuts are not made carefully. As the surgeon approaches the lateral border, the dissection slows and blunt dissection allows identification and clipping of the dorsal lingual artery and sometimes the main lingual artery (2.1). The tumor is slowly dissected from anterior/superior/medial to posterior/inferior/lateral until it is completely mobilized. All attempts are made to remove the tumor en bloc (Fig. 2.4).

Throughout resection, the surgeon should be aware of important neurovascular anatomy and landmarks. The dorsal lingual artery is commonly found in the lateral BOT and can be managed either by the primary surgeon during TLM, or the assistant surgeon during TORS, by placing 2–3 vascular clips on the patient side and one on the tumor side of the vessel prior to transection. If the vessel is cut inadvertently, pressure externally on the neck at the level of the superior thyroid cornu can slow bleeding until hemostasis can be achieved. In addition, by tracing the dorsal lingual artery laterally, the surgeon can attempt to identify the lingual artery trunk and ligate it to achieve hemostasis. While dissection may be carried across the midline, it is important to remember that if the hypoglossal nerve or lingual artery is resected on one side, the contralateral nerve and vessel must be meticulously preserved to maintain adequate function and blood flow to the oral tongue. If there is concern for lateral extension of the tumor or risk to major vasculature based on preoperative assessment or intraoperative findings, a neck dissection is recommended prior to transoral extirpation in order to identify and protect these key neurovascular structures.

During dissection, a sense of pathologic versus normal tissue response to dissection of the BOT is important to develop. Margins are often difficult to assess visually during resection, and tactile feedback cannot be relied upon during TORS. It is important to maximize the optical benefits of the DaVinci system: three-dimensional visualization and enhanced optical magnification. The camera arm is often brought closer to the operating field as the surgery progresses to adequately ensure resection of the deep surgical margin. These considerations underscore the importance of frozen-section analysis and an integrated system for personal communication between surgeon and pathologist. Once the tumor is completely freed, it is removed from the oropharynx and oriented by the surgeon. The margins of resection are carefully inspected, and the tumor is taken to the pathologist by the surgeon so that direct verbal communication and tumor inspection by both parties can ensure precise assessment of the surgical margins. Based on feedback from the pathologist, additional surgical margins may be required. These must be carefully oriented and discussed with the pathologist to ensure adequate resection. Once negative margins have been achieved, the wound is copiously irrigated with sterile saline and hemostasis is ensured. Most commonly, the wound is left to heal by secondary intention. We prefer to place thrombin-infused surgical foam to aid in postoperative hemostasis. In cases of extensive tumor resection, a nasogastric feeding tube is placed, which can be removed postoperatively as the patient demonstrates adequate swallow function. If the tumor ablation is confined to the BOT only, without the need to perform an extensive lateral wall resection, we will forgo the placement of a nasogastric feed tube.

Management of the Neck

Whenever possible, we prefer to stage the neck dissection and perform them at a separate time from the TORS resection. We feel that this can help avoid a fistula, and also affords the surgeon to return to the operating room to clear additional margins if necessary. In our experience, if there is concern for vascular injury during TORS, we prefer to perform the neck dissection first and electively ligate the ipsilateral lingual artery. Alternatively, if the nodal dissection is performed after TORS, we prefer to wait 4–6 weeks to allow the primary tumor site to heal sufficiently so as to avoid a communication into the neck.

Airway Management

All patients undergo a direct laryngoscopy after the completion of the procedure to evaluate the surgical site for bleeding and assess the status of the airway. If there is concern for airway edema such as tongue swelling, the patients remain intubated until the swelling resolves and they can be safely extubated. However, in our experience, almost all patients can be safely extubated at the completion of the case.

POSTOPERATIVE CARE

Patients who have undergone TORS for BOT disease are usually extubated in the operating room or upon transfer to the postoperative recovery unit. The patients are then managed in the hospital overnight with intravenous pain medication, as well as gastrointestinal prophylaxis with proton pump inhibitors and H2-blocker for reflux precautions. We also treat patients with sucralfate to minimize gastric acid reflux to the open wound at the BOT. The patients commence a diet on the first postoperative day. This diet usually consists of soft foods, which can be swallowed with relative ease. It should be noted that clear liquids are the most difficult to swallow in this immediate postoperative period. Patients are then free to follow any diet they can tolerate as soon as they are able to have their pain under good control. Patients are usually discharged from the hospital on the second postoperative day. All patients require intensive swallowing therapy to ensure optimal recovery after surgery.

COMPLICATIONS

Postoperative hemorrhage remains the most feared and likely complication after TORS. The risk estimates are 5–6% in most large series. There is a potential risk of injury to the lingual artery, which can result in significant bleeding. The possibility of experiencing some postoperative bleeding when the eschar that covers the surgical defect sloughs off should also be discussed with the patient. Most bleeding can be treated with observation or topical cautery if it occurs from a more anterior portion of the BOT. However, more active bleeding or bleeding from a deeper portion of the surgical wound may require control of the bleeding in the operating room. It is important to remember that the surgical robot offers transoral access to regions of the anatomy that would not be subjected to dissection in routine transoral cases. Therefore, when postoperative hemorrhage is encountered, the surgeon must remember that this is more complicated than a simple posttonsillectomy hemorrhage. We have found that interventional radiology can be helpful in these cases. However, the best strategy is to prevent the bleeding by obtaining meticulous hemostasis. The current literature suggests that transcervical ligation of the external carotid system does not reduce the bleeding rates. Therefore, it may be prudent to ensure that the end-vessels are carefully ligated during the transoral resection.

RESULTS

Patients typically experience pain and dysphagia after robotic-assisted surgery of the BOT. The pain lasts between 2 days through 2 weeks as the wound heals and granulates (Fig. 2.5). Most patients do have dysphagia, but are able to tolerate oral intake as early as postoperative first or second day. Patients typically work with a speech pathologist with some basic swallowing exercises to facilitate early resumption of swallowing. The long-term risk of feeding tube dependence is highly correlated with the modality that is used to complete the definitive treatment of these patients. Those patients who undergo extensive chemoradiotherapy for the management of the disease tend to have a higher rate of feeding-tube dependence.

Patients who have a small volume primary cancer can often be treated with surgery alone: by definitively resecting the primary cancer with clear margins and the lymph node metastasis. The neck dissection can be performed at the same time as TORS surgery; however, we prefer to have the final pathology reports so that if a close margin is identified then further resection of the primary site can be performed at the time of the neck dissection, several weeks after the primary resection.

In those patients who present with a low-volume primary cancer, it is possible to perform a robotic-assisted resection of the BOT to achieve negative margins, and subsequently clear the neck, without having to subject the patients to additional adjuvant therapy. Based on anecdotal experience, patients treated in this fashion have excellent oncologic and functional results, and return to their daily lives quickly without suffering from the long-term side effects associated with chemoradiation. However, those patients who present with a large volume cancer may in fact require adjuvant therapy with chemoradiation. The potential to deintensify the radiation fields that need to be delivered to the patient to control the cancer, may decrease treatment morbidity and long-term swallowing difficulties.

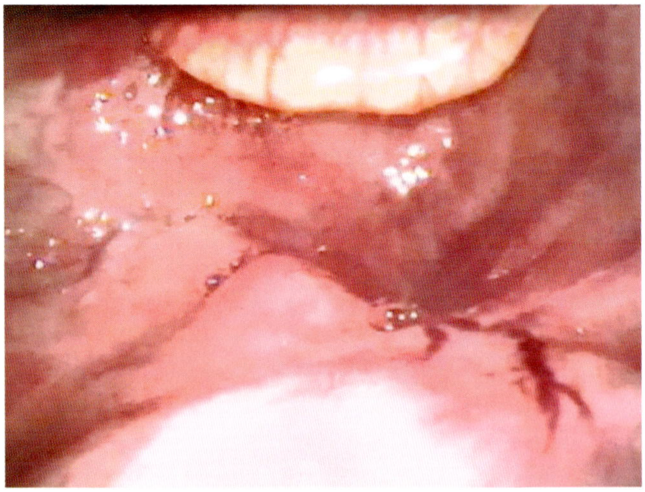

Fig. 2.5: The appearance of the BOT 2 months after robotic-assisted resection. This is the appearance prior to initiation of radiation therapy. The vallecula is preserved and the BOT is well healed.

Future Considerations

Transoral surgery for BOT malignancies has been performed for many years. The most common type of transoral surgery offered to these patients is TLM, popularized by Dr. Wolfgang Steiner and his group. Unfortunately, this surgery is technically demanding, and is often limited by the exposure of the tumor and the limitations of line-of-sight laser technology. Also, the tumors are often removed piecemeal, rather than en bloc, which makes it even more challenging for the pathologist to determine histopathologic tumor margins. For these reasons, TLM for oropharyngeal cancer has not, in general, gained the popularity it enjoyed in Europe in the rest of the world. The advent of the robotic surgical system has allowed for many surgeons to now practice TORS for BOT disease. However, this technology has only been used for the past 4–5 years, with increasing popularity. There is, therefore, a paucity of data that demonstrates the oncologic utility of performing TORS for the management of BOT malignancies.

In the USA and Canada, several randomized trials have been designed to investigate the utility and oncologic effectiveness of TORS for the management of oropharyngeal carcinoma. These trials seek to (1) use TORS to deescalate treatment for patients with low volume HPV-associated carcinoma and (2) evaluate the utility of TORS plus pathologic-guided adjuvant therapy versus definitive chemoradiation in the context of HPV-negative oropharyngeal cancer. The results of these trials will significantly enhance our understanding of when and how to apply this novel and exciting technology, with the ultimate goal of improving the survival and quality of life for our patients suffering from oropharyngeal malignancies.

Pearls and Pitfalls

- Proper history-taking and physical examination are critical for assessing the patient's risk factor(s) for harboring a HPV-related cancer.
- Careful radiographic evaluation including CT or PET/CT scan is critical for demonstrating the subsite in which the primary tumor may be located. In addition, it provides important information regarding the extent of lymph node metastasis or distant metastasis.
- Transoral robotic surgery resection allows for complete surgical extirpation of these tumors without cosmetic deformity and likely reduced morbidity. The resection must then be oriented for the pathologist to provide comments on the adequacy of recession.
- Not removing tissue from the glossotonsillar sulcus can lead to inadequate tissue removal and positive margins.
- The lingual artery can be encountered in this region and intraoperative hemorrhage can occur if the dissection is not carefully performed.
- Dysphagia and pain are the most common side effects associated with this procedure and can be managed with narcotic pain medications, as well as swallowing therapy.
- There is a small risk of postoperative hemorrhage as a consequence of this procedure, but it should be recognized early and appropriate management is required, including potential operative control of hemorrhage.

VIDEO LEGEND

Video 2.1: TORS for base of tongue cancer.

SUGGESTED READING

1. Balaker AE, Abemayor E, Elashoff D, et al. Cancer of unknown primary: does treatment modality make a difference? Laryngoscope. 2012;122(6):1279-82.
2. Begum S, Gillison ML, Nicol TL, et al. Detection of human papillomavirus-16 in fine-needle aspirates to determine tumor origin in patients with metastatic squamous cell carcinoma of the head and neck. Clin Cancer Res. 2007;13:1186-91.
3. Haas I, Hoffmann TK, Engers R, et al. Diagnostic strategies in cervical carcinoma of an unknown primary (CUP). Eur Arch Otorhinolaryngol. 2002;259:325-33.
4. Mehta V, Johnson P, Tassler A, et al. A new paradigm for the diagnosis and management of unknown primary tumors of the head and neck. Laryngoscope. 2012. Nov 14 (epub).
5. Waltonen J, Ozer E, Hall N, et al. Metastatic carcinoma of the neck of unknown primary origin: evolution and efficacy of the modern workup. Arch Otolaryngol Head Neck Surg. 2009;135:1024-9.

Chapter 3 Transoral Robotic Surgery—Hypopharynx

Eric M Genden, Eitan Prisman

INTRODUCTION

Background

Hypopharyngeal squamous cell carcinoma (SCC) is a relatively rare but aggressive malignancy associated with a poor prognosis. It accounts for 3–5% all of head and neck SCC and often presents at an advanced stage.[1] The pyriform sinus is the most common subsite involved, accounting for >85% of hypopharynx SCC.[2] Most patients are of male gender, over the age of 65 with 90% of patients presenting with a significant smoking history and 50% with associated alcohol misuse.[3,4] Not surprisingly, the rate of synchronous lesions in this subset of patients approaches 8%.[3] Due to a lack of significant symptoms in early stage disease, over 50% of patients present with advanced (stage IV) disease.[4] The rich lymphatic drainage accompanying the hypopharynx contributes to a rate of ipsilateral nodal disease in the range of 60–80%,[5] and up to 40% presenting with contralateral disease.[6] In an apparent clinically negative neck, the rate of occult ipsilateral and contralateral neck disease can be as high as 36% and 27%, respectively.[4,6] Hypopharyngeal SCC is associated with a particularly poor prognosis. Of nearly 3,000 hypopharyngeal SCC diagnosed from 1980 to 1985 and from 1990 to 1992, the 5-year disease-specific survival was 63.1%, 57.5%, 41.8% and 22% for stages I–IV, respectively.[3] Despite advances in surgical therapies, chemotherapeutic options and radiation technology, the overall prognosis in hypopharynx SSC has not significantly improved.[7]

The paradigms in treatment of hypopharynx SCC have changed several times over the past few decades. In the 1960s, laryngopharyngectomy replaced radiation therapy as the primary modality of therapy for hypopharynx SCC of the 1940s and 1950s. Primary surgery or radiation remained the primary modality in the treatment of hypopharynx SCC until the introduction of platinum-based chemotherapeutics in the 1980s and its application to the treatment of laryngeal SCC.[8,9]

Due to the trends in organ preservation, applied from the experience gained in laryngeal carcinoma, concurrent chemoradiotherapy has gained significant momentum as the primary modality of treatment for hypopharynx carcinoma. However, unlike in laryngeal carcinoma, there is a scarcity of evidence to support this treatment modality in the hypopharynx. The only randomized control trial of hypopharynx carcinoma that included a surgical arm was performed in 1996. Induction chemotherapy followed by radiation therapy (in responders) was compared with surgery followed by postoperative radiation therapy. This study found no significant difference in survival or recurrence, with a larger percentage of patients in the induction arm retaining a functioning larynx.[10] However, all patients in the surgical arm had total laryngectomy with partial pharyngectomy and not partial laryngopharyngectomies or the minimally invasive procedure that are available today. Furthermore, combined chemotherapy and radiation therapy increase toxicity to the aerodigestive tract and are associated with a likely underreported rate of detrimental effects on swallowing function.[11] The treatment options are further complicated when reviewing the results of concurrent chemotherapy versus induction chemotherapy.[9,12,13] The North American laryngeal literature suggests that as concurrent chemotherapy became the more common treatment for larynx carcinoma, the associated overall survival had decreased.[14,15] However, this suggestion is controversial as contrary results were found in similar European trials.[16]

While there have been significant technical improvements in partial laryngopharyngectomies including combined suprahyoid and lateral pharyngectomy, as well as advances in reconstructive techniques, laryngopharyngectomy with reconstruction remains associated with a significant functional impairment. Nevertheless, in advanced disease, including infiltrating tumors and those associated with significant cartilage involvement, initial radical surgery followed by adjuvant therapy, as opposed to concurrent chemoradiotherapy, is often advocated.[8,17,18] However, the optimal management remains controversial.

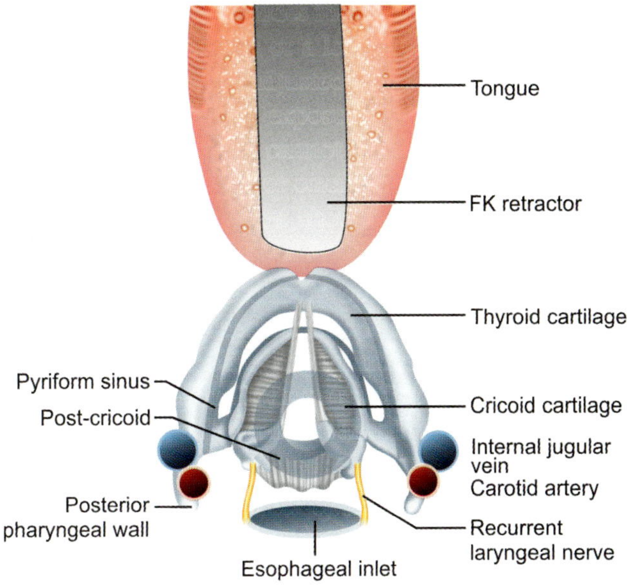

Fig. 3.1: Schematic diagram of the endoscopic hypopharyngeal anatomy from the surgeons perspective after assembling the FK retractor.

Rationale for Procedure

Over the past four decades, the surgical arena has witnessed significant advancements in the field of minimally invasive surgery. In the 1970s, transoral endoscopic laser microsurgery (TLM) was developed and soon thereafter was applied to the treatment of hypopharynx SCC.[19] In addition, the more recent development of transoral robotic surgery (TORS) presents an additional technique that has provided equivalent locoregional control without the collateral functional impairment of traditional surgery.[9,20] This is particularly true for early stage and a select group of advanced stage, hypopharynx SCC and is the focus of this chapter.

Transoral laser surgery was applied to the hypopharynx with equivalent oncological outcomes to both open surgery and organ preservation concurrent chemoradiation therapy protocols with a low rate of postoperative morbidity.[21,22] The relative advantage of TLM is the ability to gain exposure to the hypopharynx, without the need to disrupt the laryngeal framework and the inherent functional impairment associated with those traditional open approaches. Furthermore, resurfacing of the wound can take place by secondary intention, negating a bulky reconstruction.[21,23,24] However, TLM resection may be limited by the line of sight of the microscope.[25] The inherent advantages of robotic-assisted surgery, in terms of improved tissue manipulation and visualization as well as relative degrees of freedom, have provided a potentially superior technique in the treatment of hypopharynx SCC.

Applied Anatomy

The hypopharynx comprises the inferior segment of pharynx that is bounded above by the plane of the superior border of the hyoid and extends inferiorly to the plane corresponding to the lower border of the cricoid. It includes three subsites: the left and right pyriform sinuses, the posterior and lateral pharyngeal wall and the postcricoid region. The postcricoid region joins superiorly with the left and right pyriform sinuses and posteriorly with the posterior pharyngeal wall to form a circumferential segment of pharynx whose inferior border defines the esophageal inlet (Fig. 3.1).

Indications and Contraindications

Tumor Characteristics

We consider T1–T3 pyriform sinus and posterior pharyngeal wall lesions as potential candidates for TORS, provided there is at least one intact arytenoid with normal vocal cord mobility. However, we exclude lesions with significant posterior cricoid involvement or those that involve the apex of the pyriform sinus or with vocal cord fixation. Furthermore, we exclude advanced T4 stage disease and in particular those that have thyroid cartilage or prevertebral fascia involvement and those with unresectable nodal disease or carotid artery invasion.

Patient Characteristics

Particular attention to the common variables routinely applied in the anesthesiology literature to identify patients who are potentially difficult intubation is important. These variables include an interincisal distance <4 cm, neck circumference >40 cm, hyomental and sternomental distance <6.05 and 13.9 cm, respectively as well as Mallampati score.[29] Furthermore, the size of the tongue and tongue base should be assessed and have been shown to predict those patients with difficult access during TORS of hypopharynx SCC.[28] This assessment will aid in identifying suitable patients for TORS. We exclude patients who have medical contraindications to general anesthesia, those who have poor pulmonary reserve as determined based on preoperative pulmonary function test and those with preoperative radiation to the larynx/hypopharynx. It is critical to select out patients with adequate access. Those patients who on diagnostic panendoscopy have only a "fair view," as defined above, or those with advanced C-spine pathology are excluded.

Table 3.1: Inclusion and exclusion criteria for TORS

- Inclusion
  - T1–T3 pyriform sinus or posterior pharyngeal wall
  - At least one intact arytenoid with normal vocal cord mobility
- Exclusion
  - Involvement of posterior cricoid apex of the pyriform sinus
  - T4 stage disease
  - Involvement of thyroid cartilage or prevertebral fascia
  - Unresectable nodal disease or carotid artery invasion
  - Medical contraindication to general anesthesia
  - Poor pulmonary reserve
  - Preoperative radiation to larynx/hypopharynx
  - Inadequate exposure

Preoperative Workup

Investigations

Pulmonary function tests serve as an objective value of pulmonary function when a thorough history and physical examination suggests a compromised pulmonary function, and help predict patients who are at higher risk from surgical intervention.

Radiology

High-resolution computed tomography (CT) is useful to determine extent of disease including paraglottic extension and cartilage involvement.[30] Positron emission tomography CT (PET-CT) is becoming increasingly useful to rule out metastatic disease and to help in identifying potential suspicious lymph node metastases.[30] In the setting where PET-CT is not available, the lung should be imaged at least with a chest X-ray. While breathing and swallowing confound magnetic resonance imaging (MRI), it does provide superior soft tissue delineation in terms of extent of submucosal spread and prevertebral fascia involvement. When there is suspicion of submucosal spread, which can be common in hypopharyngeal carcinoma,[31] a dedicated MRI should be considered. Traditionally, barium swallow was used to image these lesions;[32] however, we do not routinely order this investigation.

Panendoscopy

In addition to obtaining tissue diagnosis, a preoperative panendoscopy provides an opportunity to determine eligibility for TORS and is highly recommended.[28] The larynx and hypopharynx are carefully examined to determine arytenoid mobility and to characterize the tumor in terms of size, subsite involvement and lateral extension. Equally important is to determine whether adequate exposure can be obtained. To this end, the pharyngolaryngoscope Feyh-Kastenbauer (FK) Retractor (Gyrus Medical Inc., Maple Grove, MN) is assembled. Exposure can be assessed based on a recent description by De Virgilio et al.[28] In particular, "good exposure" is defined as full vision of the supraglottis and an unfolded pyriform sinus; "Fair vision" as full vision of the supraglottis and a folded pyriform; while "poor vision" is defined as a limited view of the supraglottis and folded pyriform sinuses. While the 30° endoscope usually provides the most optimal view, in a select group of patients with an interincisal distance of <4 mm, it is difficult to obtain the necessary angle to view the lesion with a 30° endoscope. In these cases, a 0° telescope may be applied with laryngeal compression as discussed below.

Instrumentation

The instrumentation can be divided into three parts based on the three steps of the procedure, namely exposure, ablation and reconstruction.

Exposure

- Pharyngolaryngoscope FK retractor (Gyrus Medical Inc., Maple Grove, MN)
- 2-0 tapered silk suture
- da Vinci Si surgical robotic system (Intuitive Surgical Inc., Sunnyvale, CA)
- 8-mm 30° and 0° da Vinci Endoscope (Intuitive Surgical Inc., Sunnyvale, CA).

Ablation

- 5-mm EndoWrist monopolar spatula cautery (Intuitive Surgical Inc., Sunnyvale, CA)
- 5-mm EndoWrist Maryland forceps (Intuitive Surgical Inc., Sunnyvale, CA)
- Hand-held Yankauer suction.

Reconstruction

- Two 5-mm EndoWrist Needle Drivers (Intuitive Surgical Inc., Sunnyvale, CA)
- 4-0 Vicryl (Ethicon, Inc., Somerville, NJ).

Operative Setup with Robot

Anesthesia and Intubation

Nontraumatic nasotracheal intubation is essential to maintain the anatomic delineation of the primary malignancy and prevent unwarranted edema. At our institution, we advocate awake fiberoptic nasotracheal intubation after application of topical anesthetic. General anesthesia is then induced and an appropriate dose of induction dexamethasone is administered to limit laryngeal edema and, secondarily, postoperative nausea. An appropriate dose of muscle relaxant is essential to optimize access.

Tracheotomy

Tracheotomy at the first or second intercartilaginous space is performed through a 2-cm incision in a standard fashion. This is usually performed prophylactically prior to the TORS resection in order to optimize visualization. A decision of whether or not to decannulate is made at the end of the ablative portion based on the extent of ablation, the degree of edema as well as the patient characteristics.

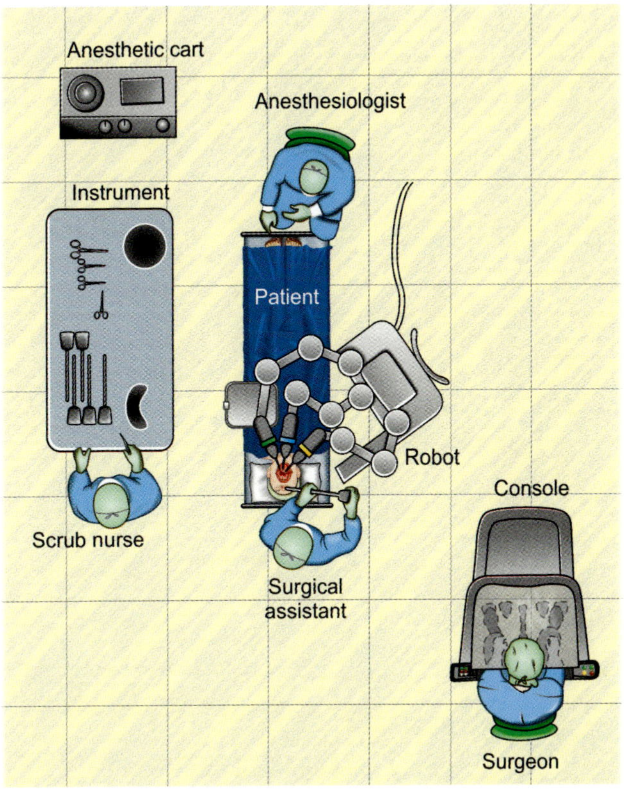

Fig. 3.2: A schematic overhead diagram of the operating room setup. Note the Robot is docked at 30° to the patient bed.

Setup

The operating room and da Vinci robot are set up in the usual fashion, with the foot of the da Vinci robot at 30° to the surgical bed, in order to optimize access of the endoscope and the two arms into the surgical field. A 30° endoscope is calibrated and balanced. While there is evidence that compared to monopolar cautery, the CO_2 laser causes less thermal damage and associated edema to adjacent structures, we have applied both techniques with equivalent results.[27] A foam doughnut is placed under the patient's head without a shoulder roll (Fig. 3.2).

Operative Technique

Optimizing Access

A 2-0 silk suture is placed in the anterior tongue, and anterior traction is applied while an appropriate blade is inserted in the FK retractor. Both the laryngeal and tongue blades should be inserted into the FK retractor to determine which one provides the most optimal exposure. In our experience, similar to that reported in the literature, the tongue blade is most useful in accessing the pyriform sinuses.[28] While some have advocated the FK-WO retractor to allow a wider lateral working space, we have successfully used the standard FK retractor.[25] It is essential that sufficient anterior traction be applied to the 2-0 silk suture in order to pull the base of tongue anteriorly, thereby extending the epiglottis and optimizing the view of the supraglottis and hypopharynx. The 12-mm sized 30° endoscope is inserted face up, followed by a 5-mm spatula monopolar cautery ipsilateral to the tumor and a 5-mm Maryland forceps to the contralateral side. In those patients with a limited view anteriorly, manual posterior compression of the larynx can be applied to improve visualization. In select patients with an enlarged or flaccid epiglottis obstructing the surgical view, a partial ipsilateral epiglottectomy has been successfully applied to aid in visualization. This is particularly useful to access the pyriform sinus and has been applied in half of pyriform sinus SCC treated with TORS[28] (Fig. 3.3).

Pyriform Sinus

The goal of surgical excision is to remove the tumor with a clear margin with minimal morbidity in terms of airway and deglutition. Transoral robotic surgery excision of a

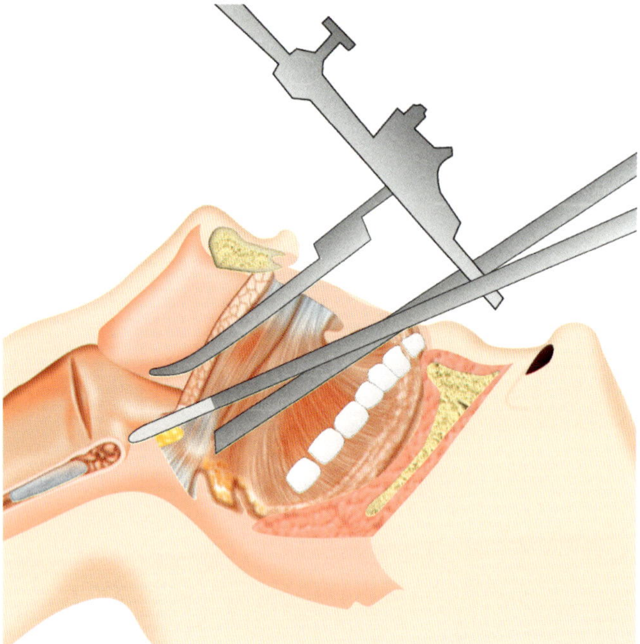

Fig. 3.3: Schematic representation of FK retractor with endoscope.

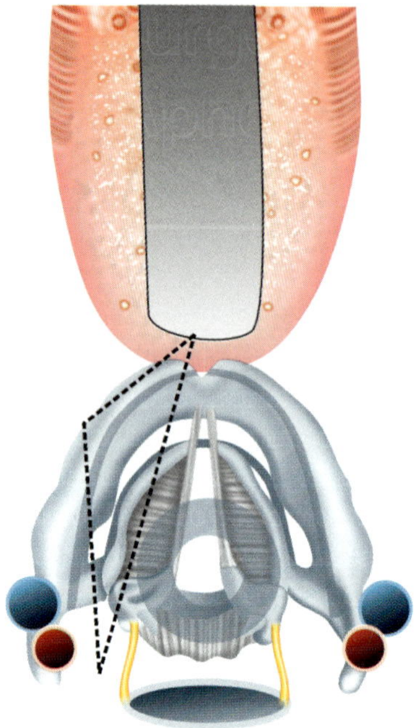

Fig. 3.4: Schematic representation of a cone resection of the left pyriform sinus as outlined but the dotted line.

pyriform sinus tumor is achieved by performing a cone-shaped resection of the pyriform, bounded superiorly at the vallecula and extending down to the apex of the cone just below the apex of the pyriform. This cone-shaped excision includes the aryepiglottic fold medially and the perichondrium of the thyroid cartilage laterally. The dissection is begun medially at the anterior aryepiglottic fold and proceeds in a posterior direction. Care is taken to preserve the integrity of the arytenoid and its vocal and muscular processes in order not to compromise laryngeal function. The dissection is then advanced laterally along the aryepiglottic fold towards the thyroid cartilage. An incision is made laterally through the perichondrium and onto the thyroid cartilage. The perichondrium is then carefully peeled inferiorly, while the cartilage remains intact. The dissection then proceeds posteriorly to posterior pharyngeal wall, where the posterior margin includes the inferior constrictor (🎥 3.1). Careful dissection in the posterolateral segment is essential to prevent inadvertent injury to the great vessels. The specimen is then pedicled on the apex of the pyriform sinus and can be removed en bloc (Figs. 3.4 and 3.5). When a large ablative defect remains in the hypopharynx, especially in the setting of prior chemoradiation therapy, primary closure of the pyriform can be accomplished with interrupted 3-0 Vicryl (Figs. 3.6A to I).

Posterior Pharyngeal Wall

Dissection of a posterior pharyngeal wall lesion is less complicated and has a similar setup as for a pyriform sinus lesion. The 30° face up telescope is used. The advantage of the robotic system is particularly appreciated during the dissection of the inferior portion of the lesion where, as opposed to the TLM, the dissection plane remains in view. The lesion is circumferentially resected with a 5 mm clear margin. The dissection is initiated superiorly, where an incision is made through the mucosa and down to the prevertebral fascia. The appropriate plane of dissection is just anterior to the prevertebral fascia. The inferior dissection is then carried out and the lesion is then approached in a circumferential pattern (Figs. 3.7A to G). These defects can be left to granulate secondarily with early initiation of oral deglutition.

Neck

The reported incidence of occult nodal metastasis is >20% and therefore ipsilateral selective neck dissection including levels II–IV is commonly indicated.[4]

Bilateral selective neck dissection should be performed for midline tumors of the posterior pharyngeal wall or postcricoid area, as well as tumors involving the medial wall of the pyriform sinus and those that cross the midline. We also consider contralateral neck dissection in

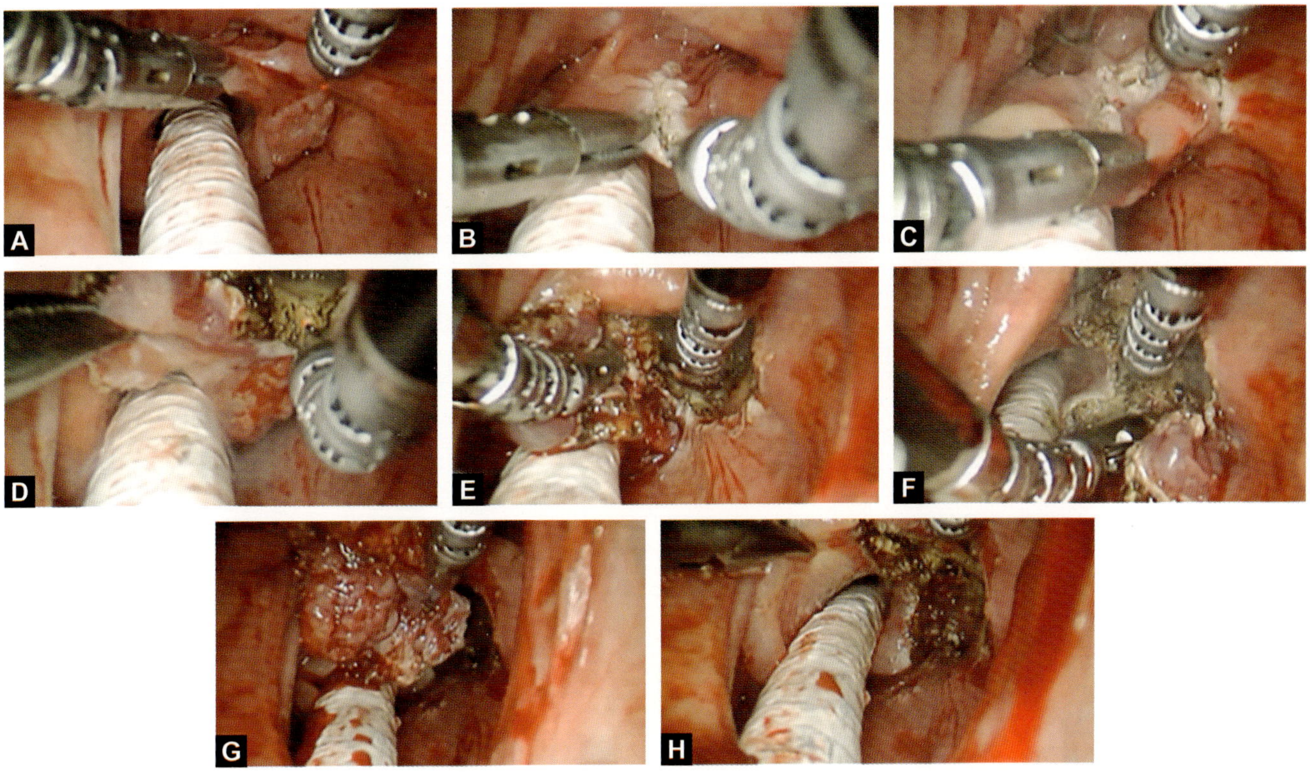

Figs. 3.5A to H: Sequential resection of a right pyriform sinus squamous cell carcinoma (A), with dissection begun medially along epiglottis (B) and continued anteriolaterally to the inner thyroid perichondrium (C to E). The specimen is then pedicled medially and removed (F) and orientation and margins are confirmed (G) and the remaining ablative defect is left to heal by secondary intention (H).

those patients with palpable ipsilateral disease or those patients presenting with advanced disease.[8] We perform all neck dissection concurrent with the TORS ablation. In advanced disease we occasionally include a level VI dissection when indicated.[33]

Complications and their Management

Careful selection of patients is integral to successful oncological and functional outcomes. The preoperative history and physical examination is essential to select out these patients. When possible, assembling the FK retractor during a diagnostic panendoscopy is useful to identify patients with adequate exposure. Maneuvers to improve exposure include anterior tongue traction, posterior laryngeal pressure and partial epiglottectomy. During surgical excision care should be taken in the posterior lateral compartment to prevent injury to the great vessels. Careful attention to tumor margins is essential, especially at the anterior lateral compartment of the pyriform, which is a particularly difficult area to obtain a clear margin. A low threshold for keeping a tracheostomy in place is important especially as one gains experience treating this disease entity. Most patients will remain with tracheostomy and nasogastric feeding tube during their postoperative recovery. It is essential to properly consent patients for this recovery period. In the case series reported to date the average time to decannulation and return to deglutition are approximately 6 and 8 days, respectively.[7] Adherence to careful patient selection and optimizing surgical access allow these results to be realistically achieved.

Follow-up

Postoperatively, patients are assessed by a formal swallow assessment prior to initiation of an oral diet. Those patients requiring a tracheostomy intraoperatively are managed postoperatively in the usual fashion with downsizing to a noncuffed tracheostomy tube on postoperative day 3 and decannulation following a successful 24-hour trial of capping. Patients are revaluated in a multidisciplinary setting at 1 week post-discharge by both the primary surgeon and a speech language pathologist. Subsequent follow-ups correspond with the National Comprehensive Cancer Network guidelines.

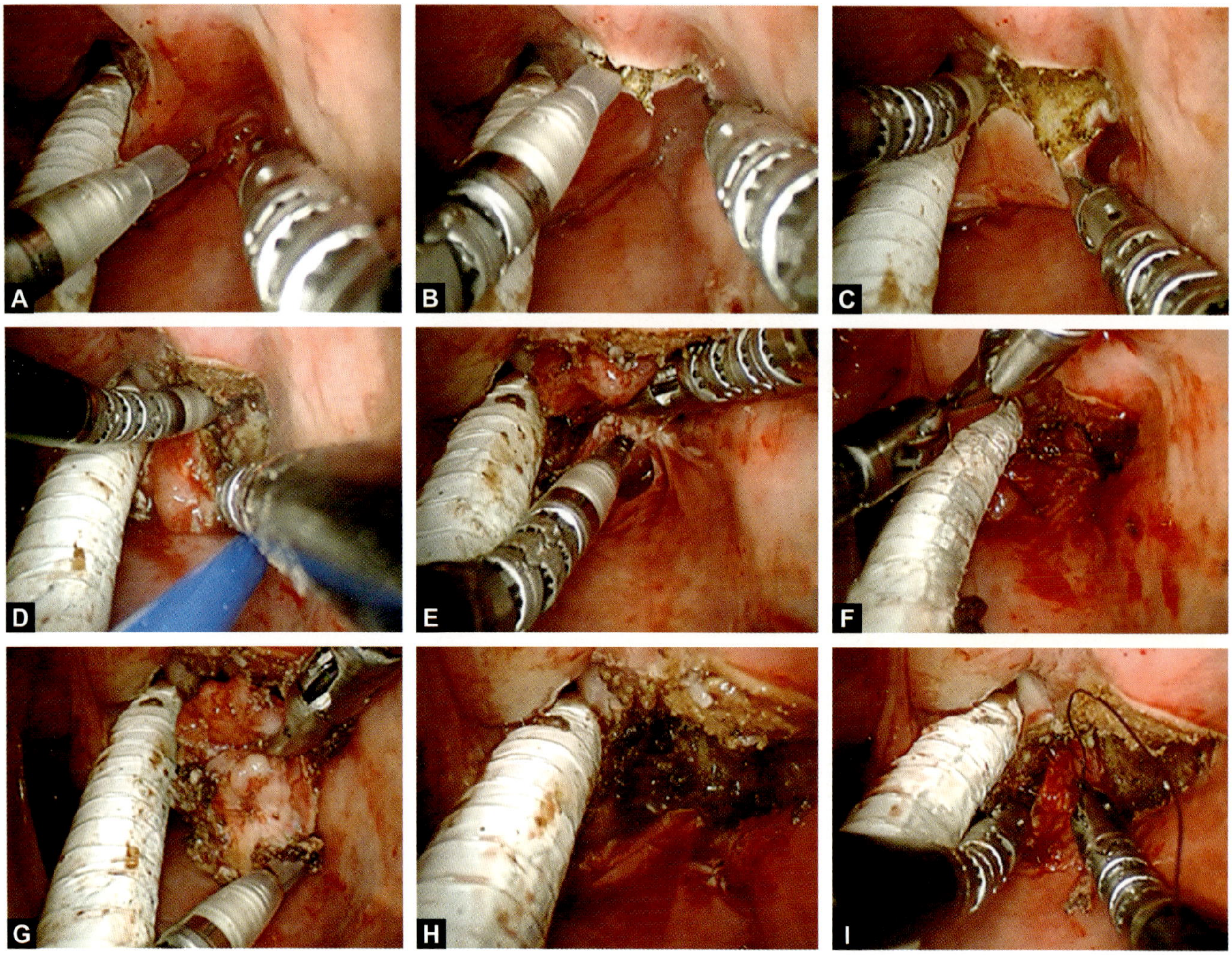

Figs. 3.6A to I: Sequential resection of a recurrent right pyriform sinus squamous cell carcinoma postchemoradiation therapy. The ablative defect is closed primarily using interrupted 3-0 Vicryl, to maintain a sensate mucosa and prevent aspiration.

RESULTS

Several early case series have reported on the successful application of TORS to the treatment of upper aerodigestive tract malignancies in terms of completeness of resection and postoperative morbidity.[26,27] Certainly, the greatest challenge in the application of TORS to treatment of the larynx and hypopharynx is access, with up to 25% of carefully selected patients having difficult exposure.[28] However, this can be overcome with maneuvers discussed below. Focusing on the hypopharynx, a prospective case series included 10 T1 or T2 pyriform sinus or posterior pharyngeal wall SCC treated successfully with TORS hypopharyngectomy were reported. All patients had clear margins without significant perioperative complications. Patients received prophylactic intraoperative tracheotomy with an average time to decannulation of 6.3 days, and a return of swallowing function within 8.3 days after surgery. These results suggested that TORS hypopharyngectomy was a feasible option with favorable morbidity.[7] In a larger prospective study of 23 patients with hypopharynx SCC, designed to determine oncological outcomes, the 3-year overall survival and disease-free survival of 89% and 84%, respectively, compared favorably to both open surgical techniques and concurrent chemotherapy. Functional outcomes of voice and swallow were objectively assessed with favorable results.[25] While these series are limited by a selection bias, they nonetheless suggest that TORS is a feasible and oncological valid option in a carefully selected group of patients.

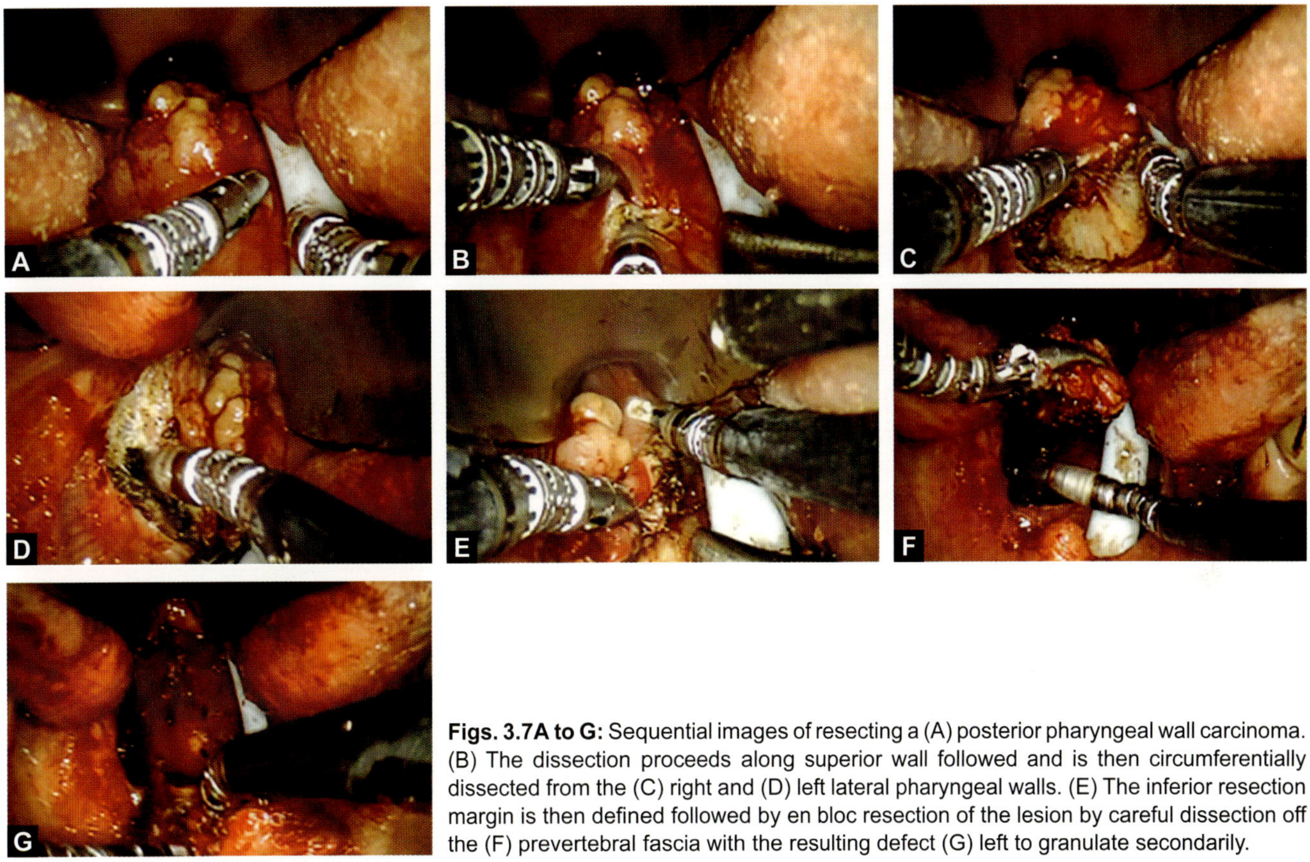

Figs. 3.7A to G: Sequential images of resecting a (A) posterior pharyngeal wall carcinoma. (B) The dissection proceeds along superior wall followed and is then circumferentially dissected from the (C) right and (D) left lateral pharyngeal walls. (E) The inferior resection margin is then defined followed by en bloc resection of the lesion by careful dissection off the (F) prevertebral fascia with the resulting defect (G) left to granulate secondarily.

FUTURE DIRECTIONS

Transoral robotic surgery is minimally invasive, safe and offers sound oncologic surgical technique, with improved functional outcomes. Careful patient selection, based on a comprehensive physical examination and preoperative imaging, is essential to obtain successful outcomes. Adequate exposure is a critical component of this technique that facilitates clear margins with minimal postoperative morbidity. Further prospective trials are required to more clearly identify patients who are better served with this technique. Certainly, TORS has emerged as a viable treatment option in the armamentarium of organ preservation therapies for hypopharynx SCC.

VIDEO LEGEND

Video 3.1: Right hypopharyngeal transoral robotic surgery.

REFERENCES

1. Cooper JS, et al. National Cancer Database report on cancer of the head and neck: 10-year update. Head Neck. 2009;31(6):748-58.
2. Kirchner JA. Pyriform sinus cancer: a clinical and laboratory study. Ann Otol Rhinol Laryngol. 1975;84(6):793-803.
3. Hoffman HT, et al. Hypopharyngeal cancer patient care evaluation. Laryngoscope. 1997;107(8):1005-17.
4. Hall SF, et al. The natural history of patients with squamous cell carcinoma of the hypopharynx. Laryngoscope. 2008;118(8):1362-71.
5. Gourin CG, Terris DJ. Carcinoma of the hypopharynx. Surg Oncol Clin North Am. 2004;13(1):81-98.
6. Buckley JG, MacLennan K. Cervical node metastases in laryngeal and hypopharyngeal cancer: a prospective analysis of prevalence and distribution. Head Neck. 2000; 22(4):380-5.
7. Park YM, et al. Feasibility of transoral robotic hypopharyngectomy for early-stage hypopharyngeal carcinoma. Oral Oncol. 2010;46(8):597-602.
8. Chan JY, Wei WI. Current management strategy of hypopharyngeal carcinoma. Auris Nasus Larynx. 2013;40(1):2-6.
9. Lefebvre JL. Surgery for laryngopharyngeal SCC in the era of organ preservation. Clin Exp Otorhinolaryngol. 2009; 2(4):159-63.
10. Lefebvre JL, et al. Larynx preservation in pyriform sinus cancer: preliminary results of a European Organization for Research and Treatment of Cancer phase III trial. EORTC Head and Neck Cancer Cooperative Group. J Natl Cancer Inst. 1996;88(13):890-9.

11. Levendag PC, et al. Dysphagia disorders in patients with cancer of the oropharynx are significantly affected by the radiation therapy dose to the superior and middle constrictor muscle: a dose-effect relationship. Radiother Oncol. 2007;85(1):64-73.
12. Forastiere AA, et al. Concurrent chemotherapy and radiotherapy for organ preservation in advanced laryngeal cancer. N Engl J Med. 2003;349(22):2091-8.
13. Forastiere AA, et al. Long-Term Results of RTOG 91-11: A Comparison of Three Nonsurgical Treatment Strategies to Preserve the Larynx in Patients With Locally Advanced Larynx Cancer. J Clin Oncol. 2013;31(7):845-52..
14. Hoffman HT, et al. Laryngeal cancer in the United States: changes in demographics, patterns of care, and survival. Laryngoscope. 2006;116(9 Pt 2 Suppl 111):1-13.
15. Chen AY, Halpern M. Factors predictive of survival in advanced laryngeal cancer. Arch Otolaryngol Head Neck Surg. 2007;133(12):1270-6.
16. Arbyn M, et al. Trends of cervical cancer mortality in the member states of the European Union. Eur J Cancer. 2009;45(15):2640-8.
17. Godballe C, et al. Hypopharyngeal cancer: results of treatment based on radiation therapy and salvage surgery. Laryngoscope. 2002;112(5):834-8.
18. Hall SF, et al. Radiotherapy or surgery for head and neck squamous cell cancer: establishing the baseline for hypopharyngeal carcinoma? Cancer. 2009;115(24):5711-22.
19. Steiner W. [Therapy of hypopharyngeal cancer. Part III: The concept of minimally invasive therapy of cancers of the upper aerodigestive tract with special reference to hypopharyngeal cancer and trans-oral laser microsurgery]. HNO. 1994;42(2):104-12.
20. Iseli TA, et al. Functional outcomes after transoral robotic surgery for head and neck cancer. Otolaryngol Head Neck Surg. 2009;141(2):166-71.
21. Rudert HH, Hoft S. Transoral carbon-dioxide laser resection of hypopharyngeal carcinoma. Eur Arch Otorhinolaryngol. 2003;260(4):198-206.
22. Steiner W, et al. Organ preservation by transoral laser microsurgery in piriform sinus carcinoma. Otolaryngol Head Neck Surg. 2001;124(1):58-67.
23. Martin A, et al. Organ preserving transoral laser microsurgery for cancer of the hypopharynx. Laryngoscope. 2008;118(3):398-402.
24. Bernal-Sprekelsen M, et al. [Complications of transoral laser surgery for malignant tumors of the larynx and hypopharynx]. Laryngorhinootologie. 2009;88(1):28-34.
25. Park YM, et al. Transoral robotic surgery for hypopharyngeal squamous cell carcinoma: 3-year oncologic and functional analysis. Oral Oncol. 2012;48(6):560-6.
26. Boudreaux BA, et al. Robot-assisted surgery for upper aerodigestive tract neoplasms. Arch Otolaryngol Head Neck Surg. 2009;135(4):397-401.
27. Genden EM, Desai S, Sung CK. Transoral robotic surgery for the management of head and neck cancer: a preliminary experience. Head Neck. 2009;31(3):283-9.
28. De Virgilio A, et al. How to optimize laryngeal and hypopharyngeal exposure in transoral robotic surgery. Auris Nasus Larynx. 2013;40(3):312-9.
29. Crosby ET, et al. The unanticipated difficult airway with recommendations for management. Can J Anaesth, 1998;45 (8):757-76.
30. Rumboldt Z, et al. Imaging in head and neck cancer. Curr Treat Options Oncol. 2006;7(1):23-34.
31. Harrison DF. Pathology of hypopharyngeal cancer in relation to surgical management. J Laryngol Otol. 1970;84(4):349-67.
32. Gedgaudas-McClees RK, McClees EC. The value of the barium-swallow technique in the evaluation of the hypopharynx. Mt Sinai J Med. 1984;51(4):455-9.
33. Harrison DF. Surgical pathology of hypopharyngeal neoplasms. J Laryngol Otol. 1971;85(12):1215-8.

Chapter 4 Transoral Robotic Supraglottic Laryngectomy (TORS-SGL)

Peter T Dziegielewski, Enver Ozer

INTRODUCTION

Laryngeal cancer confronts head and neck oncologists with the challenge of achieving cure while minimizing morbidity and preserving structure and function. This is the basis of *organ preservation*, which strives to avoid total laryngectomy. Laryngeal structures are spared where oncologically possible with the hope of preserving laryngeal function. Initial attempts to fulfill this ideal included open partial laryngectomies (OPLs), which carried variable outcomes.[1,2] To avoid the morbidity associated with open surgery, external beam radiation therapy (XRT) with chemotherapy protocols became popular organ preservation options and continue to dominate laryngeal treatment paradigms.[3-5] Unfortunately, these therapies have demonstrated significant early and late side effects including speech and swallowing disruption, tracheostomy tube dependence, gastrostomy tube (G-Tube) dependence as well as suboptimal quality of life.[6]

In the last decade, the treatment pendulum has swung back toward surgery with minimally invasive, organ preserving techniques aimed at curing disease and minimizing the toxicity and morbidity of treatment.[7-9] It has been shown that appropriately selected early and intermediate stage laryngeal cancers can be excised transorally with oncologic soundness, excellent functional outcomes and good quality of life.[7,8,10-13] Transoral techniques have included cold laryngeal microsurgery and transoral laser microsurgery.[11] Recent advances in robotic surgery have provided a third option called transoral robotic surgery (TORS), which has progressed from simple tonsillectomy to laryngectomies.[14] While TORS is quickly becoming a favorable primary treatment for oropharyngeal cancers, its history for laryngeal lesions is young.[8,12,13,15-18] In 2005, TORS supraglottic laryngectomy (TORS-SGL) was described in a dog.[18] In 2007, an early experience was described with three patients, two of whom could not be resected transorally.[17] After a publishing hiatus, three larger dedicated TORS-SGL series were released in 2012 showing successful, efficient and reproducible results.[8,12,13] This chapter illustrates TORS-SGL as a viable alternative to XRT/chemotherapy in early and intermediate supraglottic cancers.

Table 4.1: Goals of TORS-SGL

- Excise cancer with negative margins
- Preserve laryngeal function
- Avoid G-Tube
- Avoid tracheostomy
- Minimize morbidity

RATIONALE FOR PROCEDURE

Transoral minimally invasive partial laryngectomies allow the head and neck surgeon to perform an SGL without entering the neck (Table 4.1). Transoral robotic surgery offers a novel method for accomplishing this with exceptional three-dimensional (3D) high-definition (1080 p) views with powerful magnification. The cutting tools can be customized to the surgeon; scissors, Bovie cautery and CO_2 laser are all possible. Moreover, the robotic arms reduce tremor and provide 7° of freedom, giving the surgeon control in all axes, even around corners. Essentially the surgeon's hand movements are translated to a smaller scale at the level of the larynx allowing the goals of surgery to be achieved.

APPLIED ANATOMY

The supraglottis consists of the laryngeal anatomy superior to a horizontal plane passing through the lateral margin of the laryngeal ventricle at the junction with the superior vocal cord surface. The subunits of the supraglottis include (1) supra- and infrahyoid epiglottis, (2) aryepiglottic folds, (3) arytenoids and (4) false cords (including the laryngeal ventricle).

An SGL involves an en bloc subtotal resection of the supraglottic structures above the arytenoids (Table 4.2). The anterior boundary is the laryngeal surface of the thyroid cartilage at the petiole of the epiglottis. The posterior limit is the posterior aspect of the aryepiglottic folds. The inferior

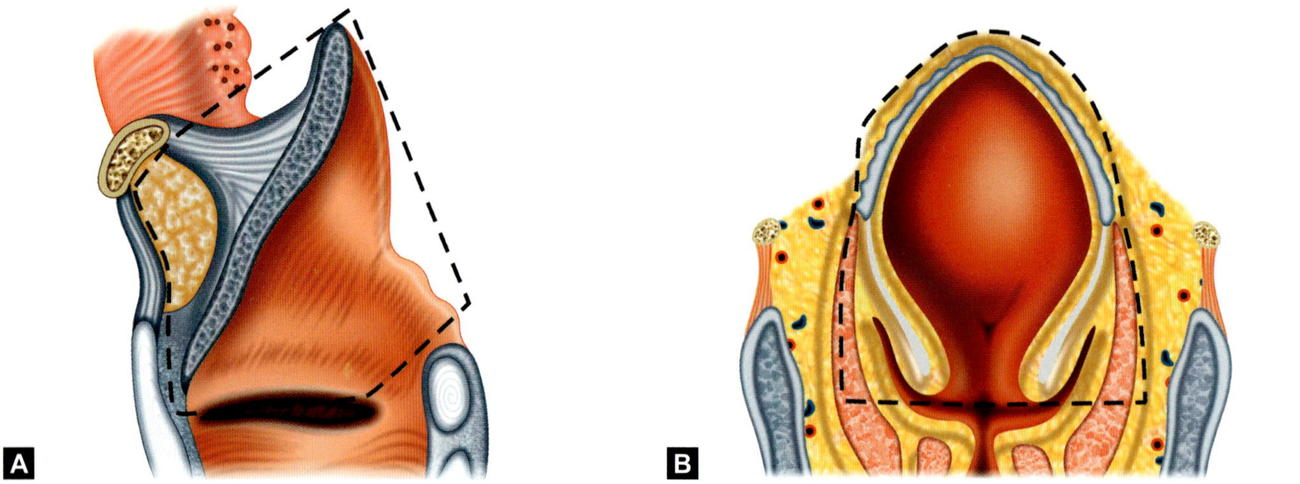

Figs. 4.1A and B: Boundaries of transoral robotic supraglottic laryngectomy (TORS-SGL). (A) Sagittal view and (B) coronal view. Dotted lines indicate TORS-SGL boundaries.

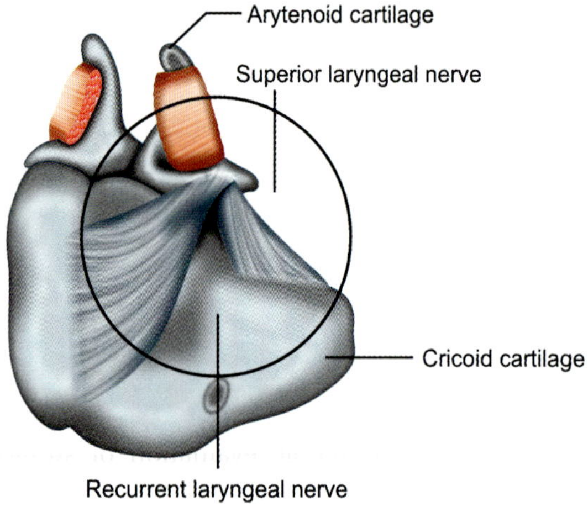

Fig. 4.2: The cricoarytenoid unit: cricoid cartilage, one arytenoid, one recurrent laryngeal nerve and one superior laryngeal nerve.

Table 4.2: Boundaries of TORS-SGL

Anterior	: Thyroid cartilage
Posterior	: Aryepiglottic folds
Superior	: Tip of epiglottis/base of tongue
Inferior	: Laryngeal ventricle
Lateral	: Thyroid cartilage/aryepiglottic mucosa

limit is a horizontal plane just above the vocal cords at the laryngeal ventricle including the aryepiglottic mucosa and the superior arytenoid mucosa. Ideally the resection will not extend deeply to include the arytenoids. Superiorly, the resection includes the entire epiglottis and may extend into the tongue base if need be. The resection may extend into other adjacent anatomic sites if necessary; however, at least one cricoarytenoid unit must be preserved to allow for tracheostomy-free breathing and optimal swallowing function (Figs. 4.1A and B). The paramount tenet of partial laryngectomy is to achieve negative margins and maintain at least one cricoarytenoid unit.[2,15,19] The cricoarytenoid unit consists of the cricoid cartilage, one arytenoid as well as one superior laryngeal nerve and recurrent laryngeal nerve (Fig. 4.2).

Table 4.3: Indications

- Adequate transoral exposure
  - Complete visualization of the tumor and its margins
  - Ability to visualize and maneuver the robotic arms without obstructing the view of the tumor
- T1 or T2 supraglottic cancer
- Select T3 supraglottic cancer
  - Pre-epiglottic space invasion
  - Ability to preserve 50% of the tongue base with an oncologic resection
  - Mobile vocal cords
- Minimal pyriform sinus involvement
- Consent for open procedure or total laryngectomy

PATIENT SELECTION

As organ conservation surgery has expounded to less invasive techniques in poorly exposed anatomical areas, appropriate patient selection has become critical to optimize functional outcomes while obtaining negative margins.[2,8,12,13,15-17,20] Previous OPLs have defined indications and contraindications. Based on these TORS-SGL, patient selection criteria are defined (Table 4.3).

Table 4.4: Contraindications

- Anterior or posterior commissure involvement
- Vocal cord fixation
- Thyroid or cricoid cartilage invasion
- Bilateral arytenoid cartilage involvement
- Poor pulmonary reserve (FEV1/FVC <50%)

Optimal functional outcomes are achieved in patients where both arytenoid cartilages can be preserved with negative tumor margins.[21] Larger tumors can be resected while avoiding a permanent tracheostomy or G-Tube; however, the risk of superior laryngeal nerve injury and postoperative scarring/strictures increases. If a T3 tumor or one with extensive pyriform sinus involvement is approached via TORS-SGL, the patient should be counseled on needing rigorous swallowing rehabilitation and potentially a temporary tracheostomy.

Transoral robotic surgery supraglottic laryngectomy is not an appropriate operation in situations that may jeopardize oncologic resection, would violate both cricoarytenoid units or leave the patient with airway compromise (Table 4.4).

The contraindications to TORS-SGL represent situations where the cricoarytenoid units would be violated or the patient would likely have poor postoperative function. Good pulmonary reserve is essential for the patient to tolerate expected transient postoperative dysphagia, aspiration and airway edema. Many patients initially experience some aspiration due to altered laryngeal sensation and loss of the epiglottis. Thus, good pulmonary reserve is needed to tolerate mild aspiration.

PREOPERATIVE WORKUP

Work for TORS-SGL consists of: lesion diagnosis, tumor mapping and staging, assessment of airway status, assessment of exposure, swallowing evaluation, metastatic work-up and treatment planning.

A suspected diagnosis is obtained from a thorough history and physical examination. Additionally, TORS exposure is assessed with attention paid to trismus/mouth opening, the height and depth of the larynx in the neck, thyromental distance, neck circumference and dental status.

Tumor mapping/staging and airway assessment are achieved with flexible nasopharyngoscopy where the upper aerodigestive tract is inspected for airway obstruction, secondary lesions and tumor extent. Further assessment of TORS exposure is made with attention paid to the tongue base size and mobility as well as visibility of the tumor and its margins.

Swallowing evaluation is begun during nasopharyngoscopy. The hypopharynx is observed for pooled secretions, and a functional endoscopic evaluation of swallowing may be performed, with a speech language pathologist present, to determine the patient's baseline safety of swallow. A video fluoroscopic examination may alternatively be used. Swallowing evaluation provides a baseline for post-operative swallowing rehabilitation.

Following the initial office examination, a staging PET-CT or CT neck and chest should be completed. The final workup includes panendoscopy and lesion biopsy under anesthesia to confirm the suspected tissue diagnosis. This can be done on the day of TORS-SGL. Additional preoperative testing may include pulmonary function testing in patients with known or suspected moderate-to-severe chronic lung disease. Prior to proceeding with surgery, it is also recommended that the patient's case be discussed at a multidisciplinary tumor board to determine all treatment options and help the patient select the optimal one for him/her.

A preoperative check list may help with preparation for surgery (Table 4.5).

Table 4.5: Example of preoperative check list

- *Suspected diagnosis*: Supraglottic cancer
- *Stage*: T1N1M0
- *Tumor extent*: Minimal base of tongue invasion
- *Airway*: Patent, difficult intubation or tracheostomy not anticipated
- *Exposure concerns*: Teeth present, deep larynx/extended thyromental distance
- *Swallowing evaluation*: Functional endoscopic evaluation of swallowing performed. Safe swallow
- *Metastatic workup*: Positron emission tomography-computed tomography = no metastases. Endoscopy on day of TORS-SGL
- *Other*: Pulmonary function tests ordered. Patient has chronic obstructive pulmonary disease
- *Tumor board*: Transoral robotic surgery supraglottic laryngectomy agreed as optimal treatment
- *Plan*: Proceed with TORS-SGL and bilateral neck dissection.

INSTRUMENTATION

To perform TORS-SGL, the following specific instruments are recommended:

1. Zeitels Suspension Gallows (Endocraft LLC, Providence, RI; Catalog Number: ZVG-100A)
2. Feyh-Kastenbauer (FK) Retractor (Gyrus ACMI, Southborough, MA; Catalog Number: 640001)
3. 5 mm Endowrist Instruments (Intuitive Surgical, Sunnyvale, CA)
   a. Monopolar Cautery ["bovie"] (Catalog Number: 420142)
   b. Maryland Dissector (Catalog Number: 420143)
4. Endoclip Hemostatic Clip Applier (Covidien, Dublin, Ireland; Catalog Number: 176620)
5. Opti-Gard Eye Protectors (Dupaco Inc., Oceanside, CA; Catalog Number: D28310)

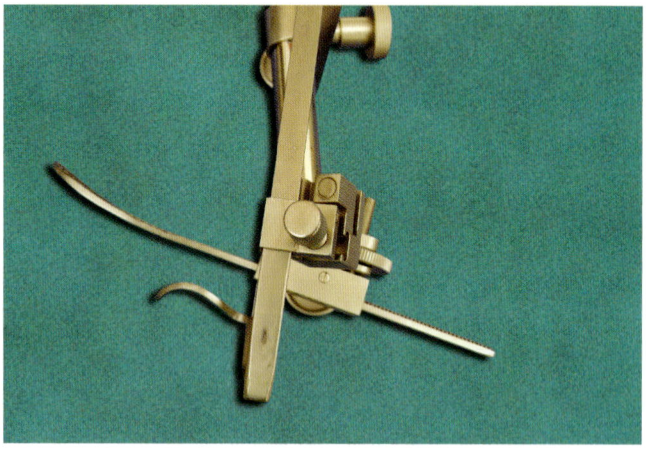

Fig. 4.3: Adjusting the Feyh-Kastenbauer (FK) retractor for transoral robotic supraglottic laryngectomy. The tongue blade is partially reversed and angled to be parallel to the tooth guard.

OPERATIVE SETUP

Anesthesia

Transoral robotic surgery is performed under general anesthesia with full paralysis to aid in oral retraction. Transnasal intubation is preferred to keep the tube posterior to the working field and lower the potential of igniting the tube with the hot Bovie cautery. To further minimize the chance of an airway fire, a laser safe endotracheal tube is employed and FiO_2 is kept at <30%, if the patient's pulmonary status allows for it.

Patient Positioning

The anesthetized patient is positioned supine with a shoulder role to extend the head. Patient's head is brought to the edge of the long end of the operating table to provide access for the robotic legs. Depending on the size of the operating theater, the operating table is then turned 90–180° to allow for the robot to come in at a 30–45° angle. Opti-Gard eye protectors are used to guard the eyes from unintentional robotic movements.

Transoral Exposure

Exposing the supraglottis and tongue base for TORS-SGL can be a challenge. A plastic tooth guard is first placed over the upper teeth. If no teeth are present, a dry gauze is used instead to provide traction for the retraction device. The FK retractor is optimally suited to exposing the base of tongue and supraglottis. It is adjusted in three axes and is first opened slightly with the tongue blade and tooth guard parallel to one another (Fig. 4.3). The FK is inserted into the oral cavity partially open and advanced so that the tongue blade enters the vallecula under direct visualization. The opening ratchet is then slightly opened and the tongue blade is slowly reversed to allow the supraglottis to drop further into view. Once adequate direct visualization is achieved the opening ratchet can be activated; however, it is cautioned that opening the retractor too far in the vertical plane may cause the tongue base to slip too far into view and obstruct the supraglottis. The best exposure is achieved with the tongue blade and tooth guard parallel to one another with 3-4 cm of opening (Fig. 4.4). The view is further adjusted with the tilting ratchet to provide a better direct angle of visualization. When the operator is satisfied with the view of the supraglottis, the FK is suspended off of a Zeitels gallows suspension device. The endotracheal tube should be inspected and adjusted at the nose to insure that it is not kinked.

da Vinci Robot Positioning

The da Vinci Surgical System (Intuitive Surgical, Sunnyvale CA) is moved to the operating table and positioned at 30–45° to the table with its legs abutting the table platform and sitting under the head of the bed. For supraglottic and base of tongue work the robot is positioned slightly farther toward the patient's head so that the arms can make very acute angles with retractor. The optimal position of the robotic equipment will depend on operating room setup and surgeon preference. A suggested setup scheme is shown in Figure 4.5. A 30° up-facing binocular robotic endoscope is calibrated and secured to the central robotic arm. The endoscope is advanced past the trochar and then inserted into the oral cavity parallel to the FK blade. It is advanced until the supraglottis (Fig. 4.6) and tumor (Fig. 4.7) can easily be visualized. The lateral robotic arms are mounted with a Maryland dissector in the non-dominant arm and monopolar spatula cautery in the dominant arm. Once the cautery is plugged in, the operator may adjust the settings (recommended = 25 watts/fulgurate). With the da Vinci Si system both cut (recommended = 15 watts/blend) and coagulate settings are possible. A fiberoptic CO_2 laser (Fiberlase, Lumenis, Santa Clara, CA) may be attached to a robotic needle driver instead of the cautery.[13,17,22] The lateral arms are positioned such that the instrument tips are visualized on the screen and easily mobile. The cannulae are kept outside the lips to prevent injury to the teeth, lips or gums. To optimize instrument mobility, the instrument arms are positioned parallel to the endoscope and angled such that they do not interfere with one another. Prior to making any mucosal cuts, the surgeon should sit at the robotic console and test the visualization and movement of the instruments.

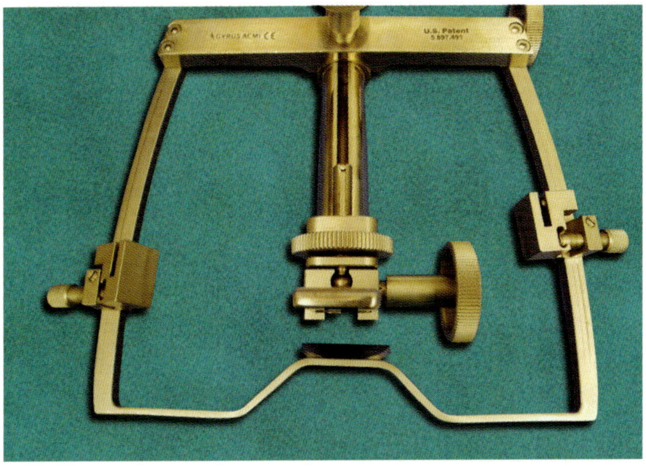

Fig. 4.4: Adjusting the Feyh-Kastenbauer retractor retractor for transoral robotic supraglottic laryngectomy. The retractor opening is kept at 3–4 cm, but enough to pass the robotic endoscope. This optimizes supraglottic and tongue base visualization.

OPERATIVE TECHNIQUE: TORS-SGL

Transoral robotic surgery allows the head and neck surgeon to perform a more traditional supraglottic resection with a cautery device in a fairly standardized and systematic manner. The approach focuses on removing the supraglottis en bloc and is similar to other tumor ablations where a functional subunit is removed to achieve negative margins.

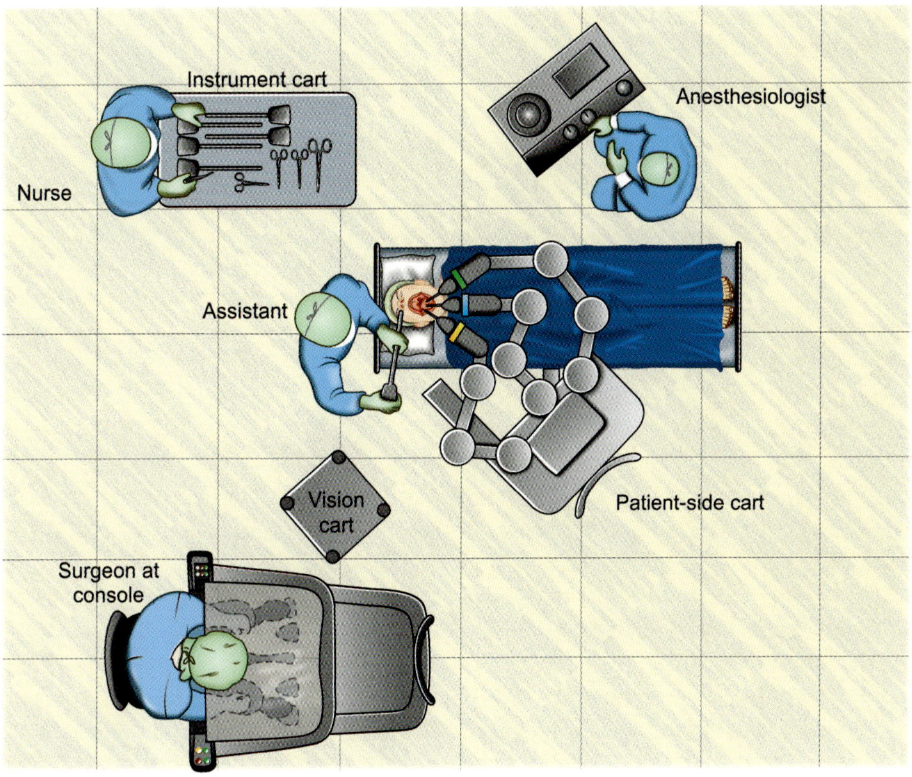

Fig. 4.5: Transoral robotic supraglottic laryngectomy operating room setup: overview.

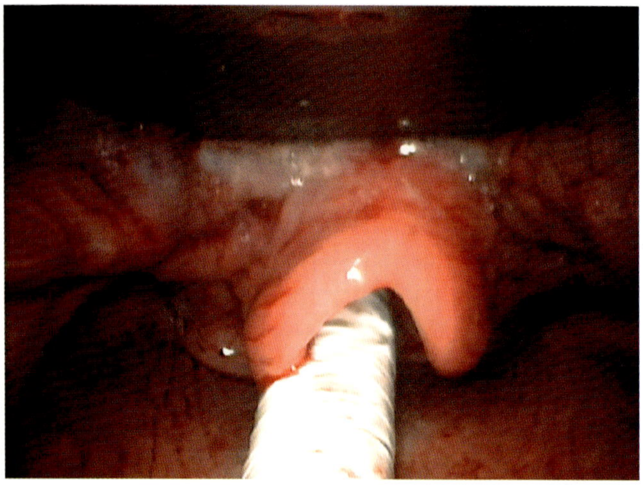

Fig. 4.6: Supraglottis view: initial view should expose the supraglottis and an adequate margin around the resection.

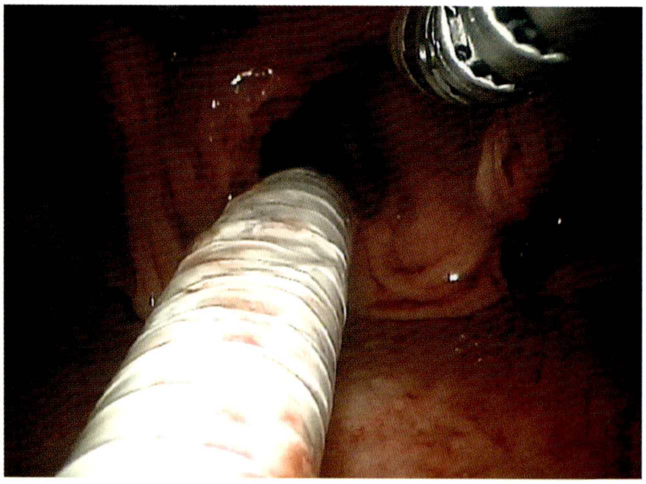

Fig. 4.7: Tumor view: the endoscope is adjusted to give full view of the tumor and its margins. A laser safe endotracheal tube remains posterior to the dissection field.

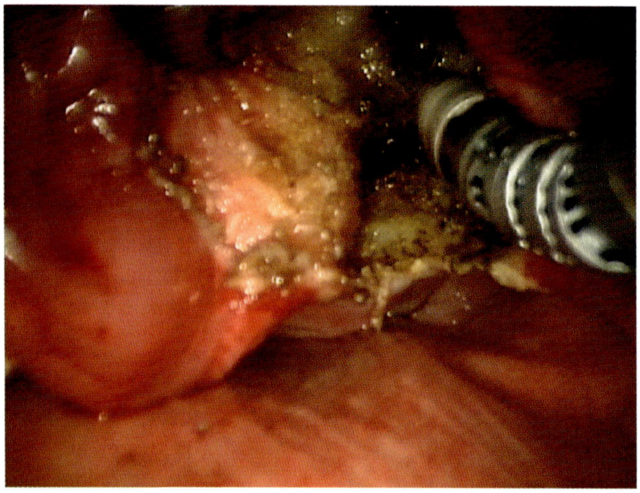

Fig. 4.8: Anterior incision: initial incisions are made anterior to the ventral surface of the epiglottis and may extend into the base of tongue.

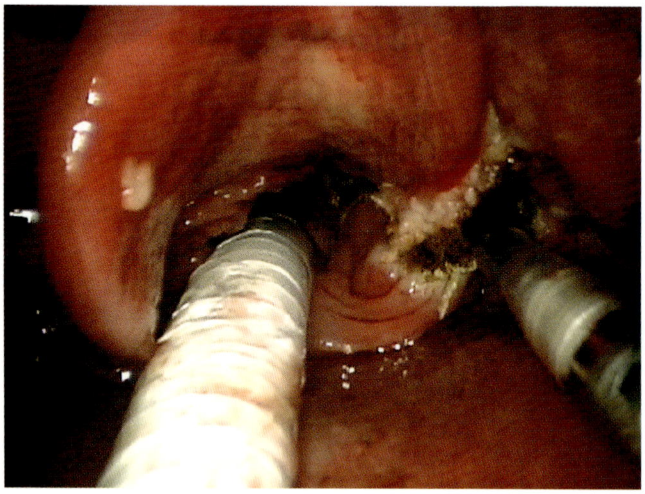

Fig. 4.9: Lateral incision: cuts are made away from the lesion and carried along the aryepiglottic folds toward the arytenoids mucosa.

The operating surgeon sits at the da Vinci robotic console with an assistant positioned at the head of the bed. The assistant's role is to eliminate smoke and blood and provide counter-tension on the resection. A pediatric Yankauer suction and suction mono-polar cautery are ideal tools for the assistant. An Endoclip hemostatic clip applier (Covidien, Dublin, Ireland) should also be available in case a larger blood vessel is encountered. Mucosal incisions are ideally made with the cautery on cut mode or with a CO_2 laser, to minimize char and allow for more accurate pathologic margin analysis. Incisions are deepened slowly with the cautery on coagulation mode.

Initial incisions are made contralateral to the side of the tumor. The first incision is superior to the ventral base of the epiglottis in a transverse direction extending laterally (Fig. 4.8). This incision may extend into the base of tongue if oncologically necessary. The specimen is pulled down by the epiglottis and the incision is deepened over the pre-epiglottic space to the hyoid bone. Due to the lack of haptic feedback on the robot arms, the Bovie is used in a "hot touch, cold touch" manner. Tissues are coagulated and the Bovie spatula tip is used as a dissector to push the tissues away. This allows for improved tissue dissection and views of upcoming structures. As the specimen is pulled down, dissection is carried along the aryepiglottic fold posteriorly to the arytenoid mucosa (Fig. 4.9). The posterior incision is then made along the arytenoid mucosa in a cranial to caudal direction encompassing

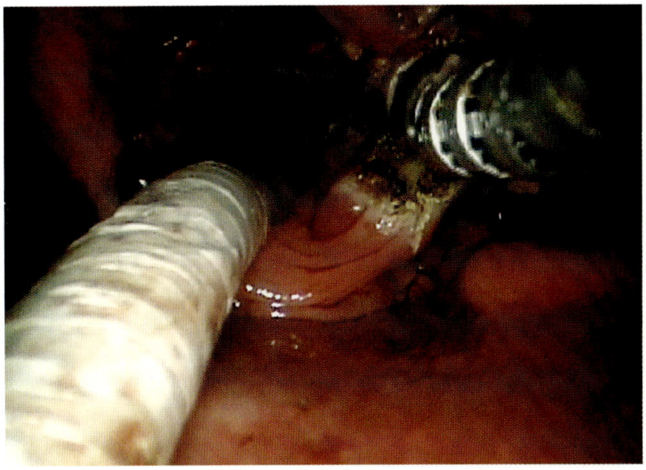

Fig. 4.10: False cord and ventricle incision: dissection is carried superior to inferior into the ventricle and then posterior to anterior parallel to the vocal cords toward the anterior commissure.

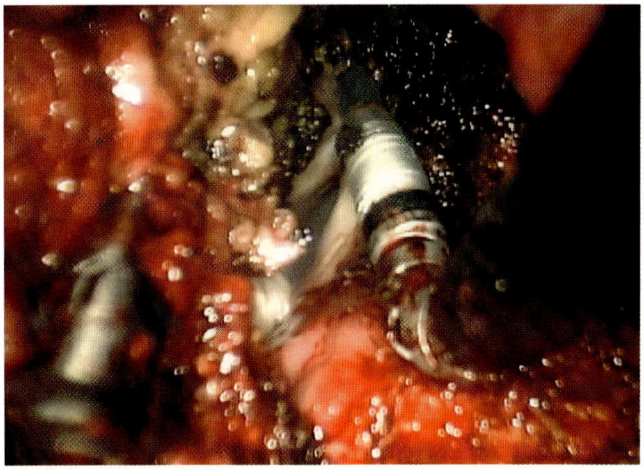

Fig. 4.11: Petiole dissection: the petiole is reached and the cut is extended to include it.

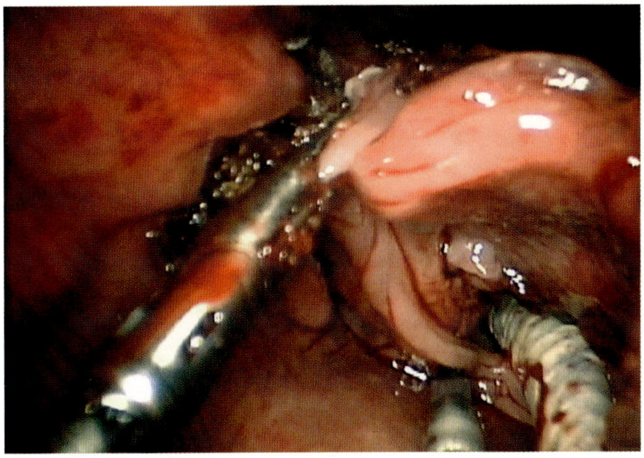

Fig. 4.12: Contralateral approach: incision is made through the contralateral aryepiglottic mucosa.

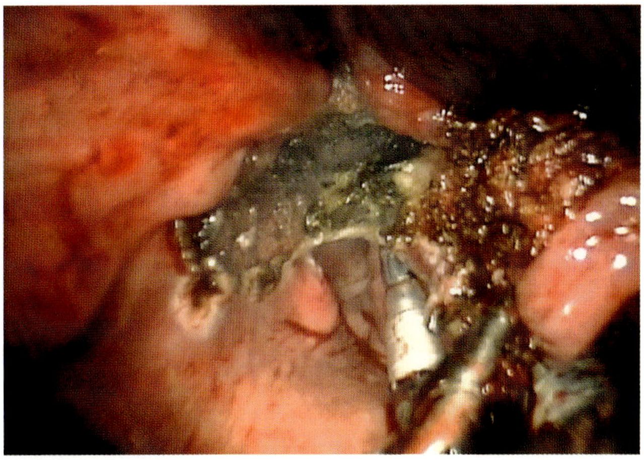

Fig. 4.13: Contralateral false cord/ventricle cuts: dissection is carried anteriorly toward the petiole.

the false vocal fold and ending in the ventricle (Fig. 4.10). Dissection is then carried anteriorly through the ventricle toward the anterior commissure to the petiole of the epiglottis (Fig. 4.11). During this step, the surgeon must be aware of the true vocal cord level and avoid burning the vocal cord mucosa. Contralateral incisions are then made around the tumor in a medial to lateral fashion along the anterior aryepiglottic mucosa (Fig. 4.12). The final dissection is carried around the arytenoid mucosa down to the level of the ventricle and anterior to the petiole (Fig. 4.13). The specimen is then detached (Fig. 4.14) and removed via the oral cavity (Fig. 4.15). The surgical bed is inspected and hemostasis is achieved with cautery or clips. Additional hemostasis is achieved with xylometazoline or topical adrenalin-soaked cottonoids. FloSeal Matrix (Baxter Healthcare Corporation, Hayward, CA) is also a useful adjunct. The tumor specimen is carefully inspected, palpated and oriented with sutures or staples. Frozen section tumor margins are sent from the surgical bed, with a focus on any areas that feel close to the tumor.

When resection is complete and frozen section margins are sent off, the robotic arms are carefully withdrawn parallel to the FK retractor. The arms are brought together and the robot is removed from the field. The FK retractor is released and removed while paying close attention to the endotracheal tube so as not to inadvertently extubate the patient. If neck dissection is planned concurrently, it is now performed. Alternatively neck dissection may be performed prior to TORS-SGL. Some surgeons may prefer this order as it would allow preemptive ligation of the superior laryngeal and lingual arteries; thus, decreasing ablative blood loss.

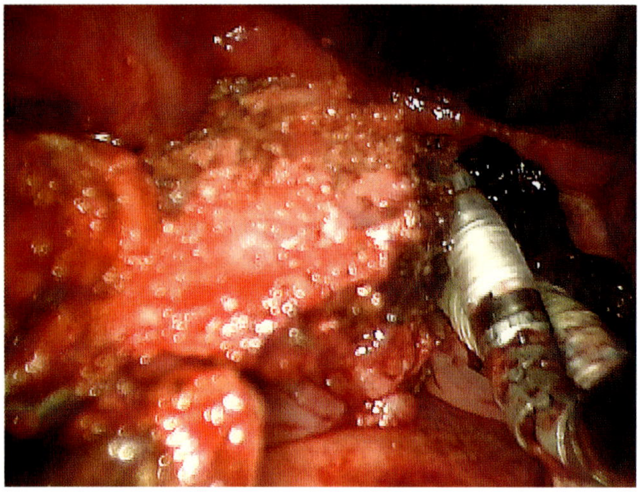

Fig. 4.14: Specimen release: the resection specimen is released at the petiole.

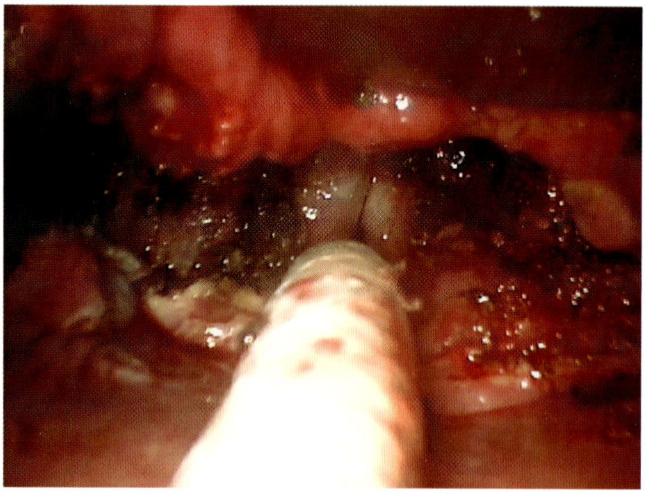

Fig. 4.15: Resection site after the tumor has been removed.

Pearls and Pitfalls

- Opening the FK retractor too much will compromise the direct line of site view of the larynx. Limit opening to 3-4 cm and adjust the axes of the retractor to improve exposure.
- Pulling too hard with the Maryland dissector can tear tissues along weak planes leading to false positive margins. For cleaner resections, use the Maryland dissector to push tissues and provide counter-tension.
- Set a timer for 1 hour. If the procedure extends longer, the FK retractor should be released for 5 minutes to prevent lingual/hypoglossal nerve neuropraxia.
- When planning the resection, consider how much of the tongue base will need to be included. If > 50% is ablated, significant swallowing dysfunction will ensue. For these patients, consider other treatment options.
- Postoperative airway edema may be reduced with an intraoperative dose of dexamethasone (10 mg IV).

POSTOPERATIVE CARE

At the completion of the case, the airway is inspected with direct laryngoscopy to guide extubation decisions. In most cases, the patient may be safely extubated in the operating room.[13] However, if the glottis appears swollen around the endotracheal tube, leaving the patient intubated overnight in a monitored setting is safer.[8] Emergency airway equipment such as a Glidescope (Verathon, Bothell, WA), rigid endoscopes, a flexible bronchoscope and a tracheotomy setup should be in the operating room and available upon extubation. Postoperative orders should include antibiotics for 3 days, a proton pump inhibitor for 6 weeks and intravenous dexamethasone for 24 hours (10 mg IV q8h).

Table 4.6: Complications are divided into intraoperative, early postoperative and late postoperative periods

Intraoperative	*Early postoperative*	*Late postoperative*
• Poor exposure • Bleeding • Premature extubation/ loss of airway • Retractor injuries • Airway fire	• Airway obstruction • Swallowing dysfunction • Hoarseness • Bleeding	• Prolonged swallowing dysfunction • Supraglottic strictures

Assessment by a speech-language pathologist on postoperative day 1 is helpful to evaluate and rehabilitate any swallowing dysfunction.[8,12,13]

Hospital discharge criteria include tolerance of an oral diet, stable vital signs and neck drains removed (if neck dissection was performed). Average length of hospital stay is expected to be approximately 4 days.[13] Follow-up visit is arranged at 2 weeks postoperatively.

COMPLICATIONS AND THEIR MANAGEMENT

Transoral robotic surgery supraglottic laryngectomy is still in its infancy, and thus, few complications have been reported. However, based on experiences with other transoral laryngeal surgery, specific complications are possible (Table 4.6).[23,24]

Intraoperative

Poor exposure: Anticipating exposure issues preoperatively is key and may preclude TORS-SGL in some patients.

Airway assessment includes inspecting for a large tongue, trismus, a small mouth or a low/anterior larynx. The FK tongue blade may be adjusted for depth, opening angle and length to improve exposure. However, if the entire tumor and its margins cannot be visualized, TORS may need to be abandoned or combined with a transcervical approach.[13,17] The patient should be consented for this possibility prior to entering the operating room.

Bleeding: Venous bleeding is best controlled with slow, purposeful cautery movements. However, if branches of the superior laryngeal or lingual arteries are violated, brisk bleeding may result. Having a suction cautery and Endo-clip hemostatic clip applier available to the assistant can be helpful.

Premature extubation/Loss of airway: The endotracheal tube cuff should be sufficiently below the glottis and slightly overinflated to resist pull back on the tube. It is also recommended that the endotracheal tube be secured to the nose with strong tape or a suture.

Retractor injuries: During the operation, the surgeon must be cognizant of the pressure the retractor can put on the tongue and oral structures. Prolonged pressure can lead to lingual nerve or hypoglossal nerve palsy, temporomandibular joint dislocation or dental injuries. If prolonged retraction is needed, it is recommended that the FK be released every 1 hour for 5 minutes.

Airway fire: Although likelihood of an airway fire in the absence of a laser is low, it is potentially the most devastating TORS-SGL complication. To minimize this risk, communication with the anesthesia team is of utmost importance. A laser safe endotracheal tube with methylene blue dyed water in the cuff along with $FiO_2 < 30\%$ will help minimize the risk. If an airway fire is detected (charred/melting tube, spark around the tube, smoke from the airway etc.), the procedure is stopped, oxygen is turned off and the endotracheal tube is quickly removed. The airway is doused with water and the patient is re-intubated with a new endotracheal tube. The airway is then inspected for damage and the patient is given steroids and antibiotics. At that point the procedure is stopped and the patient is admitted to an intensive care setting.

Laryngocervical fistula: If the thyroid membrane is violated and a neck dissection is performed, a fistula will result. This is likely recognized during the neck dissection and may not necessarily be avoided if negative margins are to be achieved during the resection. One strategy for repair includes swinging a strap muscle pedicled flap up and suturing it around the defect. Tissue glue is then applied over top. The patient is kept nothing by mouth for at least 5 days, put on antibiotics and neck drains are monitored for saliva. An oral diet trial may be pursued after 5 days. It is recommended that a neck drain be kept in until this time to allow for early detection of oral contents in the neck.

Early Postoperative

Airway obstruction: Collateral heat from the Bovie will inevitably cause some glottic edema potentially leading to stridor on extubation. Emergent reintubation may be necessary. Intermittently irrigating the field with saline will help cool tissues down and decrease unintentional burn-related edema. Additionally, reversal of anesthesia can result in coughing and blood pressure spikes, which could release airway bleeding. Ensuring hemostasis and having emergency airway equipment nearby will aid in crisis management.

Swallowing dysfunction: All TORS-SGL patients will have some swallowing difficulty postoperatively. Pain-related dysfunction is expected to resolve within days. Few patients will require a G-Tube (7.7%),[13] but many will need swallowing rehabilitation. It is recommended that all TORS-SGL patients be assessed and followed by a speech language pathologist.

Hoarseness: Transient hoarseness is common and typically resolves within 2–3 weeks. Using a proton pump inhibitor and having good vocal hygiene will help recovery.

Bleeding: Postoperative venous bleeding may manifest as blood-tinged sputum while arterial bleeds are more likely to be frank hemoptysis. Due to airway proximity, emergent reintubation or tracheostomy may be necessary. Once the airway is resecured, hemostasis is achieved as described above.

Late Postoperative

Prolonged swallowing dysfunction: While this has seldom been reported in the literature[8,13] it is conceivable that debilitated patients or those undergoing postoperative RT may encounter poor swallowing function. Continued swallowing rehabilitation therapy and follow-up is critical.

Supraglottic strictures: When opposing mucosal surfaces are cut, scarring is likely. The anterior commissure and laterally between the aryepiglottic folds/base of tongue are the two areas of greatest concern. Adhering to principles of phonomicrosurgery will minimize such outcomes.[25] Should a stricture occur, securing a safe airway is of primary importance. In some cases, a temporary tracheostomy

Table 4.7: Mean values

Perioperative measure	*Value*
Mean setup time	25 mins[2,6]
Mean operating time	25–94 mins[2,6]
Blood loss	3–40 mL[6]
Length of hospital stay	4–11 days[2,6]

may be needed. More definitive management may include TORS or transoral laser microsurgery to release the stricture with or without steroid injection.[26]

EXPECTED OUTCOMES

Perioperative Values

When planning TORS-SGL and counseling patients, it is helpful to have an idea of numeric specifics. The early literature on TORS-SGL has provided some mean values the surgeon can quote (Table 4.7).

Oncologic Outcomes

Transoral robotic surgery supraglottic laryngectomy reports have shown that obtaining negative margins is feasible and improved with the use of diligent frozen sectioning from the surgical bed.[8,12,13] Early results show low locoregional recurrence rates (0–11%), which is similar to other transoral laryngeal resections. However, long-term survival is yet to be determined.[8,12,13]

Functional Outcomes

Swallowing function is largely preserved and rehabilitable. G-Tube nutrition is rarely needed and only observed in 0-7% of patients.[8,13] Early initiation of swallowing exercises by a speech language pathologist aids in recovery. Factors delaying swallowing recovery include male gender, T3 tumors, vocal fold hypomobility or undergoing simultaneous neck dissection.[8]

Speech function is preserved if the vocal folds are not surgically entered. Tracheostomy is seldom required and has only been reported in three patients to date.[8,12,13] Transient dysphonia is often present to a mild degree in one-third of patients.[8,12,13]

CHOOSING AN SGL APPROACH

Minimally invasive approaches to early supraglottic lesions include traditional OPL, transoral endoscopic phonomicrosurgery ("cold knife"), transoral laser microsurgery and now TORS. Reasons for choosing TORS over other approaches are outlined (Table 4.8).

Table 4.8: Advantages and disadvantages of TORS-SGL

Advantages	*Disadvantages*
Three-dimensional, high definition, magnified optics	Exposure challenges
7° of movement freedom	Operating room robotic use costs
En bloc versus piece meal resection	Assistant needed
Low blood loss	
No external scar	
Shorter operating time	
Short hospitalization	
Improved swallowing and speech function versus open partial laryngectomy or RT/chemotherapy	

FUTURE DIRECTIONS

Transoral robotic surgery supraglottic laryngectomy is a promising, minimally invasive alternative surgical option for early supraglottic cancers. Complication rates can be low with excellent maintenance of swallowing and speech function. As technology progresses, it is anticipated that robotic arms and instruments will become smaller and more flexible,[27]endoscopes will become smaller and more adjustable and haptic feedback will be possible.

REFERENCES

1. Ganly I, Patel SG, Matsuo J, et al. Analysis of postoperative complications of open partial laryngectomy. Head Neck. 2009;31(3):338-45.
2. Thomas L, Drinnan M, Natesh B, et al. Open conservation partial laryngectomy for laryngeal cancer: a systematic review of English language literature. Cancer Treat Rev. 2012;38(3):203-11.
3. Hoffman HT, Porter K, Karnell LH, et al. Laryngeal cancer in the United States: changes in demographics, patterns of care, and survival. Laryngoscope. 2006;116(9 Pt 2 Suppl 111): 1-13.
4. Dziegielewski PT, O'Connell DA, Klein M, et al. Primary total laryngectomy versus organ preservation for T3/T4a laryngeal cancer: a population-based analysis of survival. J Otolaryngol Head Neck Surg. 2012;41 Suppl 1:S56-64.
5. Chen AY, Halpern M. Factors predictive of survival in advanced laryngeal cancer. Arch Otolaryngol Head Neck Surg. 2007;133(12):1270-6.
6. Hanna E, Sherman A, Cash D, et al. Quality of life for patients following total laryngectomy vs chemoradiation for laryngeal preservation. Arch Otolaryngol Head Neck Surg. 2004;130(7):875-9.

7. Iro H, Waldfahrer F, Altendorf-Hofmann A, et al. Transoral laser surgery of supraglottic cancer: follow-up of 141 patients. Arch Otolaryngol Head Neck Surg. 1998;124(11): 1245-50.
8. Mendelsohn AH, Remacle M, Van Der Vorst S, et al. Outcomes following transoral robotic surgery: supraglottic laryngectomy. Laryngoscope. 2013;123(1):208-14.
9. Strong MS, Jako GJ. Laser surgery in the larynx. Early clinical experience with continuous CO_2 laser. Ann Otol Rhinol Laryngol. 1972;81(6):791-8.
10. Cabanillas R, Rodrigo JP, Llorente JL, et al. Oncologic outcomes of transoral laser surgery of supraglottic carcinoma compared with a transcervical approach. Head Neck. 2008; 30(6):750-5.
11. Karatzanis AD, Psychogios G, Zenk J, et al. Comparison among different available surgical approaches in T1 glottic cancer. Laryngoscope. 2009;119(9):1704-8.
12. Olsen SM, Moore EJ, Koch CA, et al. Transoral robotic surgery for supraglottic squamous cell carcinoma. Am J Otolaryngol. 2012;33(4):379-84.
13. Ozer E, Alvarez B, Kakarala K, et al. Clinical outcomes of transoral robotic supraglottic laryngectomy. Head Neck. 2013;35(8):1158-61.
14. Dowthwaite S, Nichols AC, Yoo J, et al. Transoral robotic total laryngectomy: Report of 3 cases. Head Neck. 2013; 35(11):E338-42.
15. Leroux L, Maspetiol. [Partial horizontal laryngectomy in cancer of the base of the epiglottis]. Ann Otolaryngol. 1950; 67(10):663-72.
16. Park YM, Lee WJ, Lee JG, et al. Transoral robotic surgery (TORS) in laryngeal and hypopharyngeal cancer. J Laparoendosc Adv Surg Tech A. 2009;19(3):361-8.
17. Solares CA, Strome M. Transoral robot-assisted CO_2 laser supraglottic laryngectomy: experimental and clinical data. Laryngoscope. 2007;117(5):817-20.
18. Weinstein GS, O'Malley BW, Jr, Snyder W, et al. Transoral robotic surgery: supraglottic partial laryngectomy. Ann Otol Rhinol Laryngol. 2007;116(1):19-23.
19. Rizzotto G, Succo G, Lucioni M, et al. Subtotal laryngectomy with tracheohyoidopexy: a possible alternative to total laryngectomy. Laryngoscope. 2006;116(10):1907-17.
20. Genden EM, O'Malley BW, Jr, Weinstein GS, et al. Transoral robotic surgery: role in the management of upper aerodigestive tract tumors. Head Neck. 2012;34(6):886-93.
21. Brasnu DF. Supracricoid partial laryngectomy with cricohyoidopexy in the management of laryngeal carcinoma. World J Surg. 2003;27(7):817-23.
22. Remacle M, Matar N, Lawson G, et al. Combining a new CO2 laser wave guide with transoral robotic surgery: a feasibility study on four patients with malignant tumors. Eur Arch Otorhinolaryngol. 2012;269(7):1833-7.
23. Rigby MH, Reynolds LF, Hart RD, et al. T2 glottic carcinoma: analysis of recurrences in 36 cases undergoing primary transoral laser microsurgery resection. J Otolaryngol Head Neck Surg. 2012;41 Suppl 1:S85-9.
24. Rigby MH, Taylor SM. Review of transoral laser microsurgery for cancer of the upper aerodigestive tract. J Otolaryngol Head Neck Surg. 2011;40(2):113-21.
25. Matrka L, Simpson CB. Anterior Glottic Webs. Oper Tech Otolaryngol Head Neck Surg. 2012;23(2):111-16.
26. Stevens MS, Chang A, Simpson CB. Supraglottic stenosis: etiology and treatment of a rare condition. Ann Otol Rhinol Laryngol. 2013;122(3):205-9.
27. Rivera-Serrano CM, Johnson P, Zubiate B, et al. A transoral highly flexible robot: novel technology and application. Laryngoscope. 2012;122(5):1067-71.

Chapter 5 Transoral Robotic Surgery for Obstructive Sleep Apnea

Chelsey J Smith, Nilesh R Vasan

INTRODUCTION

Obstructive sleep apnea (OSA) is a disorder that can cause hypertension, cardiac disease and sudden death. Obstructive sleep apnea can be caused by many factors including obesity, as well as obstruction within the upper aerodigestive tract. Lifestyle changes to reduce weight, continuous positive airway pressure (CPAP) devices, oral appliances, and traditional surgeries such as septoplasty and uvulopalatopharyngoplasty (UPPP) may not completely resolve or reduce OSA in patients.

Transoral robotic surgery (TORS) to perform lingual tonsillectomy/base of tongue (BOT) resection has recently become another option for OSA patients. Robotic surgery for OSA allows surgery of the BOT to be easily approached through the oral cavity whereas previously, access to this area of the oropharynx was cumbersome, piecemeal and fraught with potential morbidity.

RATIONALE FOR PROCEDURE

It has been estimated that the prevalence of lingual tonsil hypertrophy is 2%, which may accentuate BOT collapse and obstruction.[1] Lingual tonsillar hypertrophy is often noted on physical exam (including both mirror and flexible nasolaryngoscope) in OSA patients. Lingual tonsil hypertrophy can contribute to apneas by reducing the anterior to posterior diameter of the oropharynx as well as obstruction via retroflexion of the epiglottis. This can often be suggested during clinical examination while the patient is upright, awake and performing a Müllers maneuver (reverse Valsalva), mimicking the degree of obstruction while asleep and particularly during rapid eye movement (REM) sleep. This anterior to posterior oropharyngeal collapse can be accompanied by lateral pharyngeal wall collapse that is currently not able to be adequately addressed surgically. In these patients, CPAP devices are recommended for circumferential collapse due to poor surgical outcomes.

Transoral robotic surgery has become an ideal surgical option for BOT resection as it allows better visualization and surgical access without the morbidity of other surgeries that required transcervical or mandibulotomy to access BOT cancers for example.

Superior visualization of the anatomy within the oropharynx is obtained by the use of high definition 1080p 3D camera endoscopes that are positioned within the posterior oropharynx as compared to transcervical routes or approaches using a laryngoscope with a distal microscope.

This robotic approach is also complementary to traditional OSA surgeries in helping to decrease CPAP pressure or possibly alleviating a particular subset of patients with OSA from using CPAP altogether. At our institution, TORS is used alone if no other areas of obstruction are identified. However, in most patients other sources of obstruction are noted such as nasal obstruction or tonsillar hypertrophy and this is addressed surgically first. Patients are evaluated postoperatively for approximately 3 months, and if they have not improved from their previous surgeries by sleep study, then the option of TORS are further explored.

APPLIED ANATOMY

The BOT along with its lymphoid tissue has well-delineated borders. The sulcus terminalis along with the circumvallate papilla on the dorsal posterior tongue serves as the division between oral tongue and the BOT. The lingual arteries that enter the BOT medial to the paired hyoglossus muscles are the major blood supply to the tongue (Figs. 5.1 and 5.2). These arteries are within the BOT and oral tongue musculature. The hypoglossal nerve courses superficial to the lingual arteries lateral to the hyoglossus muscle.

The vallecula is a transitional area between the tongue base and the epiglottis, indicating the posterior boundary of the BOT. The lingual tonsils are often "U"-shaped created by the posterior downward roll of the BOT and upward scroll of the epiglottis. The lingual tonsils are a part of Waldeyer's ring and do not have an underlying capsule at its junction with the tongue musculature. They are usually described as being partially encapsulated.

The lateral boundary of the BOT is indicated anteriorly by the palatine tonsils and posteriorly by the glossoepiglottic folds that confluence into the vallecula and epiglottis.

There is also a midline fold, the median glossoepiglottic fold. When lingual tonsil hypertrophy exists, this tissue can fill the trough of the vallecula and can cause posterior obstruction of the airway directly or indirectly via retroflexion of the epiglottis.

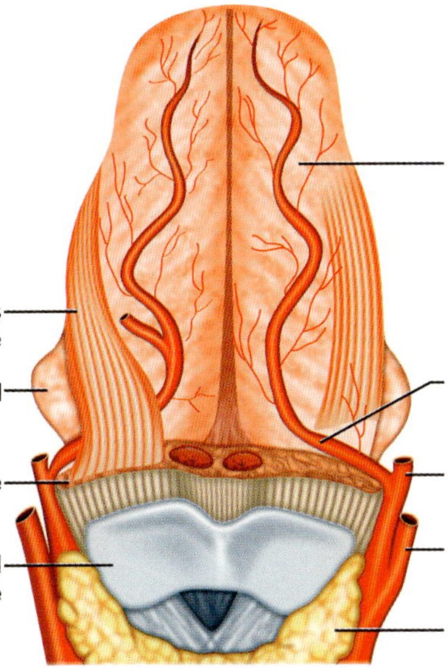

Fig. 5.1: Ventral view of the anatomical landmarks of the tongue.

INDICATIONS AND CONTRAINDICATIONS

Guidelines and algorithms for TORS lingual tonsillectomy/BOT resection do not currently exist due to the novelty of the technique and sparse literature. We have developed a workup and timeline for our patients to perform TORS as the last surgical option for the OSA patient, save tracheostomy placement.

Indications for TORS include patients who have undergone previous procedures to treat OSA and/or trial of CPAP but continue to have documented OSA on polysomnography (PSG) and also continue to have reported subjective signs and symptoms of OSA including hypersomnolence. Patients intolerant of CPAP may also be candidates. The most common examples of previous OSA operations include septoplasty, tonsillectomy, turbinate reduction and UPPP. Following a PSG (with persistent symptoms with CPAP or CPAP intolerance) and if the patient has not yet had any prior surgical intervention, we recommend the patient first undergo sedated sleep fiberoptic nasendoscopy in the operative suite coupled with surgical treatment of obstruction in the nose and oropharynx (palatine

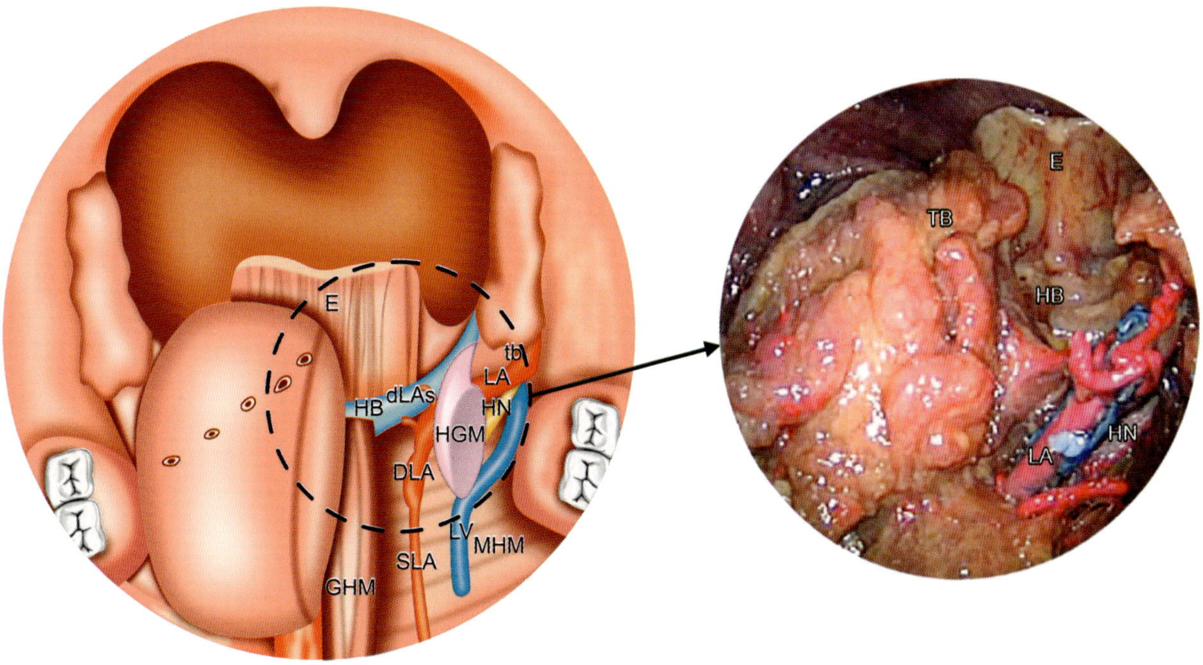

Fig. 5.2: Anterior to posterior view of base of tongue anatomy: (E: Epiglottis; HB: Hyoid bone; GHM: Geniohyoid muscle; HGM: Hyoglossus muscle; LA: Lingual artery; SLA: Superior laryngeal artery; MHM: Mylohyoid muscle; HN: Hypoglossal nerve; TB: Tongue base; DLA: Distal lingual artery; dLAs: Branches of distal lingual artery).

Source: Vinici C, et al. Transoral robotic surgery of the tongue base in obstructive sleep apnea-hypopnea syndrome: Anatomic considerations and clinical experience. Head Neck. 2012; 34:15-22 (with permission).

tonsils/palate) before proceeding with TORS at a later date if need be. After a minimum postoperative period of approximately 3 months from the initial surgery, and if the patient continues to have both OSA findings on repeat PSG and also subjective complaints of OSA, the patient has the option to proceed with TORS if they have findings of BOT obstruction/lingual tonsil hypertrophy upon fiberoptic sleep nasendoscopy (Table 5.1).

We have not performed TORS of the BOT at the time of any other oropharyngeal surgery such as tonsillectomy or UPPP to avoid the theoretical risk of circumferential scarring within the oropharynx. Other case series have performed this combined procedure however with no complication.[2,3]

The degree of BOT obstruction during sleep endoscopy is highly variable, and currently there is no standardized staging system, but the authors have used the degree of visual obstruction of the glottic larynx during sleep nasendoscopy to give a measure of BOT obstruction. A jaw thrust by the anesthesiologist should allow visualization of the entire glottic larynx anatomy (Table 5.1, Figs. 5.3 to 5.6 and 5.1).

Contraindications to TORS include poor physical health, bleeding disorders and comorbidities that preclude general anesthesia. Patients with craniofacial abnormalities, microstomia, severe trismus and those with anatomical features that will not allow appropriate intraoral access for robotic surgery are also excluded. Those

Table 5.1: Base of tongue obstruction staging system

Stage 0	Entire glottis seen (no jaw thrust required)
Stage 1	Anterior one-third of glottis obstructed
Stage 2	Anterior two-third of glottis obstructed
Stage 3	Total obstruction of glottis

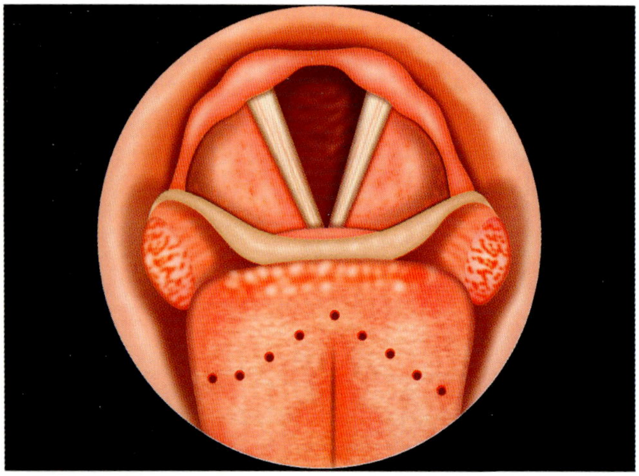

Fig. 5.3: Stage 0 base of tongue obstruction.

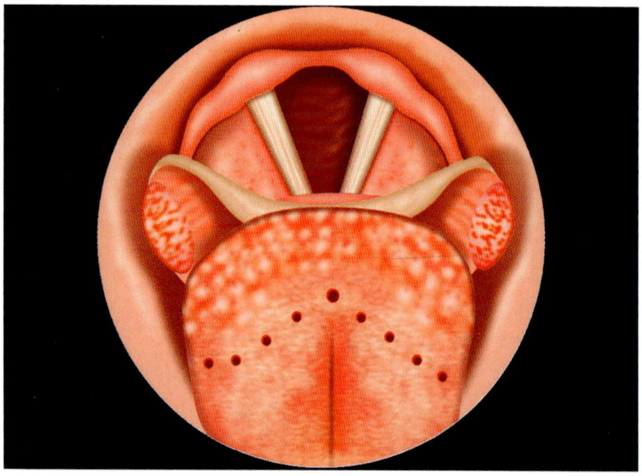

Fig. 5.4: Stage 1 base of tongue obstruction.

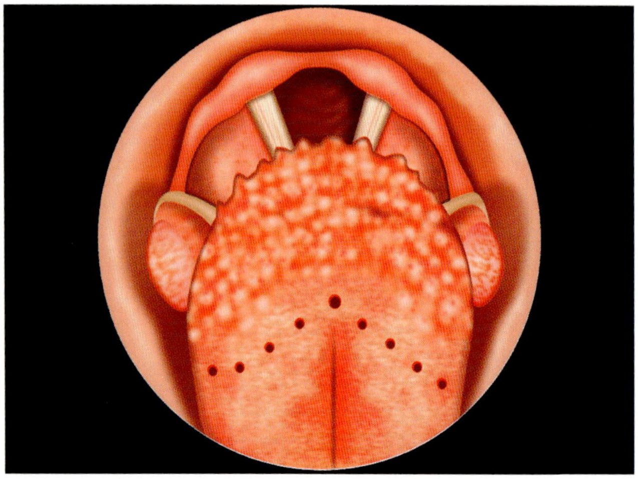

Fig. 5.5: Stage 5 base of tongue obstruction.

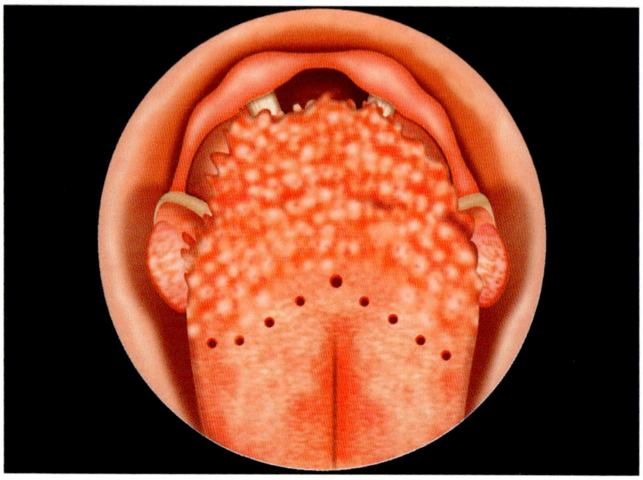

Fig. 5.6: Stage 4 base of tongue obstruction.

patients with extreme morbid obesity are suggested to seek gastric bypass consultation prior to undergoing TORS as previous studies have shown that morbidly obese individuals may not receive much benefit from upper airway surgical intervention besides placement of a tracheostomy for OSA (Table 5.2).

All patients are counseled prior to surgery that TORS may not relieve all symptoms of OSA or prevent the use of a CPAP device. The hope is to improve quality of life, decrease associated comorbidities, and decrease CPAP pressure, making it more tolerable. It is imperative that the patient understands this so that expectations remain realistic. In a small subset of patients, we have completely alleviated OSA on postoperative PSG and discontinued their CPAP use altogether. The overweight or obese patient is also informed that their cooperation with appropriate diet and exercise is of the utmost importance to achieve optimum results in conjunction with surgery.

Table 5.2: Indications and contraindications for transoral robotic lingual tonsillectomy/BOT surgery

Indications	*Contraindications*
• Lingual tonsil/base of tongue (BOT) hypertrophy	• Body mass index > 40 (relative)
• Failure of other obstructive sleep apnea procedures	• Microstomia
• Continuous positive airway pressure intolerance	• Unable to "receive" general anesthesia
• Persistent subjective symptoms	• Bleeding disorders
• Documented glottic obstruction by the BOT on sleep endoscopy	• Severe retrognathia
	• Craniofacial anomalies
	• Severe trismus

PREOPERATIVE WORKUP

Most patients diagnosed with OSA have multilevel airway obstruction, and each of these levels should be addressed in an appropriate manner. Oftentimes, OSA is accompanied by the complaints of nasal obstruction, snoring and weight gain. We generally do not consider lingual tonsillectomy as a first line procedure for patients with complex multilevel obstruction.

Once a complete history and physical examination have been performed, a PSG obtained and the degree of multilevel obstruction has been established, the patient will be consented for flexible fiberoptic sleep nasendoscopy and other indicated surgical procedures such as septoplasty, turbinate reduction, tonsillectomy, and/or UPPP. Surgical planning includes first having a sedated fiberoptic sleep endoscopy (Figs. 5.7, 5.8 and 5.1). This must be performed with an anesthesiologist who is adept at administering a slow titration of propofol to induce snoring and avoid complete airway obstruction. The degree of lingual tonsil obstruction in relation to visual glottic obstruction with and without mandible thrust during sleep endoscopy is documented in the operative note for future reference.

Approximately 3 months or later after the initial surgery, repeat PSG is performed as well as postoperative clinic visits to document the subjective progress of the patient. After the initial surgical procedures, if the patient continues to have documented OSA on PSG as well as subjective sleep issues, TORS for lingual tonsillectomy/BOT resection is revisited. Patients are advised of at least

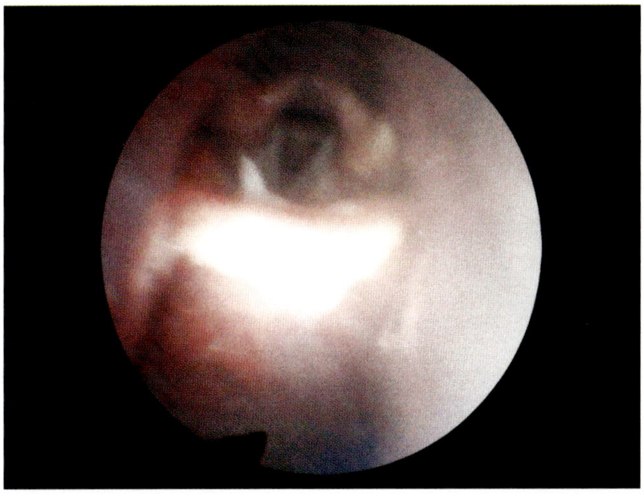

Fig. 5.7: Fiberoptic sleep endoscopy depicting a patient with Stage 0 base of tongue obstruction.

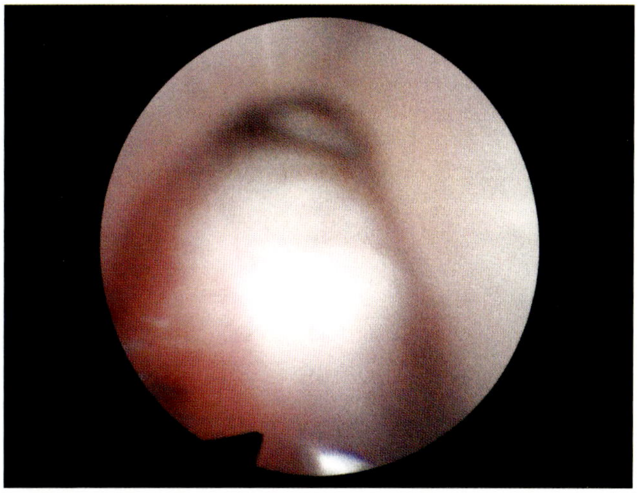

Fig. 5.8: Fiberoptic sleep endoscopy depicting a patient with Stage 4 base of tongue obstruction.

an overnight stay in the intensive care unit (most of our patients go home within the 23-hour observation period), the possibility of tracheostomy in the case of significant BOT/airway edema, bleeding, sore throat and also a continued discussion about weight loss with appropriate diet/exercise and/or gastric bypass surgery referral if indicated. Patients should be counseled that depending on the degree of tongue edema that they may require prolonged intubation, steroid administration, and hospital stay until the edema diminishes. None of our patients have required tracheostomy.

INSTRUMENTATION

Instruments needed for tonsillectomy/BOT resection TORS lingual tonsillectomy include the following:

- da Vinci Si Robotic System and Console (Intuitive Surgical, Sunnyvale, CA)
- 5 mm Maryland Forceps (Intuitive Surgical, Sunnyvale, CA)
- 5 mm Spatula Monopolar Cautery (Intuitive Surgical, Sunnyvale, CA)
- Crowe-Davis retractor or
- Modular Oral Retraction (MOR) System (Marina Medical, Miami FL) versus any modified retractor for robotic surgery that allows exposure of the BOT (with built-in dental guard)
- Davis-Meyer tongue blades (have suction for plume)
- Yankauer suction tip
- Suction Cautery Valley Lab/Covidien
- If CO_2 laser used—OmniGuide Fiber using 5 mm grasping forceps to hold and manipulate the OmniGuide (Cambridge, MA) sheath at 10 W
- Protective eye goggles (including laser)
- Mayo stand for suspension of retractor
- 2-0 silk suture.

OPERATIVE SETUP

Operative setup when performing robotic surgery is paramount. If there is inadequate space in the operative suite or if the room is set upincorrectly, this can prolong the operative and anesthesia time because of frequent pauses to reposition surgical instruments and/or the patient. Figure 5.9 and 5.1 show an example of the author's operative setup, illustrating optimal position of the patient in conjunction with the robot, the robot arms, the surgeon, anesthesia and surgical assistants. This setup allows for ample space for the robotic arms to move.

Initially, the patient is positioned with the head toward anesthesia. After intubation, the bed is turned 180°. The scrub nurse positions his/herself on the patient's left. The surgical assistant is seated at the head of the patient, and the robot's base is positioned to the right of the patient with its three arms perched superior to the patient's head (the camera head in the median position). Overhead monitors are positioned toward the assistant and nursing staff to help in assisting the surgeon at the console.

Eye protection goggles, circular headrest and a small shoulder roll are placed on the patient. A 2-0 silk suture is used to suture the endotracheal tube to the left or right retromolar trigone, depending on the surgeon's preference. Once the endotracheal tube is secured, the tongue retractor of choice is inserted to allow wide access to the BOT with dental protection (Figs. 5.10 and 5.11). The retractor is suspended using a number of options. This may include a Mayo stand, Draffin rods or a suspension arm used with the MOR system. The MOR system utilizes a choice of suspension devices including an arm similar to laryngoscopy suspension or a Martin's arm (Marina Medical Miami, FL). Sometimes it is helpful to place a silk suture through the mid anterior portion of the tongue to help retract it out of the mouth while positioning the retractor. Tongue retraction, however, can cause significant tongue edema in patients with lower dentition as the tongue is pressed against the lower teeth. Placing a tooth guard over the lower teeth is helpful in avoiding tongue injury and edema from compression against the lower teeth. The MOR system was devised to allow more options for access within the upper aerodigestive tract for oncologic procedures as well as benign conditions such as OSA (Figs. 5.12 and 5.13). The authors have used the MOR system without retraction of the tongue in some patients.

Docking of the robot is performed at a 30–45° angle to the patient. The camera, fitted with a 30° endoscope positioned upward, is then placed into the patient's oral cavity and oropharynx (camera in the median position), in line with the tongue retractor. Next, the two robotic arms are inserted with the Maryland forceps and Monopolar cautery. The Maryland forceps is usually positioned for the surgeon's dominant hand. Both instruments have 5 mm articulated arms and are angled at 45° from the camera that is in the midline. Instrument positioning is aided not only by direct vision of the arms, but a tower/screen of the endoscope video, positioned to the left of the surgical assistant. The primary surgeon adjusts the arms for maximum visualization of the tongue base in its entirety.

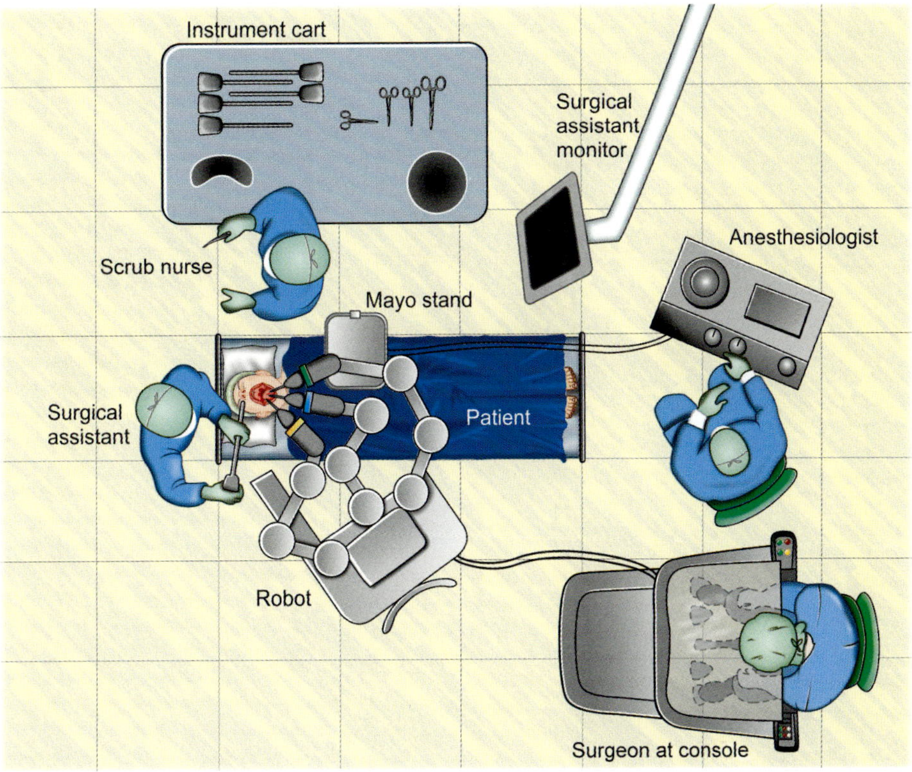

Fig. 5.9: Example of optimal room setup and spacing for transoral robotic surgery with the anesthesiologist seated at the foot of the patient, the surgical assistant at the head with a clear view of a surgical monitor and the robotic arms. The scrub is adjacent to the surgical assistant for ease of passing instruments. The primary surgeon is seated at the console with use of microphone for clear communication.

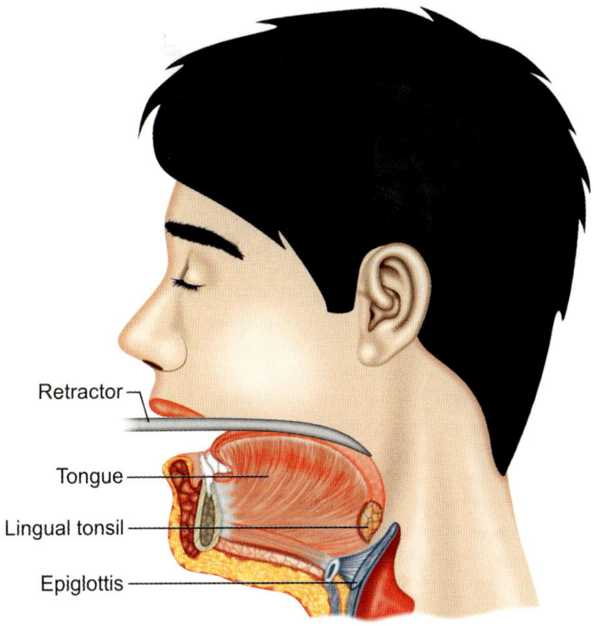

Fig. 5.10: The tongue retractor is inserted onto the tongue, allowing the base of tongue/lingual tonsils to bulge into the surgical field to allow for easier access with robotic instruments.

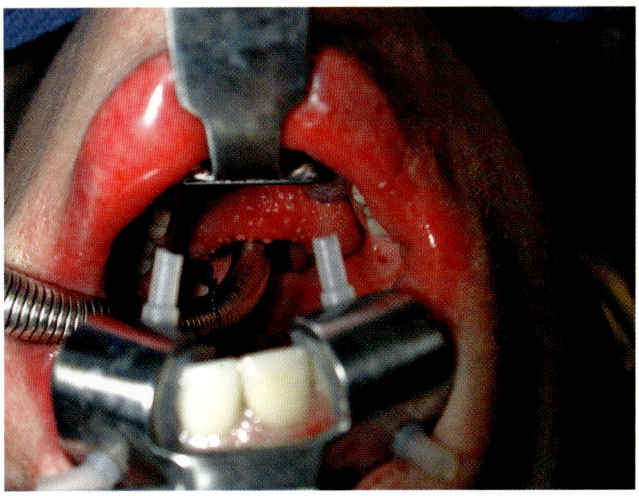

Fig. 5.11: Anterior view of the MOR system showing the endotracheal tube sutured into place as well as the appropriate dental guard. The retractor has the tongue retracted inferiorly and the portion of the tongue seen posteriorly is at the level of the circumvallate papillae.

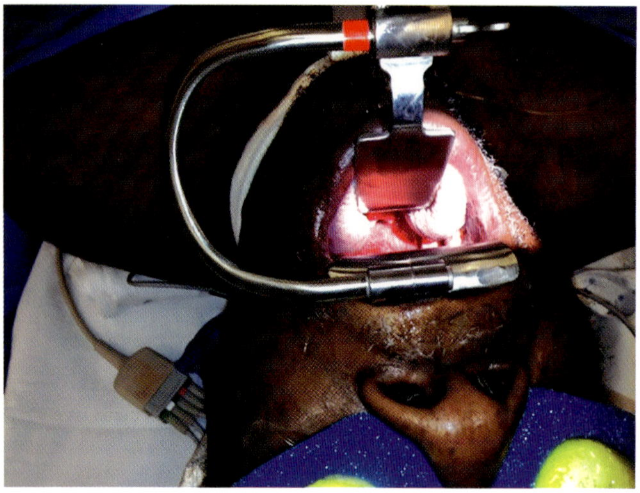

Fig. 5.12: Suspended MOR system showing a clear view of the epiglottis. This system has allowed a wider surgical field for robotic arms as surgical landmarks are clearly exposed. Note the upper tooth brace which completely covers the upper teeth to protect them from robotic arm collisions.

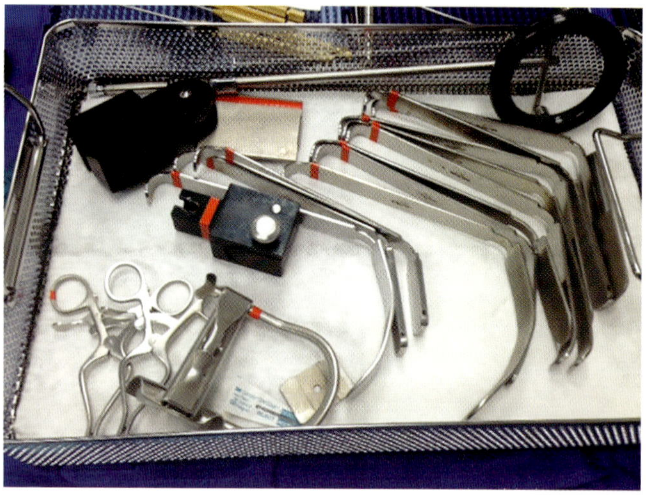

Fig. 5.13: Prototype MOR system with suspension arm (top) and modified rigid suspension brace for blades (black block, center).

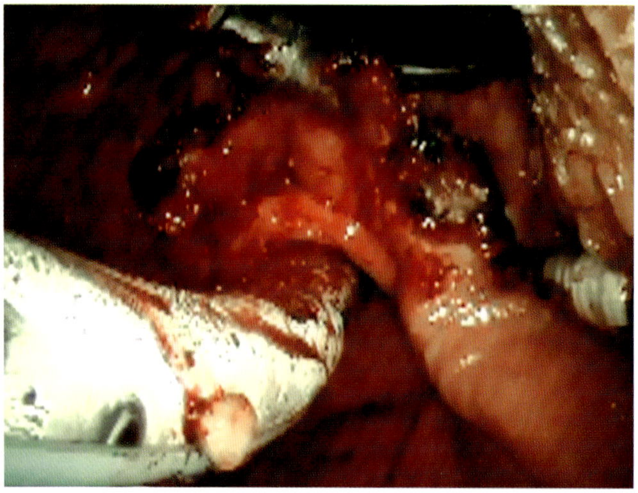

Fig. 5.14: When grasping the lingual tonsils, the direction of retraction should be posterosuperiorly

After docking, the assistant is seated at the head of the patient to ensure correct positioning of the arms, avoidance of arm collisions, suction and to apply countertraction.

OPERATIVE TECHNIQUE

Upon induction of anesthesia, 10 mg IV dexamethasone is administered. No antibiotics are needed. Once the patient and robot are positioned satisfactorily with the tongue base exposed in its entirety, the lingual tonsillectomy commences. The Maryland forceps are angled slightly upward to grasp the right lateral edge of the lingual tonsil. This angling of the forceps allows for better exposure for the surgeon. The forceps are the driving force behind this surgery, as they allow retraction needed to remove the lingual tonsils en bloc. Retraction is performed at a left posterior angle. For adequate BOT tissue excision, the monopolar instrument or laser if used should be angled superiorly (Fig. 5.14 and 5.1).

The monopolar cautery is placed at the right edge of the lingual tonsil, just lateral to the retracting forceps. The tongue can be palpated with the cautery, and dissection (using the coagulation setting 20 (Covidien) is performed in a straight line along the superior aspect of the BOT. The tonsils are removed usually en bloc in a strip like fashion from the underlying tongue musculature. A avascular plane can be created between the lingual tonsil and tongue muscle. In cases with lingual tonsil hypertrophy, the muscles of the tongue remain uninterrupted as well as the nearby lingual arteries (Fig. 5.15). In some patients, BOT muscle may require excision and in these cases the surgeon must be cognizant of lingual artery branches that may require clips for hemostasis. Dissection should not disrupt the palatine tonsil pillars and the surgical assistant may help in retracting the pillars and epiglottis away from the surgical site (5.1).

Throughout the procedure the surgical assistant uses a plastic Yankauer suction and/or suction cautery for removal of cautery/laser plume and blood. These tools can also be helpful in providing retraction. Hemostatic clips and ties along with forceps should be available to the assistant to address bleeding. Again, it should be reiterated that the assistant must be vigilant about the protection of surrounding anatomy and dentition as well as ensuring correct placement of the endotracheal tube and tongue retractor. If the tongue should become dusky or in the event that the surgery should last longer than 30 minutes, the primary surgeon should be alerted and the oral retractor released, as prolonged time under retraction can lead to increased tongue edema and postoperative discomfort.

Dissection can proceed in a right to left direction oftentimes removing this tissue as a single piece (Fig. 5.16). Tissue is then weighed. The most inferior aspect of the dissection is usually the vallecula. The surgeon must be aware that the epiglottis mucosa is quickly approached and the mucosa over the lingual aspect of the epiglottis can easily be degloved. In patients with significant BOT bulk, the retractor may need to be repositioned from time to time during the case for the best exposure.

In patients with pedunculated lingual tonsils on the right and left, these may need to be excised separately.

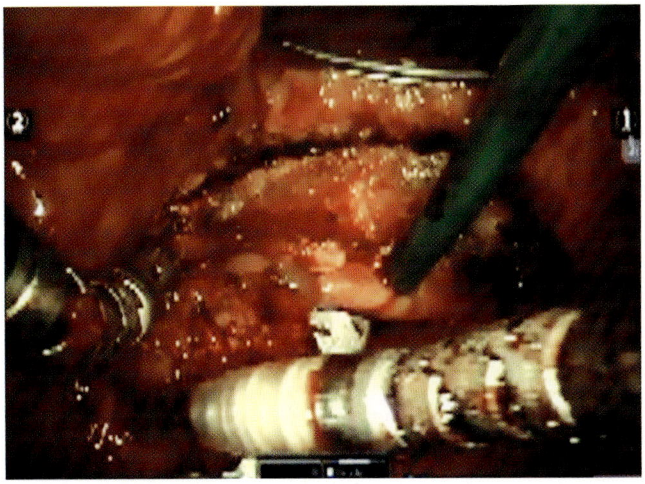

Fig. 5.15: The lingual tonsils are removed in a linear fashion away from the underlying tongue musculature.

COMPLICATIONS AND THEIR MANAGEMENT

Many complications associated with TORS BOT resection/lingual tonsillectomy can be avoided by careful placement and monitoring of the da Vinci robotic arms, suspension apparatus and endotracheal tube. The endotracheal tube is positioned laterally left or right and sutured to the retromolar trigone using a 2-0 silk suture to aid against accidental extubation and to keep the tube from obstructing the surgical view. If laser is used, then a laser endotracheal tube is required. When using the Crow Davis retractor, FK, or the MOR system, it is helpful to insert a shoulder roll to facilitate access. Whichever retraction apparatus is used, an appropriate tooth guard is paramount in protecting the dentition from the apparatus itself, the da Vinci arms, and the assistant surgeon who will be seated at the head of the patient. The MOR system utilizes a rotating mechanism for the upper teeth to help secure the retractor as well as proving protection. This upper dental guard is also stable in edentulous individuals. The assistant surgeon must also be trained to keep a constant watch over the placement of the da Vinci instruments throughout the procedure and alert the primary surgeon when dentition or other structures are impinged upon.

Tongue edema or complaints of numbness due to prolonged retraction is common. Taking the patient out of suspension intermittently can lessen the likelihood of oral tongue edema and decrease the need for prolonged postoperative intubation and steroid use or possibly tracheostomy. As the robotic surgeon becomes more experienced, intraoperative time will shorten, thereby lessening

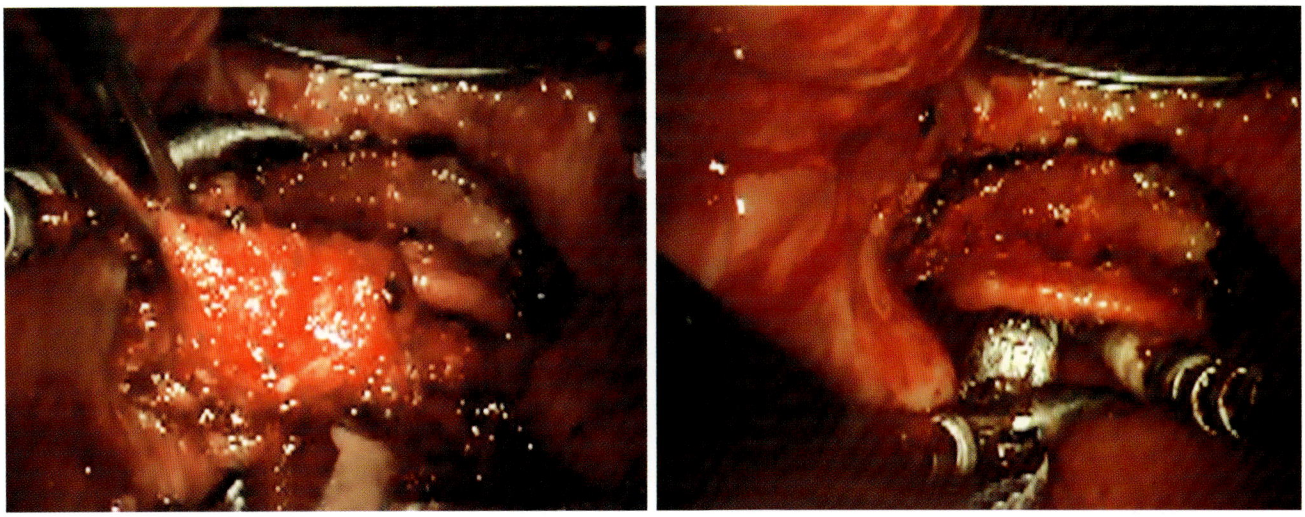

Fig. 5.16: En bloc resection of lingual tonsils.

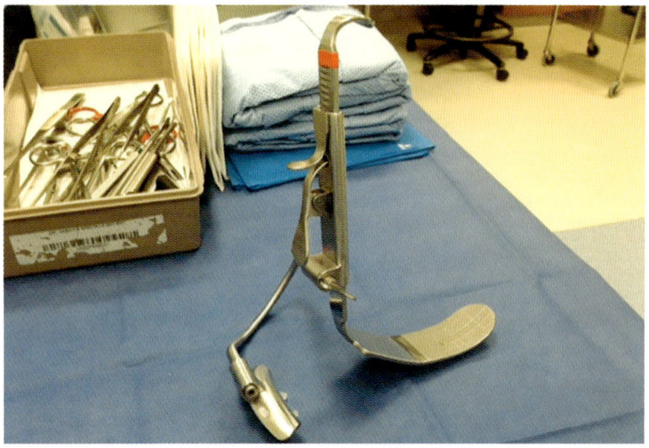

Fig. 5.17: MOR system, displaying tooth guard and curvilinear tongue blade.

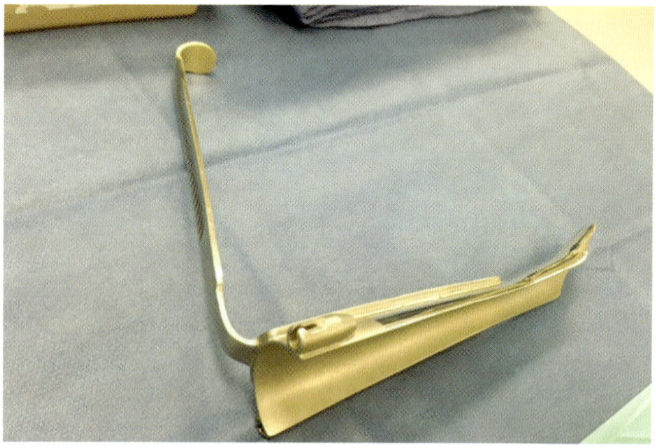

Fig. 5.18: The rigid suspension brace can be used with modifications to laryngoscope blades such as this one to allow for access to the hypopharynx or glottis.

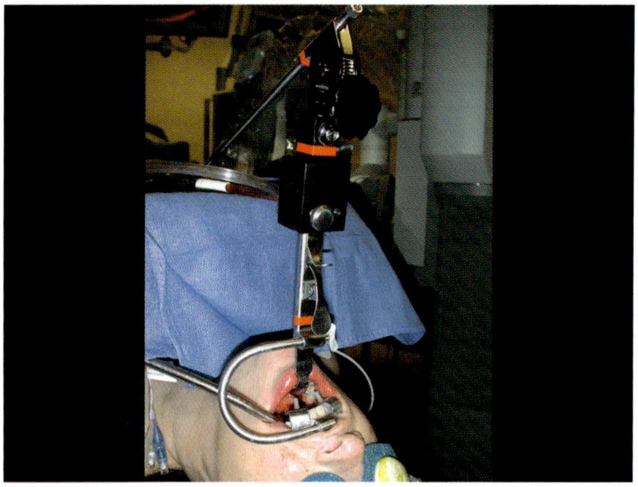

Fig. 5.19: Anteriolateral view of the rigid suspension brace.

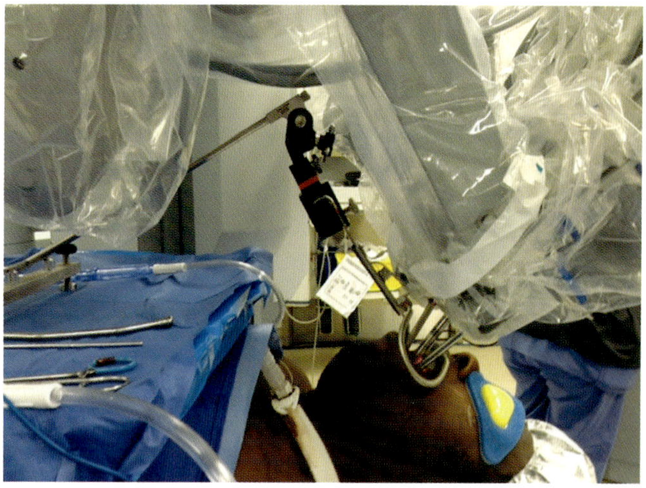

Fig. 5.20: Lateral view of the rigid suspension brace with robotic arms docked.

the likelihood of these two problems. In our experience, postoperative tongue sensation can return within days to months and there has not been any permanent deficit. None of our patients required tracheostomy. To decrease edema, the patient is medicated with both pre and postoperative IV steroids. However, the patient is educated preoperatively that postsurgical swelling cannot always be controlled with steroids or meticulous placement of the tongue retractor and that tracheostomy or prolonged intubation may be required until an appropriate airway is established and edema has subsided. Of course, with the risk of prolonged intubation there are other associated risks such as pneumonia and nutrition via nasal small bore feeding tube. The MOR system was created and utilized through an Internal Review Board (IRB) approved protocol to facilitate BOT/oropharyngeal surgery with the tongue remaining within the oral cavity and not retracted out of the mouth. This is patient-dependent and in some cases the patient's tongue will need to be retracted for adequate access. The MOR system (patent pending) is a modular system that allows customization of tongue blades inserted into a retractor for which pre-existing Crow-Davis tongue blades can also be used. The upper tooth guard is also adjustable and interchangeable to help obtain favorable angles within the oropharynx. The system includes a more rigid suspension brace to be used in conjunction with pre-existing laryngoscope suspension arms (Figs. 5.17 to 5.20). This system allows for improved access to the oropharynx, hypopharynx and larynx (including glottic larynx).

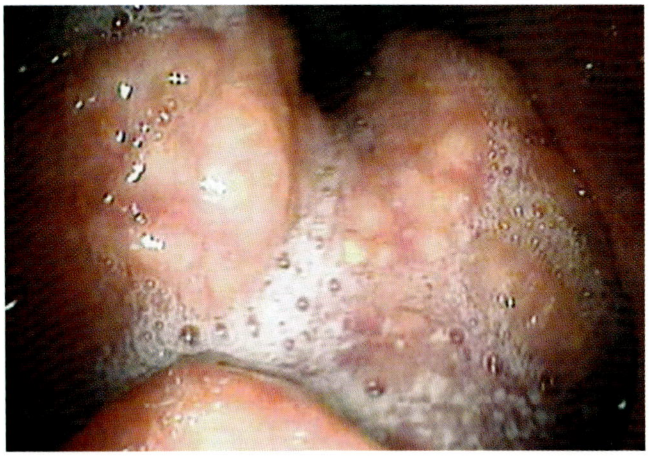

Fig. 5.21: Significant, obstructive lingual tonsil hypertrophy in a preoperative patient.
Source: Vinici C, et al. Transoral robotic surgery of the tongue base in obstructive sleep apnea-hypopnea syndrome: Anatomic considerations and clinical experience. Head Neck. 2012; 34:15-22 (with permission).

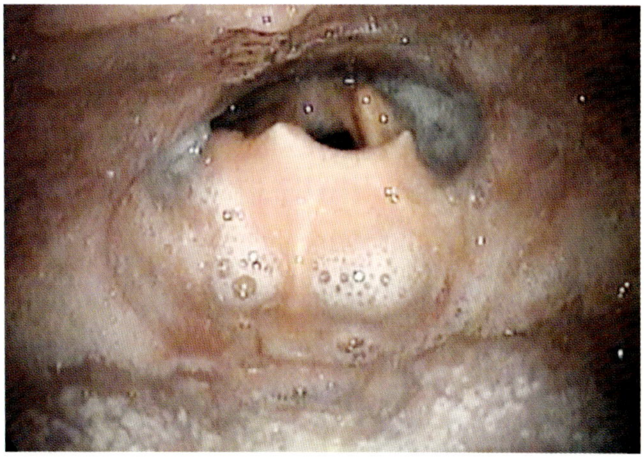

Fig. 5.22: Postoperative photo of the same patient in Figure 5.21 after transoral robotic surgery lingual tonsillectomy (with permission).

Postoperative hemorrhage is uncommon, but it is one of the most feared complications. Bleeding from the lingual, tonsillar, and/or pharyngeal arteries postoperatively is rare but can occur, and the resultant bleed is similar to that of a postsurgical tonsillectomy bleed. Patients are educated to return immediately to the emergency department in the event of bloody emesis or frank bleeding in preparation to return to the operative room for cauterization/control. The percentage of TORS postoperative bleeds after lingual tonsillectomy is not yet known due to its novelty, but in our subset of TORS OSA patients, only one patient experienced a small bleed at home approximately 10 days after the operation, which spontaneously resolved. No OSA patient has required readmission for bleeding.

FOLLOW-UP

Once the patient is able to tolerate liquids, pain is controlled and there are no signs or symptoms of airway edema; the patient is discharged home with appropriate pain prescriptions. A 2-week follow-up appointment is scheduled for postoperative wound check with mirror and/or flexible endoscope. The appearance is similar to that of the tonsil fossa after tonsillectomy but with less slough. The next postoperative visit is then scheduled in 4 weeks unless the patient is experiencing any sort of concern such as persistent pain or difficulty swallowing. After the second postoperative visit, the third and final PSG is scheduled and timed at a minimum of 3 months following surgery. This period allows for adequate healing time of the BOT prior to sleep study, and also allows the surgeon to monitor the patient's subjective symptoms over the period of 3 months as the patient heals and scar contracture occurs (Figs. 5.21 and 5.22).

RESULTS

Our early experience in 10 TORS lingual tonsillectomy patients included those that had undergone surgeries for sleep apnea previously including septoplasty, UPPP and/or tonsillectomy. All had persistent OSA after these primary surgeries and despite lifestyle changes. The pre- and postoperative PSG data have been compared for eight of these patients thus far.

Pre- and postoperative PSG comparisons (pre, post, *p*-value respectively) showed statistically nonsignificant improvements in the median apnea hyponea index (AHI) (49.8, 19.5, $p = 0.84$), sleep onset latency (11.8 minutes, 17.5 minutes, $p = 0.84$), sleep efficiency (80.5%, 92.3%, $p = 0.2$), and Epworth Sleepiness Scale (14.5, 10, $p = 0.88$). All eight patients have had subjective improvement in symptoms and quality of life. None of our patients required tracheotomy. One patient that underwent tracheostomy elsewhere for severe OSA was able to be successfully decannulated after our series of procedures including TORS lingual resection. Only one patient experienced a small bleed at home after TORS OSA surgery approximately 10 days after the operation with spontaneous resolution. No return visit to the operative suite was necessary. This study is limited by a small sample size with associated limited statistical power. These results are also preliminary as patient data is still being collected and long-term outcomes are yet to be established.

Other studies have demonstrated similar results.[2-6] Lin[5] included 12 patients' status post-TORS with statistically significant mean postoperative AHI improvement as compared to preoperative values (17.6 vs. 43.9, $p = 0.007$). The average AHI reduction was 56.2. Subjective symptoms were also significantly improved via Epworth Sleepiness Scale. Body mass index and minimum oxygen saturation were also compared, but there was no significant difference in these categories. Patients who had previous sleep apnea surgery were excluded from this study however.

Vicini et al.[2,3,4] reported a case series of 10 patients undergoing TORS with a mean reduction of AHI from 38.3 to 20.6. This study described complications as "rare and of minor importance." Another manuscript evolved from this study, including a total of 20 TORS patients showing a significant mean AHI improvement of 24.6 and improved Epworth scale.

In a case series that included 40 OSA patients who had TORS, Hamilton et al.[6] noted "no major bleeding or airway complications." Of these 40 patients, 27 underwent concomitant z-palatoplasty. These 27 were compared with another cohort receiving radiofrequency BOT reduction or submucosal minimally invasive lingual excision. Postoperative pain and length of hospital stay were similar. Reduction in mean AHI was 60.5% versus 37% versus 32%, respectively. Transoral robotic surgery was the only procedure to significantly improve minimum oxygen saturation, however, those who underwent TORS experienced a longer period to resume regular diet and normal activity. No TORS patients required a tracheostomy. The method of robotic BOT resection was also different in that a midline vertical trough was excised as compared to truncating the BOT as we have described.

FUTURE DIRECTIONS

The future concerning TORS BOT/lingual tonsillectomy for OSA is still in the process of investigation and long-term efficacy has not yet been established. With sleep apnea becoming more prevalent in society, the otolaryngologist has more options to treat OSA, and robotic lingual tonsillectomy is one more tool in the surgical armamentarium. We feel at this time that TORS is not a first line therapy for this multilevel disease, although there are case studies from other institutions that have used it as a first line therapy with apparent success.[5] In our experience, coupled with the correct adjuvant treatment, it has the ability to improve PSG findings and more importantly, improve quality of life for both the patients and their significant others.

While there may be debate about TORS as a first line OSA treatment, there are also differences in surgical technique. While the author dissects the lingual tonsils in a linear fashion from right to left across the BOT, other techniques have been described such as that in Hamilton et al.[6] This case series, one of the largest described in the literature, performed dissection in an inverted "V" fashion. Cauterization was angled toward the lingual septum, therefore removing a larger portion of the midline tongue base along with the lingual tonsils. They also showed significant declines in AHI and increases in minimum oxygen saturations on postoperative PSG. This operation, however, was not performed in isolation and a palate procedure was also performed concurrently.

The literature concerning TORS for OSA is sparse, and we continue to work toward evidence-based, quantitative studies to better delineate the benefits of TORS for OSA. As more robotic surgeons endeavor to use this as a surgical treatment option and publish their data, larger powered studies with long-term outcomes will be established.

VIDEO LEGEND

Video 5.1: TORS-Lingual tonsillectomy and sleep nasoendoscopy.

REFERENCES

1. Sanchez-Morillo J, Gómez-Diago L, Rodríguez-Gimillo P, et al. Airway evaluation by indirect laryngoscopy in patients with lingual tonsillar hypertrophy. Acta Otorrinolaringol Esp. 2013;64(5):345-51.
2. Vicini C, Dallan I, Canzi P, et al. Transoral robotic tongue base resection in obstructive sleep apnoea-hypopnoea syndrome: a preliminary report. ORL J Otorhinolaryngol Relat Spec. 2010;72(1):22-7.
3. Vicini C, Dallan I, Canzi P, et al. Transoral robotic surgery of the tongue base in obstructive sleep apnea-hypopnea syndrome: anatomic considerations and clinical experience. Head Neck. 2012;34(1):15-22.
4. Vicini C, Montevecchi F, Pang K, et al. Combined transoral robotic tongue base surgery and palate surgery in obstructive sleep apnea-hypopnea syndrome: expansion sphincter pharyngoplasty versus uvulopalatopharyngoplasty. Head Neck. 2014;36(1):77-83.
5. Lin HS, Rowley JA, Badr MS, et al. Transoral robotic surgery for treatment of obstructive sleep apnea-hypopnea syndrome. Laryngoscope. 2013;123(7):1811-6.
6. Friedman M, Hamilton C, Samuelson CG, et al. Transoral robotic glossectomy for the treatment of obstructive sleep apnea-hypopnea syndrome. Otolaryngol Head Neck Surg. 2012;146(5):854-62.

Section 2

Thyroid

Chapter Outline

Chapter 6 Transaxillary Robotic Thyroidectomy

Jandee Lee, Woong Youn Chung

INTRODUCTION

Technical advances have clearly improved endoscopic techniques in head and neck surgery. These advances include high-intensity light sources, improved hand instrumentation and electrosurgical devices. Occasionally, technical advances profoundly change a particular field and, therefore, the management of associated clinical conditions. A prime example is the evolution of thyroidectomy from a conventional cervical approach. Since the first published case report of endoscopic parathyroidectomy in 1996,[1] various methods of endoscopic surgery have been introduced. Endoscopic surgery yields excellent cosmetic outcomes with faster recovery from sensory changes in the neck and less postoperative pain.[2,3]

Despite the technical advances and proven benefits of endoscopic thyroidectomy for thyroid tumors, complex procedures, such as the management of advanced thyroid cancer and operations that require radical neck dissection, are typically still managed by conventional open approaches. Despite the benefits of the endoscopic approach, these procedures are difficult to perform in the neck due to space limitations. The limited workspace of the neck has delayed the widespread application of various endoscopic techniques in head and neck surgery. Another factor preventing the more widespread acceptance and application of endoscopic techniques to thyroid surgery has been the steep learning curve required by surgeons and the longer operative times associated with many of these advanced procedures. Other limitations encountered with endoscopic thyroidectomy include counterintuitive hand movements, two-dimensional visualization, limited degrees of instrument motion within the body and ergonomic difficulties and tremor amplification.[4,5] Therefore, although endoscopic thyroidectomy has been regarded as suitable for some benign tumors, its applicability to thyroid cancer has been investigated in only a small number of pilot studies. Overall, it is unclear whether resident and attending surgeons are uncomfortable with endoscopic head and neck surgery because of their unfamiliarity with these techniques, due to having too few patients for an adequate learning curve, or because there are inherent limitations to endoscopic thyroidectomy that make thyroid surgeons choose other routes of surgery.

RATIONALE FOR PROCEDURE

To overcome these obstacles, the da Vinci Surgical Robot System (Intuitive Surgical, Sunnyvale, CA, USA) was recently applied to the area of head and neck surgery. As this robot technology is further refined and improved, more precise and less invasive surgical options beyond endoscopy may become available. In 2007, 100 years after Theodor Kocher received the Nobel Prize for his work on the thyroid gland, Chung's group presented its first experience with robotic thyroidectomy performed via a gasless transaxillary approach.[6] From October 2007 to December 2011, >6,000 robotic thyroidectomies were performed in Korea. Robotic surgery has the potential to transform endoscopic surgery by providing, for the first time, instruments with distal ends that mimic the intricate movements of the human hand while at the same time providing the surgeon with a high-definition, three-dimensional view of the operative field.[4,5] Studies to date have shown that the short-term oncologic effectiveness of robotic thyroidectomy, assessed by measuring serum thyroglobulin (Tg) concentration by 131-radioactive iodine (^{131}RAI) scanning, as well as its morbidity rate and safety, compare favorably with those of conventional open thyroidectomy.[7-18] Moreover, as endoscopic surgery is problematic for complex and difficult procedures such as radical neck dissection for thyroid cancer, this surgical robot system promises more precise and improved endoscopic surgical techniques and enables compartment-oriented anatomical neck dissection. Robotic modified radical neck dissection (MRND) using a gasless transaxillary approach has also been introduced for patients with papillary thyroid carcinoma (PTC) and lateral lymph node (LN) metastases (N1b),[19,20] with similar oncologic effectiveness and safety as conventional open MRND.

In addition, this new technique was found to enhance quality of life (QoL) outcomes relative to conventional open thyroidectomy.[21-26] Among the QoL benefits of robotic surgery are excellent cosmetic results and reductions in neck sensory changes, voice and swallowing discomfort after surgery. For surgeons, robotic surgery has improved ergonomics and has a shorter learning curve than open or endoscopic surgery.[12,13]

Further analyses of surgeons' experience with robotic thyroidectomy including long-term follow-up as well as randomized controlled trials remain important. In this chapter, we define the indications and contraindications for robotic thyroid surgery and introduce the most upgraded surgical skills required for robotic thyroidectomy and radical neck dissection. We also discuss recent surgical literature, focusing on the impact of these developments on thyroid cancer management including the benefits and limitations of robotic thyroidectomy.

APPLIED ANATOMY FOR ROBOTIC THYROID SURGERY

To begin to understand the complexities of robotic thyroid surgery, surgeons must first comprehensively review the overall anatomy of the thyroid gland and adjacent regional LN compartments. The neck has been divided into anatomical areas to facilitate an organized approach to surgical procedures in given areas. Therefore, detailed knowledge of the anatomy of the neck is the foundation that will allow successful completion of robotic thyroidectomy and radical neck dissection.

Our approach for remote access robotic thyroid surgery uses an incision in the axillary fold and proceeds to the neck via a dissection along the fascia of the pectoralis muscle. In our practice, a working space is created under direct vision in the plane between the subcutaneous tissue and the pectoralis major muscle. The sufficient dissection is required to maintain a working space after setting the external retractor. The operative field can be successfully performed by making an adequate working space as follows. The border of the outer space is formed by the subcutaneous and subplatysmal skin flaps, and its bottom by the clavicle, pectoralis major muscle and soft tissues of the lateral neck. The border of the inner space consists of the sternal head of the sternocleidomastoid (SCM) and strap muscles, and the bottom by major vessels and the clavicular head of the SCM muscles (Fig. 6.1).[27]

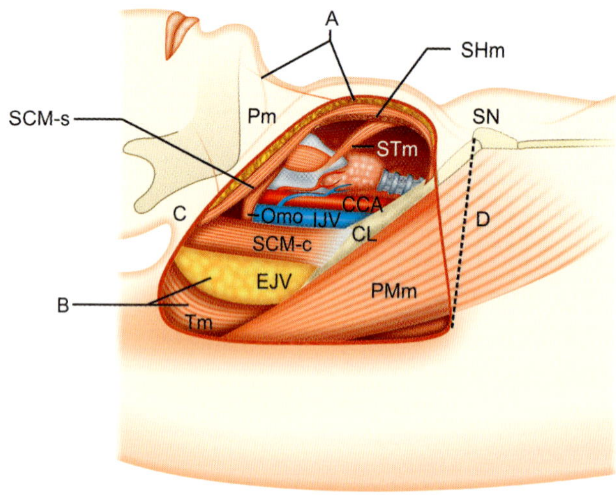

Fig. 6.1: The outer space—(1) Ceiling: subcutaneous and subplatysmal skin flap (A). (2) Bottom: clavicle (CL), pectoralis major muscle (PMm), and soft tissues of the lateral neck (B) including the external jugular vein (EJV) and the anterior border of the trapezius muscle (Tm). (3) Superior border: subplatysmal skin flap of neck level V area (C). (4) Inferior border: sternal notch (SN) and an imaginary line from the sternal notch to the lower border of the axillary incision (D). The inner space—(1) Apex: sternal head of the SCM (SCM-s), strap (sternohyoid muscle (SHm) and sternothyroid (STm) muscles. (2) Bottom: common carotid artery (CCA), internal jugular vein (IJV), and clavicular head of the SCM muscles (SCM-c). (3) Superior border: omohyoid muscle (Omo) and the junction of the two SCM muscle branches. (4) Inferior border: strap muscles (STm, SHm) attached to the sternum.

INDICATIONS AND CONTRAINDICATIONS FOR ROBOTIC THYROIDECTOMY WITH OR WITHOUT RADICAL NECK DISSECTION

Preoperative Workup

Patient workup consists of a physical examination and imaging modalities including high-resolution ultrasonography (US) and neck computed tomography. Preoperative diagnosis of thyroid nodules based on the results of US-guided fine needle aspiration cytology (FNAC). Tumor characteristics assessed include size, location, presence of extrathyroid invasion, multiplicity, bilaterality and presence of cervical LN metastasis (Table 6.1).

The extent of thyroidectomy and radical neck dissection is based on American Thyroid Association guidelines.[28] All patients with thyroid cancer also undergo prophylactic central compartment neck dissection (CCND). Patients

Table 6.1: Indications and contraindications for robotic thyroidectomy with or without radical neck dissection

Indications	• Benign thyroid nodule without substernal extension • Differentiated thyroid cancer without the following contraindications
Contraindications	• A history of previous head-and-neck surgery or irradiation • Uncontrolled thyrotoxicosis • Unrelated pathologic conditions of the neck or shoulder • Lesions located in the dorsal thyroid area, especially in the region adjacent to the tracheoesophageal groove (because of possible injury during surgery to the trachea, esophagus or recurrent laryngeal nerve). • Suspicious perinodal infiltration to adjacent structures such as the internal jugular vein or major nerves at lateral metastatic lymph nodes • Distant metastasis

with lateral neck LNs that are clinically palpable or appear suspicious on preoperative staging US and are assessed by FNAC also undergo TT (total thyroidectomy) with MRND. The preoperative presence of lateral LN metastasis is based on Tg concentrations in US-guided FNAC wash out fluid. In patients with N1b tumors, we follow the prescribed extent of MRND for PTC (levels IIA, III, IV and VB), whereas LNs at levels IIB and VA are not routinely dissected. However, if palpation or preoperative imaging show evidence of an enlarged or suspicious LN at level I, IIB or VA, these compartments are included in en bloc dissection.[19,20]

INSTRUMENTATION

A. Recommended camera and Endowrist instrumentation
   - Harmonic ACE, 5 mm/8 mm: 420275/420274 with insert 400272 or
   - Harmonic curved shears, 5 mm/8 mm: 420173/420174 with insert 400169
   - ProGrasp forceps: 420093
   - Maryland dissector, 5 mm: 420143
   - Intuitive Surgical camera head
   - Intuitive Surgical 30° endoscope
   - Basic accessory kit and drapes

B. Recommended endoscopic instrumentation and accessories.
   - Retractor (Chung's retractor) consisting of Elevator Set (#SJM-10-1) and Lifter Set (#SJM-10-3) by Biorobotics, Inc.
   - Fibro-optic retractor-2
   - Army/navy retractors
   - Neck pillow
   - Arm board
   - Monopolar cautery pen with short, medium and long tips.

OPERATIVE SETUP WITH ROBOT

Robotic Thyroidectomy Setup

Robotic thyroidectomy using a gasless transaxillary approach has been considered an advanced method of thyroid surgery since 2009. This procedure utilizes three robotic arms and a single camera (Fig. 6.2). In robotic thyroidectomy, port (cannula) placement and the location of the camera are of major concern as it is important to avoid collisions among robotic instruments as well as to provide free access to the thyroid bed.

Due to its visual perspective of surgical anatomy, the gasless transaxillary approach has many advantages. First, the operative view is the same as that in open surgery. Therefore, the upper and lower poles of the thyroid gland, major vessels and neck LNs can be easily viewed and manipulated. Second, the parathyroid glands and recurrent laryngeal nerve (RLN) are directly exposed in the lateral view, allowing dissection near these organs and neck LN dissection to be safely and completely performed without injuring important organs. Third, the working space can be stably and safely established without gas and maintained by continuous negative pressure suction of the air and blood.[9]

Patient Positioning

Patient preparation: Under the general anesthesia, the patient is placed in a supine position on a small shoulder roll with the neck slightly extended. The arm is extended and a 5- and 6-cm vertical incision is marked in the anterior aspect of the ipsilateral axilla (Fig. 6.3A). The arm of the lesion-side is raised to minimize the distance between the axilla and the anterior neck. This setup rotates the clavicle, lowering its medial aspect and providing excellent access to the thyroid. Initially, we found that some patients experienced transient traction injuries

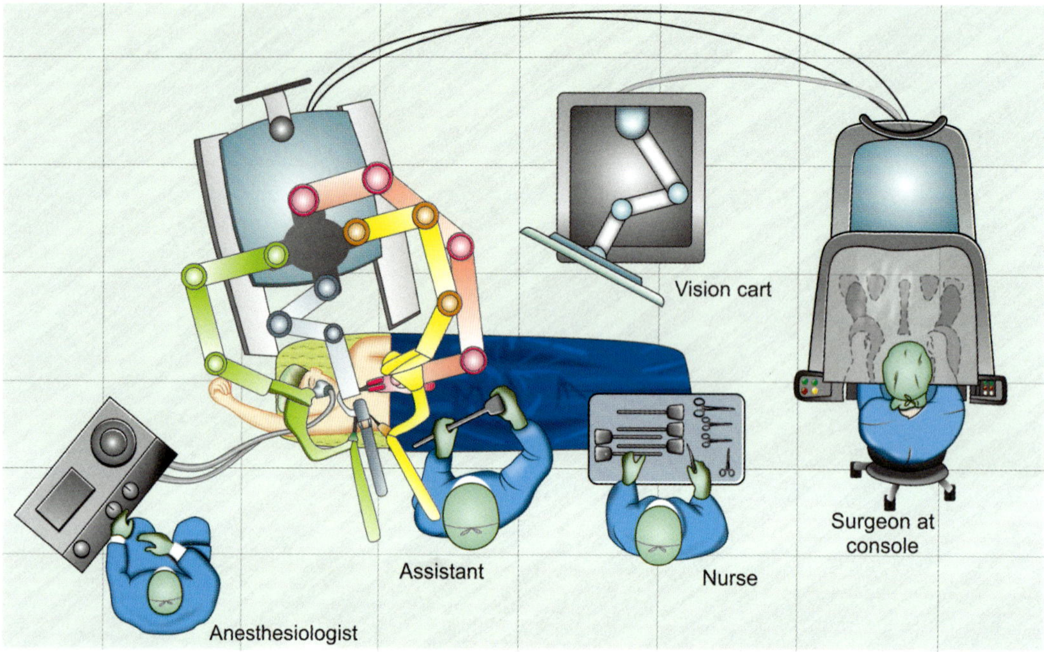

Fig. 6.2: Operating room setup (for a right-sided lesion). View from the ceiling of a standard operating room with outlines for robotic thyroidectomy. The patient cart should always be placed contralateral to the location of the thyroid lesion. For a left-sided lesion the patient and anesthesiologist should be rotated 180° and the scrub nurse should be on the left side of the assistant.
Source: Lee J, Chung WY. Robotic thyroidectomy and neck dissection: past, present, and future. Cancer J. 2013;19(2):151-61.

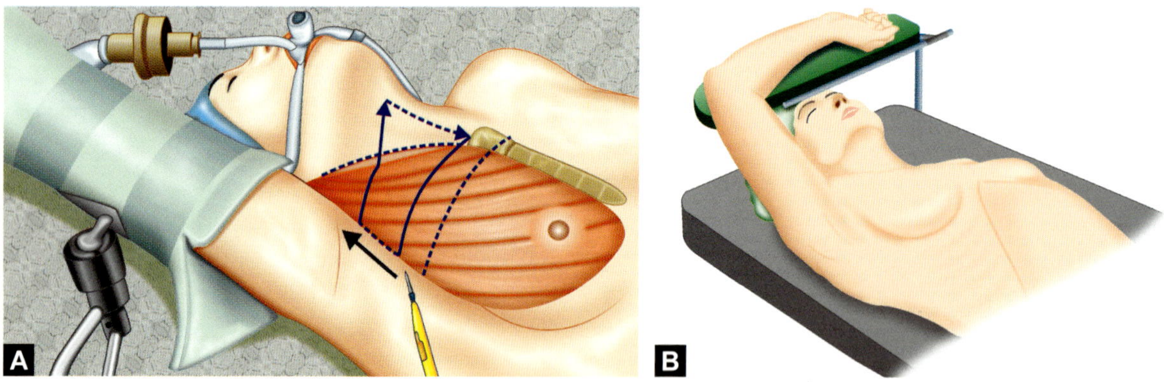

Figs. 6.3A and B: Procedures during robotic thyroidectomy. (A) Patient position and skin incision line. The incision was made along the axillary skin crease on the lateral border of the pectoralis major muscle. (B) Modified arm position. The lesion-side arm was extended to expose the axillary area at the shoulder and flexed at the elbow at an angle of approximately 90° to avoid brachial plexus neuropraxia.
Source: (A) Kang SW, Lee SC, Lee SH, Lee KY, Jeong JJ, Lee YS, et al. Robotic thyroid surgery using a gasless, transaxillary approach and the da Vinci S system: the operative outcomes of 338 consecutive patients. Surgery 2009; 146:1048-55; (B) Courtesy of Intuitive Surgical International.

from brachial plexus neuropraxia due to the position of the patient's arm. To avoid these injuries, the arm of the lesion-side is raised straight superiorly but naturally within the range of shoulder motion.[29] To avoid these injuries, the patient's arm should not be hyperextended. Modified patient positioning has been developed in the United States, especially for patients with obstacles due to a large body habitus.[11,27,30,31] In this alternative positioning, the lesion-side arm is extended to expose the patient's axillary area at the shoulder, followed by flexing the elbow to an angle of approximately 90°, such that the wrist is above the forehead of the patient with the palm facing the ceiling. The arm is then padded and fixed to an arm board overlying the forehead (Fig. 6.3B).

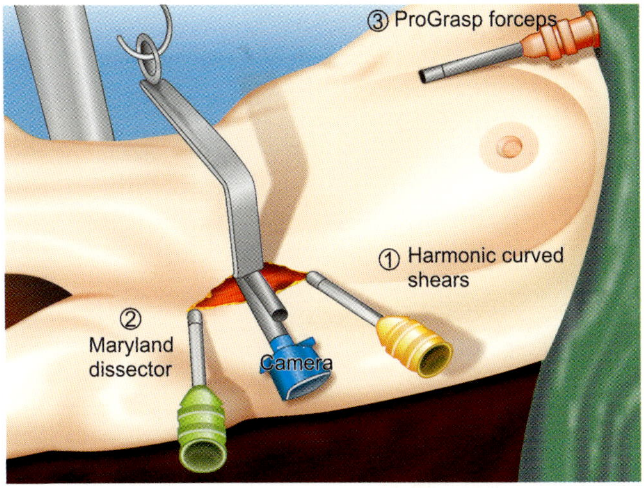

Fig. 6.4: Schematic representation of a two-incision thyroidectomy docking. A second 0.6–0.8 cm skin incision was created on the tumor side of the anterior chest wall to allow insertion of the fourth robotic arm (with ProGrasp forceps)
Source: Courtesy of Intuitive Surgical International.

Creation of working space: A 5- to 6-cm vertical skin incision along the lateral border of the pectoralis major muscle is made in the axilla, and a working space is then created in the plane between the subcutaneous tissue and the pectoralis major muscle by electrical cautery under direct vision. A subplatysmal skin flap is made beyond the clavicle, and until the bifurcation of the SCM muscles (between the sternal head and the clavicular head) is exposed. The dissection is approached through the avascular space of the two heads of SCM muscles and beneath the strap muscles. The carotid sheath is separated down from the strap muscle, taking care not to injure the internal jugular vein (IJV) and the common carotid artery (CCA), and the omohyoid muscle is retracted superficially and posterolaterally. After exposing the contralateral thyroid gland, an external retractor (Chung's thyroid retractor) is inserted to maintain an adequate working space, consisting of sufficient outer and inner spaces. To achieve an adequate working space, the incision entrance should be maintained to provide a height of > 4 cm and the retractor blade should be > 1cm from the anterior surface of the thyroid gland (🎥 6.1).

Robot Positioning and Docking

Robot positioning: After creation of working space, the patient cart is placed on the lateral side of the patient (opposite side to the skin incision). The operative table should be positioned slightly oblique with respect to the direction of the robotic column to allow the straight line between the robotic column and the surgical approach route (direction of retractor insertion). The camera arm is positioned with its set-up joint towards the patient's head to ensure maximum clearance for the instrument arm. The camera arm should be positioned in the middle of the incision of the patient's axilla, such that the camera arm is in line with the camera cannula and center column of the patient cart. If the camera arm is located correctly within its proper range, the patient cart wheel is locked. Proper introduction angles are important to prevent collisions between robotic arms (🎥 6.1).

Docking stage (Two-incision technique): The novel method of robotic thyroidectomy using a gasless transaxillary approach requires two skin incisions; axillary incision for camera, first and second robot arm access and an anterior chest incision for the third robotic arm. In two-incision robotic thyroidectomy, a second skin incision (0.6–0.8 cm long) is made on the medial side of the anterior chest wall to insert the third robot arm, 2-cm superiorly and 6-8 cm medially from the nipple (Fig. 6.4). A 12-mm cannula for the 30°-down dual channel telescope is placed on the central arm, and Harmonic curved shears, together with a Maryland dissector, are placed on both lateral sides of the scope. The edge of the camera cannula is positioned to view the target anatomy by clutching the camera and extending tilting the back of the arm towards the floor. With the 30° down scope, this provides a good view of the thyroid. A ProGrasp forceps is inserted through the anterior chest wall incision. It is important that the angle and position of the da Vinci arm joints are optimized during this setup. The camera arm starts parallel with the retractor and centered above the thyroid. The instrument arms should come in at the edges of the incision and angle out away from the camera. If the setup has performed correctly, the Maryland dissector arm, the camera arm and the ProGrasp forceps arm will form an inverted triangle externally with the insertion axis, and make a triangle internally with the instrument tips (Figs. 6.5A and B).

Docking stage (single-incision technique): After performing >700 robotic thyroidectomies using a two-incision technique, we found that we were able to perform robotic thyroidectomy using a single incision.[32] According to single incision technique, four robotic arms are inserted through a single axillary incision. For the conduit of the robotic thyroidectomy via a single axillary incision, dual-channel telescope is inserted in an upward direction, and centered at the bottom of the incision. Before the 8-mm cannula

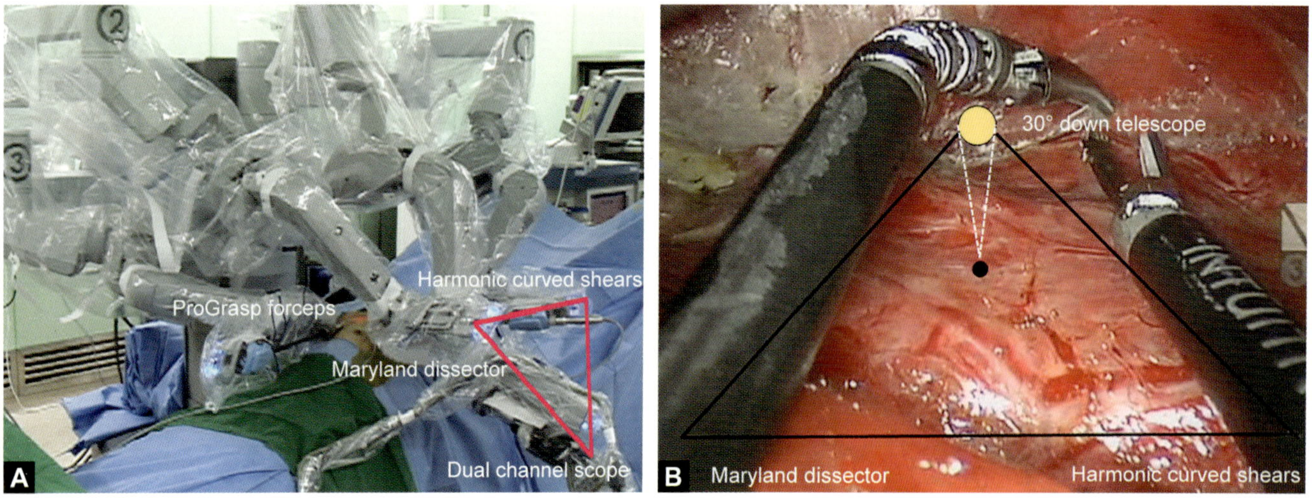

Figs. 6.5A and B: Positions following a correct final external setup of the robot. (A) The Maryland dissection arm, camera arm and ProGrasp forceps arm should form an inverted triangle external to the insertion axis. (B) The instrument and camera tips should form a normal triangle internal to the site of the operation.
Source: Lee J, Chung WY. Robotic surgery for thyroid disease. Eur Thyroid J. 2013 Jun;2(2):93-101.

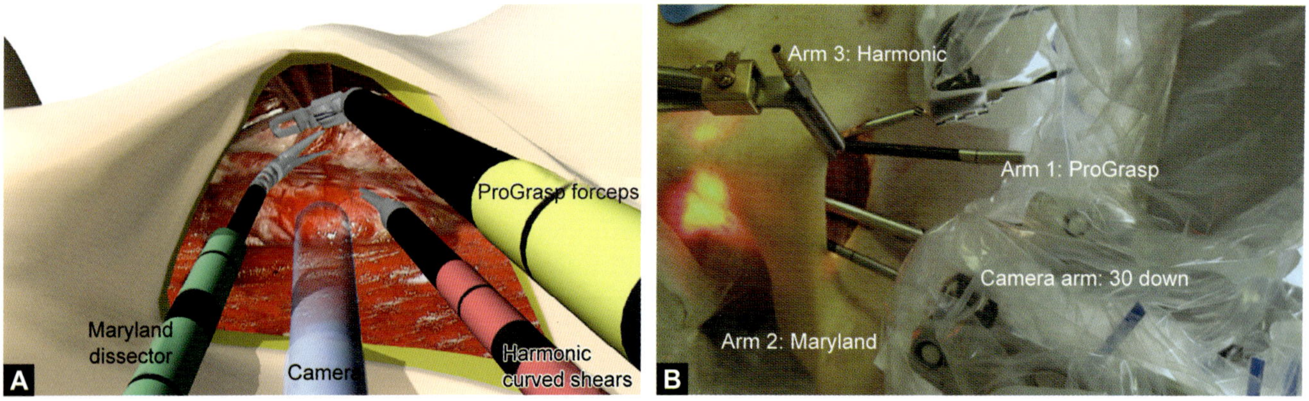

Figs. 6.6A and B: Single incision robotic thyroidectomy. (A) Schematic of a single-incision thyroidectomy docking. All four robotic instruments and the camera were inserted through the axillary incision. (B) External view after port placement and instrument insertion. All instruments should be as far from each other as possible.
Source: Courtesy of Intuitive Surgical International.

is positioned in the incision, attach the ProGrasp forceps to robot arm and insert the instrument through the cannula until it is at full insertion. The tip of ProGrasp forceps is then positioned beneath the anterior part of the skin incision parallel to the retractor blade. The 5-mm cannula for the Harmonic curved shears at the lesion side of the camera, and the 5-mm cannula of a Maryland dissector is then positioned on the opposite edge of the incision. Therefore, all three instruments and the camera are inserted through the axillary incision (Figs. 6.6A and B). At this point, the ProGrasp forceps must be located as close as possible to the ceiling of the working space (the retractor blade). Instruments should be as far apart as possible. The arms must be spaced and positioned in a manner minimizing collisions between the instruments and the camera. If most movements could not be at the wrists during single-incision technique, large internal movements may cause external collisions (6.1).

Robotic Radical Neck Dissection Setup

Cervical LN metastases occur early and often in PTC. Extensive neck dissection coupled with meticulous pathologic examination reveal locoregional LN metastases in 12–81% of patients with PTCs.[33] Standard guidelines for the treatment of patients with PTC and lateral cervical LN metastases (N1b) recommend bilateral total thyroidectomy and MRND at all levels (levels II–V) due to the possibility of skip metastases.

Since the introduction of Crile's method of en bloc dissection of head-and-neck cancers, the conventional open method using a long cervical incision has been adopted worldwide and has remained the most efficient technique for neck dissection in these patients. To overcome displeasing cosmetic outcomes resulting from the long cervical scar, several endoscopic approaches to neck dissection have been developed using remote skin incision. However, endoscopic surgery is more demanding and requires more time than open surgery, primarily because of instrumental and anatomical limitations. Moreover, endoscopic surgery is particularly problematic for complex and difficult procedures such as radical neck dissection for head and neck cancer, in keeping with the principles of oncologic safety. Use of the robot system in radical neck dissection eliminates these technical pitfalls and limitations of endoscopic surgery. Robotic radical neck dissection in patients with N1b PTC is a more precise and improved endoscopic technique, enabling compartment-oriented anatomical neck dissection.[19,20] This robotic technique has other advantages including the increased dexterity achieved using the multiarticulated endowrist, a steady camera platform, a three-dimensional magnified operative view and scaled and tremor-filtered movements. Accordingly, the meticulous and precise motions of modern robotic instruments have introduced new levels of technical safety and feasibility to robotic radical neck dissection.

Patient Positioning

Patient preparation: The patient under general anesthesia is placed in a supine position on a small shoulder roll with the neck slightly extended. The lesion-side arm is abducted to expose axilla and lateral neck and the head is tilted and rotated to face the non-lesion side (Fig. 6.7A). The landmarks for flap dissection are bounded by the sternal notch and the midline of the anterior neck medially, the anterior border of the trapezius muscle laterally and the submandibular gland superiorly.

Creation of working space: A 7-8 cm vertical skin incision is placed in the axilla along the anterior axillary fold and the lateral border of the pectoralis major muscle. The subcutaneous flap from the axilla to the midline of the anterior neck is dissected over the anterior surface of the pectoralis major muscle and clavicle by electrical cautery under direct vision. After exposing the clavicle, subplatysmal flap dissection proceeds to the midline of the anterior neck medially, to the upper point where the external jugular vein (EJV) and greater auricular nerve cross the lateral border of the SCM muscle superiorly. The EJV is ligated at the crossing point of the SCM muscle. Laterally, the trapezius muscle is identified and dissected upwards along its anterior border. During the flap dissection in the posterior neck area, the spinal accessory nerve is identified and exposed along its course. After subplatysmal flap dissection, the clavicular head of the SCM is divided at the level of its attachment to the clavicle to expose the junction area between the IJV and the subclavian vein, and the dissection proceeds upwards along with the posterior surface of the SCM to expose the submandibular gland and the posterior belly of the digastric muscle. The proximal EJV is then clipped and divided at the crossing point of the SCM lateral border, and soft tissue detachment from the posterior surface of the SCM is continued lateral to medial until the IJV and CCA are exposed. After flap dissection, the patient's head is returned to the neutral position. A spatula-shaped wide external retractor (Chung's retractor) is then used to raise and tent the skin flap at the anterior chest wall, the SCM, and the strap muscles to create a working space. The entire neck levels (level II–V areas) are fully exposed by elevating the SCM muscle and the strap muscles (Fig. 6.7B). A second skin incision (0.6–0.8 cm long) is then made on the medial side of the anterior chest wall to allow the fourth robotic arm to be inserted (2-cm superiorly and 6-8 cm medially from the nipple).

Robot Positioning and Docking

The robotic column is placed on the lateral side of the patient contralateral to the main lesion, and the operative table is positioned slightly obliquely with respect to the direction of the robotic column to allow direct alignment between the axis of the robotic camera arm and the operative approach. Proper introduction angles are important to prevent collisions between robotic arms. Four robotic arms are used during the operation. Three arms are inserted through the axillary incision. A 30° dual channel camera is placed on the camera arm through a 12-mm cannula that should be placed in the center of the axillary skin incision. In particular, the camera arm has to be inserted to face upward that means the external third joint should be placed in the lower portion (floor) of the incision entrance, and the camera tip should be directed upward.

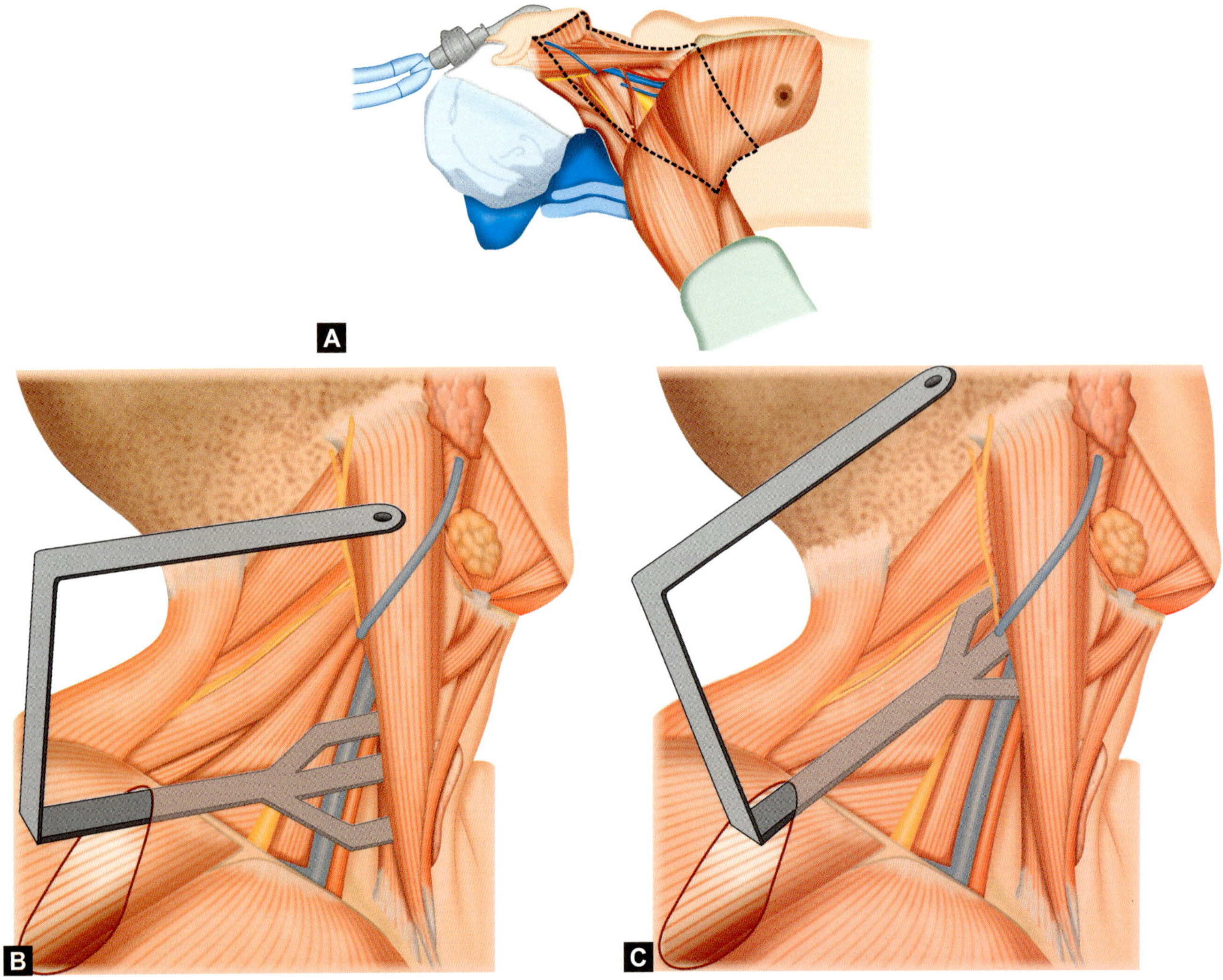

Figs. 6.7A to C: Protocol for robotic modified radical neck dissection (MRND). (A) Patient position during robotic MRND. The neck was extended slightly, with the face turned away from the lesion. (B) Initial position of the external retractor during robotic MRND of levels III, IV and V. The external retractor was placed between the thyroid and strap muscle, with the direction of the blade from the axilla to the anterior neck. (C) Repositioning of the external retractor during robotic MRND. For level II dissection, the blade of the external retractor was reinserted toward the submandibular gland.

Source: Kang SW, Lee SH, Ryu HR, Lee KY, Jeong JJ, Nam KH, et al. Initial experience with robot-assisted modified radical neck dissection for the management of thyroid carcinoma with lateral neck node metastasis. Surgery. 2010;148(6):1214-21.

The 5-mm Maryland dissector is installed on the left side of the camera and the Harmonic curved shears on the right side through 8-mm cannula. A ProGrasp forceps is placed on the fourth arm and inserted through the 8-mm anterior chest cannula. The Harmonic curved shear and the Maryland dissector arms should be inserted in the opposite manner to the camera arm (to face downward). Finally, the external three joints of the robotic arms should form an inverted triangle. These proper positioning of angles are important to prevent collisions between robotic arms.

OPERATIVE TECHNIQUE

Actual Operation Procedure for Robotic Thyroidectomy

After completing the docking procedure, thyroidectomy is performed in the same manner as conventional open thyroidectomy. The thyroid gland is retracted using a ProGrasp forceps on the fourth robotic arm and dissection is performed employing a Harmonic curved shears and a Maryland dissector. This procedure allows the surgeon

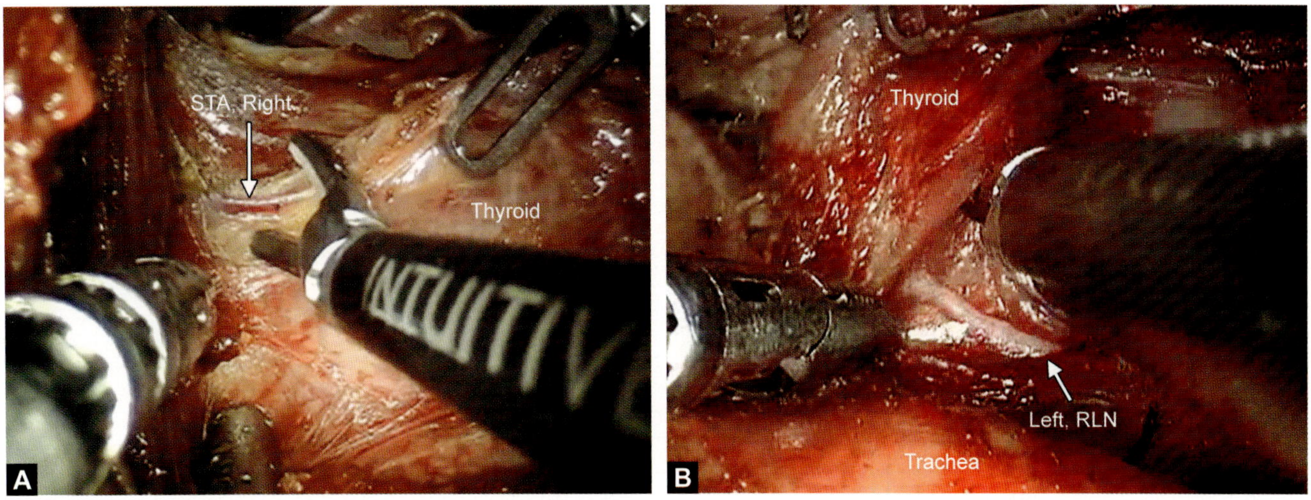

Figs. 6.8A and B: Operative findings of robotic total thyroidectomy by right transaxillary approach. (A) Identification and individual ligation of the superior thyroid artery using a Maryland dissector and dissection with Harmonic curved shears (STA, Rt: Superior thyroid artery, right). (B) After completing ipsilateral (Right) lobectomy, dissection around tracheoesophageal groove and preservation of the contralateral(Left) recurrent laryngeal nerve (Lt, RLN: Recurrent laryngeal nerve, Left).

to use three robotic arms during thyroidectomy. The dissection of superior pole of the thyroid gland using the ProGrasp forceps was initiated to retract the thyroid downward and Maryland dissector to create traction on the thyroid tissue. The superior thyroid gland vessels are identified and individually ligated close to the thyroid gland to avoid injury of the external branch of superior laryngeal nerve using Harmonic curved shears. The upper pole of thyroid gland is separated from the cricopharyngeal and cricothyroid muscles until the superior parathyroid gland is exposed and preserved (Fig. 6.8A). The thyroid gland is then pulled in a superior and medial direction using the ProGrasp forceps, and the lateral side of the CCND is performed from the CCA to the inferior thyroid artery superiorly and to the substernal notch inferiorly. All dissections and ligations of vessels are performed using the Harmonic curved shears. After exposing the CCA to the inferior thyroid artery, soft tissue and central compartment nodes are detached to the substernal notch until the anterior surface of trachea is exposed (Fig. 6.8B). The inferior thyroid artery is divided close to the thyroid gland using the Harmonic curved shears, and the whole cervical course of the RLN is traced. In the Berry ligament area, the thyroid gland is meticulously detached from the trachea to avoid direct or indirect thermal injury of the RLN. In cases of bilateral total thyroidectomy, contralateral lobectomy was usually performed after completing ipsilateral lobectomy. The removal of the contralateral lobe was done by capsular dissection through the thyroid capsule with adequate retraction of the thyroid lobe and trachea. The blood vessels were divided close to the thyroid capsule. The contralateral Berry's ligament was divided by Harmonic curved shear close to the thyroid capsule while retracting the contralateral lobe laterally and taking care to preserve the contralateral RLN. In patients with a prominent trachea and a deeply located contralateral thyroid, the surgical table can be tilted by 10–15°, which provides optimal exposure of the contralateral trachea-esophageal groove. The resected specimen is removed through an axillary skin incision. A 3-mm closed suction drain is inserted through a separate skin incision under the axillary skin incision (Fig. 6.9). Wounds are closed cosmetically. The axillary incision scar is completely covered when the arm is in its natural position. Apart from docking of the robotic arms, during console stage, the two-incision and single-incision robotic thyroidectomy procedures are the same (6.1).

Actual Operation Procedure for Robotic Modified Radical Neck Dissection

Actually, the robotic MRND procedure is similar to conventional open technique. Lateral neck dissection is initiated from the level III and IV area around the IJV. The IJV is handled medially using the ProGrasp forceps, and soft tissues and LNs are pulled laterally using a Maryland dissector. Careful dissection is needed during the detachment of the LNs from the posterior aspect of the IJV to avoid injury to the CCA and the vagus nerve. The dissection of

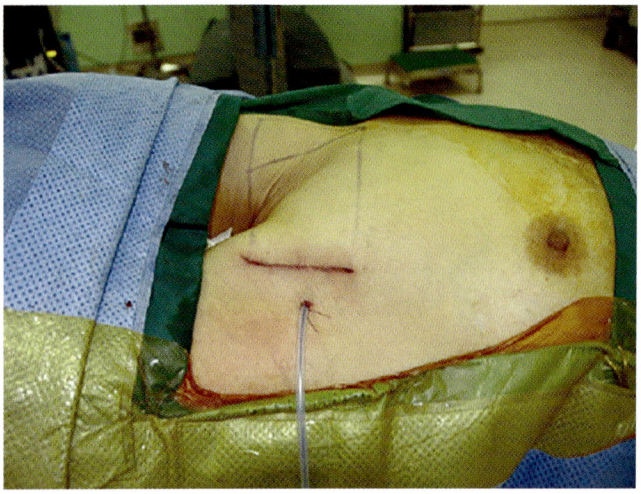

Fig. 6.9: Immediate postoperative scar after transaxillary single-incision robotic thyroidectomy.

the IJV is progressed upward from level IV to the upper level III area. During this procedure, the superior belly of the omohyoid muscle is cut at the thyroid cartilage level. Bundle of LNs are then drawn superiorly using the ProGrasp forceps, and the LNs are meticulously detached from the junction of the IJV and subclavian vein. In general, the transverse cervical artery as a branch of the thyrocervical trunk courses laterally across the anterior scalene muscle, anterior to the phrenic nerve. Using this anatomic landmark, the phrenic nerve and transverse cervical artery can be preserved without injury or ligation. Further dissection is followed along the subclavian vein laterally. The inferior belly of omohyoid muscle is cut where it meets the trapezius muscle. The distal EJV is then clipped and divided at its connection with the subclavian vein. Level V dissection in the posterior neck area proceeds along the spinal accessory nerve in the superomedial direction, and is followed by level IV dissection, while preserving the brachial nerve plexus, the phrenic nerve and the thoracic duct. The dissection proceeds by making turns at levels V, IV and III, and then by proceeding upward to the level II area. The individual nerves of the cervical plexus are sensory nerves, and when encountered during dissection some small branches of them might be sacrificed to ensure complete node dissection, while preserving the phrenic nerve and ansa cervicalis.

After performing the level III, IV and VB node dissection, re-docking is needed for a better operating view to dissect the level II LN. The external retractor is then reinserted through the axillary incision and directed toward the submandibular gland (Fig. 6.7C). The operating table should also be repositioned more obliquely with respect to the direction of the robotic column to allow the same alignment between the axis of the robotic camera arm and the direction of retractor blade insertion. Drawing the specimen tissue inferolaterally, soft tissues and LNs are detached from the lateral border of the sternohyoid muscle, the submandibular gland and the anterior surfaces of the carotid artery and the IJV. Level IIA dissection is advanced until the posterior belly of the digastric muscle is exposed superiorly. After removing the specimen, fibrin glue is sprayed around the area of the thoracic duct and minor lymphatics, and a 3-mm closed suction drain is inserted just under the axillary skin incision. Wounds are closed cosmetically. The incision scar in the axilla is completely covered when the arm is in its neutral position (Figs. 6.10A to C).

PRESENT STATUS OF ROBOTIC THYROID SURGERY

Master-slave-type robotic surgical systems are increasingly used to perform robotic thyroid surgery, including in patients with thyroid cancer. The da Vinci Surgical System was first used clinically in 2007 for thyroidectomy.[6] Since our group demonstrated the feasibility of robotic thyroidectomy in 2009, many other centers have adopted a robotic platform and continue to improve surgical methods, and the number of publications describing the robotic thyroidectomy has markedly increased. Moreover, a recent series of systematic reviews has analyzed each of these surgical outcomes.[34] Comparative studies of robotic and conventional open thyroidectomy have reported that robotic thyroidectomy is safe and feasible, but is associated with longer operation times and higher costs than conventional open surgery.[7-18] Overall morbidity rates, mean number of retrieved LNs, mean blood loss and mean length of hospital stay were similar for robotic and conventional open surgery, as were oncologic outcomes, as determined by measuring serum Tg concentrations using ^{131}RAI scanning. However, robotic thyroid surgery in its present form entails longer operation times and higher costs than conventional open thyroid surgery. Studies comparing robotic with conventional endoscopic thyroidectomy have shown similar postoperative complication rates and mean length of hospital stay, but the number of LNs retrieved was higher during robotic than endoscopic surgery.[7-9,12,15] These findings suggested that robotic thyroidectomy is feasible and safe, and can overcome some of the technical limitations associated with conventional endoscopic

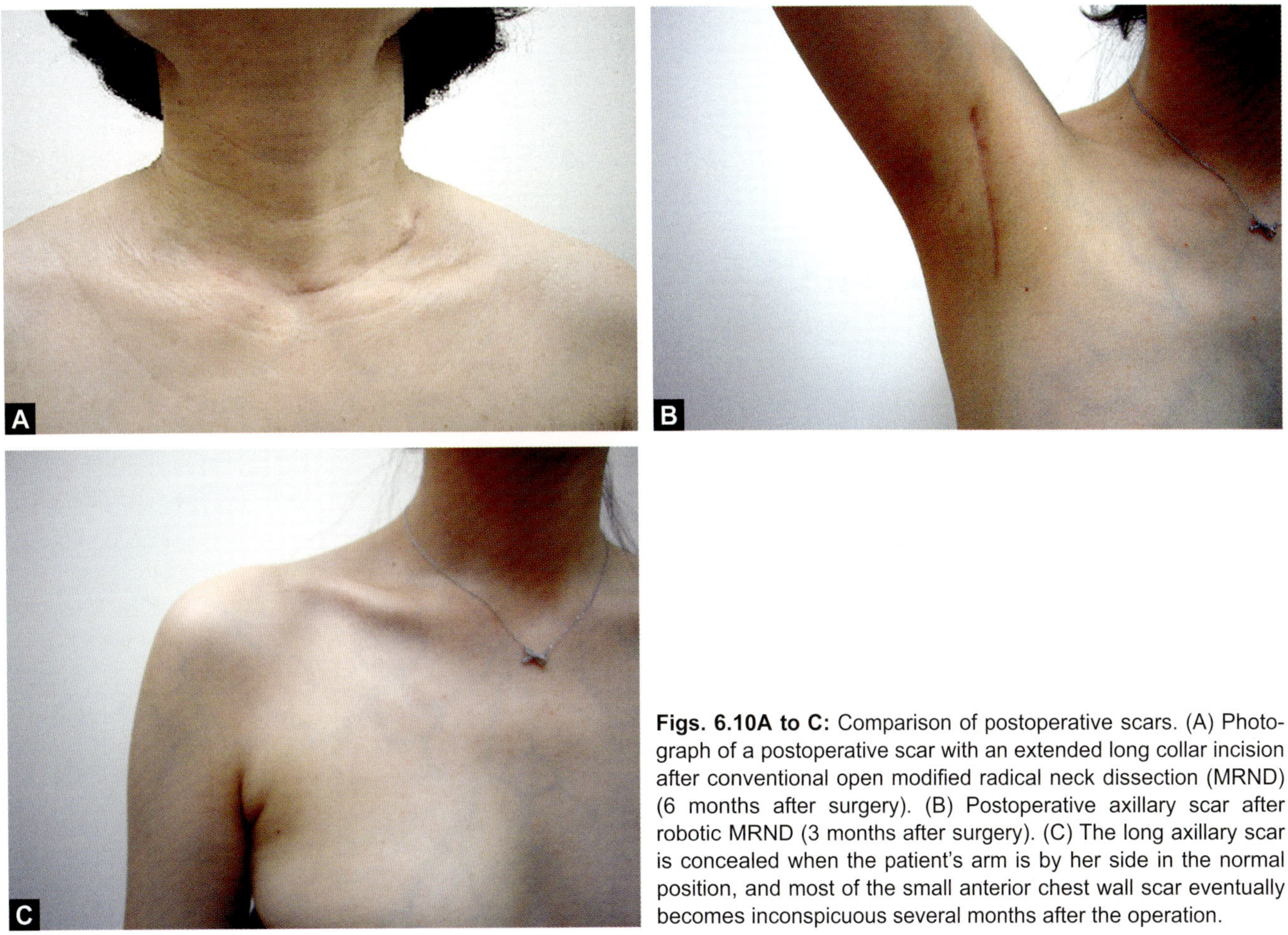

Figs. 6.10A to C: Comparison of postoperative scars. (A) Photograph of a postoperative scar with an extended long collar incision after conventional open modified radical neck dissection (MRND) (6 months after surgery). (B) Postoperative axillary scar after robotic MRND (3 months after surgery). (C) The long axillary scar is concealed when the patient's arm is by her side in the normal position, and most of the small anterior chest wall scar eventually becomes inconspicuous several months after the operation.

procedures. Due to the recent introduction of robotic thyroid surgery, its long-term outcomes cannot be compared with those of open or endoscopic thyroid surgery, but the short-term outcomes and oncologic adequacy of robotic thyroidectomy have been satisfactory. Further investigations and randomized trials are needed to establish a role for robotic thyroid surgery.

Early phases of robotic thyroid surgery were characterized by the rapid development of robotic surgical techniques and better perioperative assessments of oncologic outcomes and morbidity rates. The next phase of development should be directed toward improving QoL for both patients and surgeons. Several reports from Korea of QoL after robotic thyroidectomy have been published.[7-9,21-26] These studies have found lower levels of dissatisfaction and regret in patients undergoing robotic than conventional open thyroid surgery, largely due to differences in cosmetic outcomes. Prospective trials evaluating functional parameters including pain, neck discomfort and sensory changes in the neck, as well as cosmetic outcomes, showed favorable outcomes for robotic compared with conventional open thyroid surgery. Similarly, objective and subjective voice and swallowing discomfort after surgery were improved in patients undergoing robotic thyroidectomy than in patients undergoing conventional open surgery. Therefore, use of robotic surgery results in an overall increase in cosmetic satisfaction and decreases in several measures of postoperative discomfort among patients.

To determine the effects of robotic thyroidectomy on surgeons, a recent survey compared the type and magnitude of musculoskeletal stress during open, endoscopic and robotic thyroidectomy. These three approaches involved different physical tasks and differences in the type and magnitude of musculoskeletal stress.[13] Use of the robotic technique reduced musculoskeletal discomfort, compared with discomfort experienced during open or endoscopic thyroidectomy. Moreover, robotic thyroidectomy was associated with a shorter operation time than conventional endoscopic thyroidectomy and learning robotic surgical techniques was less complicated than adapting conventional endoscopic techniques.[12] Multicenter trials evaluated surgeon learning curves for robotic thyroidectomy by analyzing a range of perioperative parameters, including operation time, complication rate, intraoperative blood loss, length of hospital stay, number of dissected LNs and extent of complete resection.[35,36] These study results indicated that, to become proficient in robotic total thyroidectomy with CCND and subtotal thyroidectomy with CCND, a surgeon must perform 55-70 and 35-45 operations respectively. Moreover, beginning surgeons acquired the necessary technical skills, similar to those of experienced surgeons, once the learning curve was completed.

The widespread adoption of robotic thyroidectomy has increased interest in using the robotic system to perform radical neck dissection in thyroid cancer patients with lateral neck node metastasis. However, wide acceptance and implementation of robotic techniques in advanced thyroid cancer patients with lateral neck node metastasis have been slow because of the complexity and sophisticated surgical procedures required. Recent reports showed that robotic methods have been found feasible and safe in these patients, both for complete thyroid resection and adequate LN dissection.[19,20,37] Moreover, robotic MRND provides more satisfactory cosmetic outcomes than open MRND, due to the long neck scar resulting from the latter. A recent comparative analysis of QoL after robotic and MRND showed that both yielded similar oncologic and safety outcomes and similarly excellent QoL.[37] However, robotic MRND remains at an early stage, and the advantages and disadvantages of this new technique require further evaluation.

QUESTIONS AND SOLUTIONS

The main drawbacks of robotic surgery are its costs, limited availability within some health systems, the large size of the robot and console, the lack of tactile feedback or haptics and the need to train residents, attending surgeons and operating room personnel on the use of this technology.[4]

The costs of robotic surgery depend on the model of each nation's health care system. In some countries, reimbursement is greater for robotic than for conventional open surgery, whereas, in other countries, reimbursement is according to a flat fee schedule, regardless of the approach used. Data based on urologic procedures such as prostatectomies and pyeloplasties, have shown that the robotic technique becomes cost-effective once the learning curve has been overcome and the surgeon can efficiently perform an operation within a specific time limit. Other main cost benefits result from a shorter duration of hospital stay and a decreased incidence of complications. Therefore, robotic technology is most cost-effective in settings in which the volume of patients is high enough to overcome the initial learning curve. To date, only one study, in the United States, has compared the cost effectiveness of endoscopic and robotic thyroidectomy with that of conventional open surgery.[38] That study showed that endoscopic and robotic thyroidectomies were significantly more expensive than standard open surgery, but that increasing the number of endoscopic and robotic thyroidectomies performed per year reduced their unit cost. However, the number of robotic thyroidectomies per year required to make the robotic technique cost-effective for thyroid surgery has not been determined. In addition, the proper modification of robotic systems in some publicly funded systems and in many private care systems remains very challenging.

Current robotic systems are composed of three parts: a patient-side robot, a vision cart and the robotic master console, which together take up a huge area in an operating theater. The robot surgical cart may be too large to fit into some operating rooms. In addition, a relatively limited number of surgical instruments are available for robotic surgical systems. During some robotic surgical procedures, it may be necessary to reposition the robot system. In these cases, the robot should be dedocked after completing the initial portion of the surgery, the patient's bed turned, new ports inserted and the robot redocked in another position. Future robot systems will need to be much smaller to lessen the complexity of their use.[39,40]

Another significant consideration in robotic thyroidectomy is the loss of haptics and imaging feedback. Thus, all the training surgeons go through to understand the reactions of tissues to the applications of various instruments is not applicable to the use of a robot. Therefore, for beginning robotic surgeons, the lack of haptics or tactile feedback may often result in injury to adjacent organs or rupture of blood vessels. Despite this initial limitation, most beginning robotic surgeons quickly adapt to and compensate for the lack of haptics or tactile feedback by using the improved visual feedback of the magnified, three-dimensional display. That is, the high-resolution stereoscopic images of current robot systems clearly constitute an additional compensatory mechanism. Experienced robotic surgeons have realized that this ability to use visual clues is easily learned, and that the loss of tactile feedback is no longer a hindrance. Future robot systems may improve surgical performance by, e.g. overlaying color markings on tissues to denote the amount of force applied to certain predetermined thresholds. Moreover, information about the forces applied by a surgical robot during surgery may be converted to electrical signals, which can distort the shape of telemanipulators being handled by the surgeon, allowing the surgeon to receive some form of touch sensation feedback about the interactions of the robot with the tissues.[39]

Another current limitation of robotic surgery is the need to train teams, including attending surgeons, surgical assistant(s) and nurses, to improve their proficiency.[40] The surgical team must understand the spatial relationships of the instruments outside the operative field of vision to minimize collisions between instruments and inadvertent tissue injury. To overcome these new challenges, training pathways have been created for surgeons and surgical team members. The first assistant and nurse specialist are important members of the robotic operative team. Robot systems are more challenging for the first assistant and nurse because the robotic arms move over the patient at the same time. Although robotic instrument exchange can become quite efficient, it still requires attachment of the robotic instruments to the instrument arms before insertion. Responsibilities include timely docking of the patient cart, safe exchange of instruments and port repositioning to avoid collisions. In addition, the first assistant is the initial responder to any potential complications and is vital to providing adequate visualization for surgeons. Proficiency can only be obtained by commitment of the entire team. Success of initial robotic surgeries is dependent on patient selection, the complexity of the procedure and maintaining proper operative decisions. For a proper initial learning curve, the first 30-40 robotic thyroid surgeries performed by a surgical team should be relatively simple.[40] These operations will allow the surgical team to become familiar with port placement, patient positioning and docking. Once the learning curve has been overcome, the team can progress to more complex operations. Maintenance of proficiency is obtained by regular and successful completion of these operations. Furthermore, the surgeon and the operative team should be self-critical and should periodically assess operation time, blood loss and complication rate, followed by discussions of the most suitable instruments and equipment and the proper indications for robotic surgery.

FUTURE DIRECTIONS

Robotic thyroidectomy and radical neck dissection have revolutionized the surgical management of thyroid cancer. We found that robotic thyroidectomy and radical neck dissection using a gasless transaxillary approach were safe and feasible in thyroid cancer patients, showing the same oncologic outcomes as conventional open surgery, as determined by postoperative ^{131}RAI scans, Tg concentrations and number of retrieved cervical LNs. For surgeons, the use of a robot offers a shorter operation time and a shorter learning curve compared with conventional endoscopic thyroidectomy, and causes less musculoskeletal discomfort than open or endoscopic thyroidectomy. For patients, this technique provides excellent cosmetic results, a reduction in pain, improvements in sensory changes and decreased postoperative voice changes and swallowing discomfort. However, large volume studies with long-term follow-up periods are needed to determine whether the robotic procedure results in superior oncologic and QoL outcomes compared with endoscopic or open thyroidectomy.

VIDEO LEGEND

Video 6.1: Robotic total thyroidectomy/central node dissection via right axillary approach.

REFERENCES

1. Gagner M. Endoscopic subtotal parathyroidectomy in patients with primary hyperparathyroidism. Br J Surg. 1996; 83:875.
2. Ikeda Y, Takami H, Sasaki Y, et al. Clinical benefits in endoscopic thyroidectomy by the axillary approach. J Am Coll Surg. 2003;196:189-95.
3. Ikeda Y, Takami H, Sasaki Y, et al. Are there significant benefits of minimally invasive endoscopic thyroidectomy? World J Surg. 2004;28:1075-8.
4. Visco AG, Advincula AP. Robotic gynecologic surgery. Obstet Gynecol. 2008;112:1369-84.
5. Stylopoulos N, Rattner D. Robotics and ergonomics. Surg Clin North Am. 2003;83:1321,37.
6. Kang SW, Jeong JJ, Yun JS, et al. Robot-assisted endoscopic surgery for thyroid cancer: experience with the first 100 patients. Surg Endosc. 2009;23:2399-2406.
7. Lee J, Chung WY. Current status of robotic thyroidectomy and neck dissection using gasless transaxillary approach. Curr Opin Oncol. 2012;24:7-15.
8. Lee J, Chung WY. Robotic thyroidectomy and neck dissection: past, present and future. Cancer J. 2013;19(2):151-61.
9. Lee J, Chung WY. Robotic surgery for thyroid disease. Eur Thyroid J. 2013 April 26 [Epub ahead of print], [DOI: 10.1159/000350209]

10. Kang SW, Lee SC, Lee SH, et al. Robotic thyroid surgery using a gasless, transaxillary approach and the da Vinci S system: the operative outcomes of 338 consecutive patients. Surgery. 2009;146:1048-55.
11. Kuppersmith RB, Holsinger FC. Robotic thyroid surgery: an initial experience with North American patients. Laryngoscope. 2011;121:521-6.
12. Lee J, Lee JH, Nah KY, et al. Comparison of endoscopic and robotic thyroidectomy. Ann Surg Oncol. 2011;18:1439-46.
13. Lee J, Kang SW, Jung JJ, et al. Multicenter study of robotic thyroidectomy: short-term postoperative outcomes and surgeon ergonomic considerations. Ann Surg Oncol. 18: 2538-47.
14. Lee S, Ryu HR, Park JH, et al. Early surgical outcomes comparison between robotic and conventional open thyroid surgery for papillary thyroid microcarcinoma. Surgery. 2012;151:724-30.
15. Lee S, Ryu HR, Park JH, et al. Excellence in robotic thyroid surgery; a comparative study of robot-assisted versus conventional endoscopic thyroidectomy in papillary thyroid microcarcinoma patients. Ann Surg. 2011;253:1060-6.
16. Landry CS, Grubbs EG, Morris GS, et al. Robot assisted transaxillary surgery (RATS) for the removal of thyroid and parathyroid glands. Surgery. 2011;149:549-55.
17. Kandil EH, Noureldine SI, Yao L, et al. Robotic transaxillary thyroidectomy: an examination of the first one hundred cases. J Am Coll Surg. 2012;214:558-64.
18. Tae K, Ji YB, Cho SH, et al. Early surgical outcomes of robotic thyroidectomy by a gasless unilateral axillo-breast or axillary approach for papillary thyroid carcinoma: 2 years' experience. Head Neck 2012;34:617-25.
19. Kang SW, Lee SH, Ryu HR, et al. Initial experience with robot-assisted modified radical neck dissection for the management of thyroid carcinoma with lateral neck node metastasis. Surgery. 2010;148:1214-21.
20. Kang SW, Lee SH, Park JH, et al. A comparative study of the surgical outcomes of robotic and conventional open modified radical neck dissection for papillary thyroid carcinoma with lateral neck node metastasis. Surg Endosc. 2012;26:3251-7.
21. Lee J, Nah KY, Kim RM, et al. Differences in postoperative outcomes, function, and cosmesis: open versus robotic thyroidectomy. Surg Endosc. 2010;24:186-94.
22. Tae K, Ji YB, Jeong JH, et al. Robotic thyroidectomy by a gasless unilateral axillo-breast or axillary approach: our early experiences. Surg Endosc. 2011;25:221-8.
23. Tae K, Kim KY, Yun BR, et al. Functional voice and swallowing outcomes after robotic thyroidectomy by a gasless unilateral axillo-breast approach: comparison with open thyroidectomy. Surg Endosc. 2012;26:1871-7.
24. Lee J, Na KY, Kim RM, et al. Postoperative functional voice changes after conventional open or robotic thyroidectomy: a prospective trial. Ann Surg Oncol. 2012;19:2963-70.
25. Tae K, Ji YB, Jeong JH, et al. Comparative study of robotic versus endoscopic thyroidectomy by a gasless unilateral axillo-breast or axillary approach. Head Neck. 2013;35:477-84.
26. Ryu HR, Lee J, Park JH, et al. A comparison of postoperative pain after conventional open thyroidectomy and transaxillary single-incision robotic thyroidectomy: a prospective study. Ann Surg Oncol. 2013 Mar 26 [Epub ahead of print].
27. Lee S, Park S, Lee CR, et al. The impact of body habitus on the surgical outcomes of transaxillary single-incision robotic thyroidectomy in papillary thyroid carcinoma patients. Surg Endosc. 2013 Jan 24 [Epub ahead of print].
28. American Thyroid Association (ATA) Guidelines Taskforce on Thyroid Nodules and Differentiated Thyroid Cancer, Cooper DS, Doherty GM, Haugen BR, et al. Revised American Thyroid Association management guidelines for patients with thyroid nodules and differentiated thyroid cancer. Thyroid. 2009;19:1167-214.
29. Lee J, Yun JH, Nam KH, et al. Perioperative clinical outcomes after robotic thyroidectomy for thyroid carcinoma: a multicenter study. Surg Endosc. 2011;25:906-12.
30. Holsinger FC, Terris DJ, Kuppersmith RB. Robotic thyroidectomy: operative technique using a transaxillary endoscopic approach without CO_2 insufflation. Otolaryngol Clin North Am. 2010;43:381-8.
31. Berber E, Heiden K, Akyildiz H, et al. Robotic transaxillary thyroidectomy: report of 2 cases and description of the technique. Surg Laparosc Endosc Percutan Tech. 2010;20:e60-3.
32. Ryu HR, Kang SW, Lee SH, et al. Feasibility and safety of a new robotic thyroidectomy through a gasless, transaxillary single-incision approach. J Am Coll Surg. 2010;211:e13-9.
33. Randolph GW, Duh QY, Heller KS, et al.; American Thyroid Association Surgical Affairs Committee'SuTaskforce on Thyroid Cancer Nodal Surgery. The prognostic significance of nodal metastases from papillary thyroid carcinoma can be stratified based on the size and number of metastatic lymph nodes, as well as the presence of extranodal extension. Thyroid. 2012;22:1144-52.
34. Jackson NR, Yao L, Tufano RP, et al. Safety of robotic thyroidectomy approaches: meta-analysis and systemic review. Head Neck. 2012 Mar 8 [Epub ahead of print].
35. Lee J, Yun JH, Nam KH, et al. The learning curve for robotic thyroidectomy: a multicenter study. Ann Surg Oncol. 2011; 18:226-32.
36. Lee J, Yun JH, Choi UJ, et al. Robotic versus endoscopic thyroidectomy for thyroid cancer: a multi-institutional analysis of early postoperative outcomes and surgical learning curves. J Oncol. 2012; 734541 [DOI: 10.1155/2012/734541].
37. Lee J, Kwon IS, Bae EH, et al. Comparative analysis of oncological outcomes and quality of life after robotic versus conventional open thyroidectomy with modified radical neck dissection in patients with papillary thyroid carcinoma and lateral neck node metastases. J Clin Endocrinol Metab. 2013 May 15 [Epub ahead of print].
38. Cabot JC, Lee CR, Brunaud L, et al. Robotic and endoscopic transaxillary thyroidectomies may be cost prohibitive when compared to standard cervical thyroidectomy: a cost analysis. Surgery. 2012;152:1016-24.
39. Lendvay TS, Hannaford B, Satava RM. Future of robotic surgery. Cancer J. 2013;19:109-19.
40. Ben-Or S, Nifong LW, Chitwood WR, Jr. Robotic surgical training. Cancer J. 2013;19:120-3.

Chapter 7 Robotic Thyroidectomy for American (Western) Patients

Salah E Mohamed, Emad Kandil

INTRODUCTION

The Czech author Karel Capek first introduced the term "robot" in 1920 as a name for artificial people.[1] People throughout history have conceived "robots" as automated machines that improve the quality of work. Fortunately, surgical robots have evolved following a similar pattern. In 1995, Intuitive Surgical Inc. designed a robot that could improve surgeons' proficiency. Later in the 1990s, there were three surgical robotic systems that were being used in academic institutions: the Aesop endoscope robotic control system, Zeus robotic system made by Computer Motion and the da Vinci surgical system made by Intuitive Surgical. The Zeus system was used in the University of Pittsburg to perform the first robotic surgery—a beating-heart coronary artery bypass graft procedure in the late 1990s. However, the da Vinci surgical system is the only commercially available surgical robot that is being used by surgeons today. During the last decade, robotic surgery has evolved to the preferred surgical method in cardiothoracic, thoracic, urologic, gynecologic and gastrointestinal procedures.

The incidence of thyroid cancer has increased with papillary thyroid cancer accounting for 70%. Thyroid surgery back in the sixth century A.D. had catastrophic results. They were being predominantly performed in the treatment of thyroid goiters in relieving obstructive symptoms. In 1850, thyroid operations were accompanied by a mortality rate reaching 41%. However, with the evolution of technology, thyroid surgery today has become one of the safest surgical procedures. Different approaches are currently being used in thyroid surgery, each carrying its own limitations and advantages. With Kocher's contribution to thyroid surgery, conventional thyroidectomy approach remains the gold standard at many centers today, and is associated with a very low rate of morbidity. Kocher initially employed a vertical incision thyroidectomy, and then finally with more operative experience he transitioned to a low transverse cervical incision. Surgeons today use a small, high cervical incision in the skin crease in the anterior neck creating a mycocutaneous flap to gain access to the thyroid compartment. Nonetheless, this approach left patients with a visible cervical scar, which is concerning especially for the population of young women who want to preserve their neck appearance. Furthermore, some patients develop a hypertrophic or keloid scars that leave patients devastated with the cosmetic results.

Surgeons as a result have developed alternate methods to minimize the surgical incisions or to relocate them to an extracervical location to avoid a conspicuous cervical scar. Some advantages of these approaches are cosmetic and some provide better visualization and magnification of the operative field with the robotic or videoscopic approach. Furthermore, with significant improvements in endoscopic instrumentation and better understanding of endoscopic cervical anatomy, there has been further growth of head and neck endoscopic surgery in the management of thyroid and parathyroid disease. However, this approach has limitations in obtaining adequate surgical views and in the manipulation of the endoscopic instruments, resulting from the two-dimensional operative views of the surgical area and the narrow working space. In 1996, Gagner reported the first endoscopic parathyroidectomy.[2] Then, later on the following year Huscher et al. described the first endoscopic right thyroid lobectomy.[3]

The initial experience with endoscopic thyroidectomy included the use of gas insufflation to overcome the limited visualization of the surgical space through the small incision.[2,3] Unfortunately, this technique presented its own complications, such as subcutaneous emphysema, systemic absorption of carbon dioxide and severe tachycardia as reported in the literature.[4,5] After these initial experiences, further techniques such as breast, axillary, axillobreast and anterior chest approaches have been reported.

Some surgeons have turned to robotic surgery to overcome some of these limitations of endoscopic remote access thyroidectomy (Figs. 7.1A and B).[6-9] This system offered the possibility of reducing the limitations of conventional endoscopy by providing a three-dimensional,

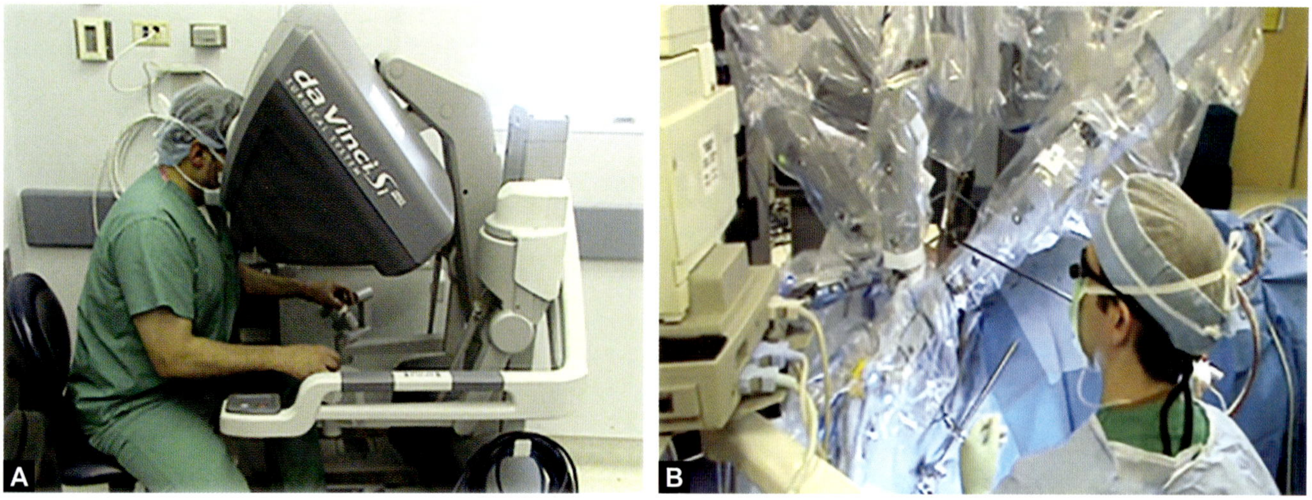

Figs. 7.1A and B: (A) Surgeon operating the robot. (B) An assistant helping the surgeon.

stable, magnified picture, providing the surgeon with an ergonomically perfect position at a site remote from the patient, improving freedom of motion through the use of multi-articulated instruments and enabling surgeons to perform precise, minute movements and dissection and providing a hand-tremor filtration system.[10-18] Additionally, Lee et al. in their experience found that robotic thyroidectomy yielded similar oncological outcome and safety as the conventional open procedure. Furthermore, robotic thyroidectomy resulted in better cosmetic results and reduction in sensory changes in the neck and dysphagia.[19]

The robotic approach was developed to avoid an external scar however surgeons have noted improved visualization of structures such as the recurrent laryngeal nerve with the high definition optics. The complication rate when performing robotic thyroidectomy by high volume robotic surgeons is similar to the traditional approach.

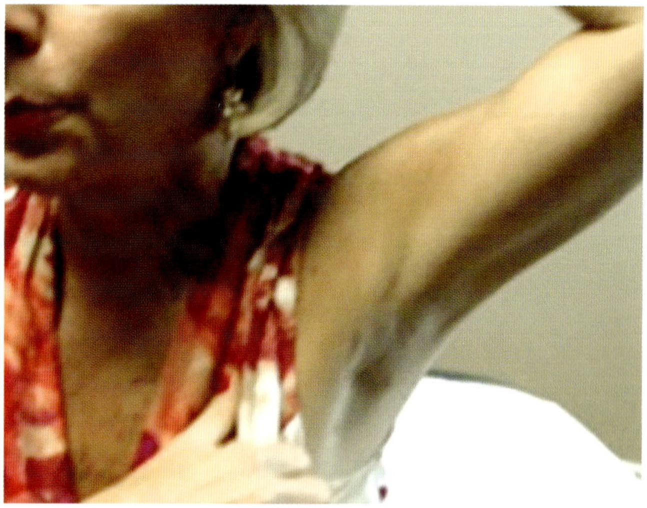

Fig. 7.2: Two months postoperative cosmetic results after the transaxillary thyroidectomy approach.

ROBOTIC THYROIDECTOMY

In 2001, Kang et al. adopted the gasless endoscopic thyroidectomy using the transaxillary approach to treat over 700 patients with thyroid disease. However, the application of the robotic technique was difficult due to the bulky robotic arms as well as the narrow and deep working space.[8] In 2007, robotic assisted surgery was reported to overcome the difficulties with the older technique. The benefit of the endoscopic thyroid operation using the transaxillary approach are: the operative view is the same as that of conventional surgery allowing easy manipulation of the upper and lower thyroid poles, elimination of postoperative hyperesthesia and fibrotic contractures in the anterior neck area, and it allows central compartment neck dissection to be performed[4, 20-22] with a excellent cosmetic result leaving the incision well concealed in the axillary fold when the arm is at rest (Fig. 7.2). Kang later in 2009 reported his experience with the application of the robotic system to his endoscopic approach.[8] He used a combination of a unilateral transaxillary incision and anterior chest incision to access the thyroid space.[8,22,23] This approach had equivalent oncological outcomes in a large number of patients when compared to those using the conventional (open) approach.[22,24] Furthermore, the addition of the robot to his endoscopic approach provided additional benefits such as easier identification and preservation of the recurrent laryngeal nerve (RLN) and the parathyroid glands (Fig. 7.3); complete and safe thyroid resection, easier lymph node dissection and improved surgeon comfort;[8] and less pain and faster return to functional activity for the patient. This remote-access technique is not considered minimally invasive; nevertheless it has rapidly gained popularity in North American practice.[25-30]

Terris et al. in 2011 developed a hybrid technique, the robotic facelift approach using a retroauricular incision. They utilized the robotic technology to gain remote access to the thyroid space without having a visible cervical scar (Figs. 7.4A and B).[31] Terris experienced easier positioning of the patient and a shorter distance to the thyroid when compared to the transaxillary approach.[32] One drawback to the robotic facelift thyroidectomy approach is the inability to perform a total thyroidectomy from a single unilateral incision, whereas this can be done in the robotic transaxillary approach.

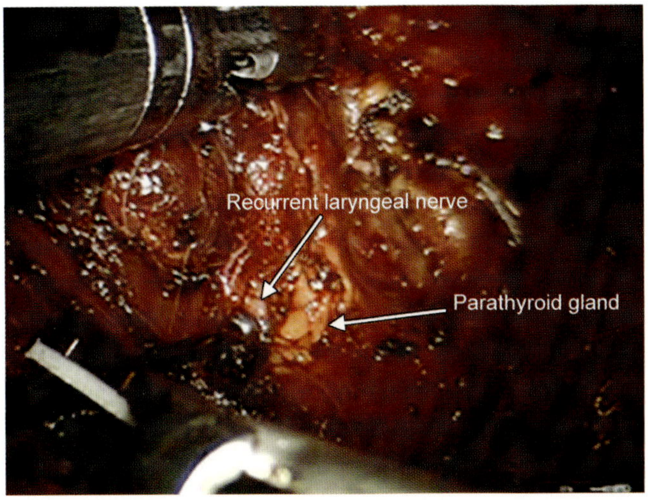

Fig. 7.3: Identification and preservation of the recurrent laryngeal nerve (RLN) and the parathyroid glands during the transaxillary and the facelift thyroidectomy approach. The RLN is stimulated intraoperatively to ensure its integrity.

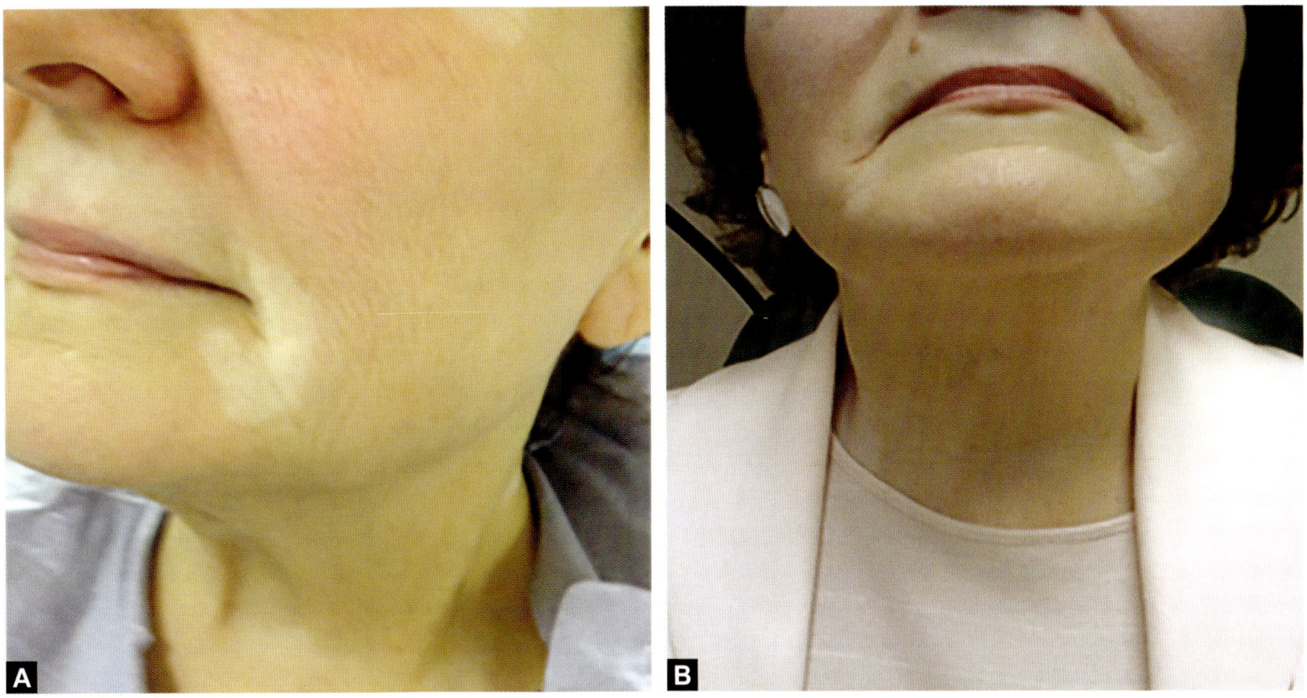

Figs. 7.4A and B: (A) Preoperative facelift thyroidectomy approach patient. (B) The facelift thyroidectomy approach is used to gain remote access to the thyroid space without leaving a visible cervical scar.

Table 7.1: Indications and relative contraindications for minimally invasive video-assisted thyroid surgery

Indications	*Relative contraindications*
• Total thyroid volume <30 mL • T1 papillary thyroid cancer • A thyroid nodule <3 cm in diameter	• History of thyroiditis • History of neck radiation • Total thyroid volume > 30 mL • Minimally invasive video-assisted thyroid surgery (MIVAT) • History of MIVAT • Graves' disease (in early experience) • Hashimoto's thyroiditis

INDICATION AND PATIENT SELECTION

The surgeon must be aware that young female patients will focus on the location and length of the incision in the assessment of the overall quality of the surgery. Nonetheless, it is essential to establish guiding principles that can serve as the framework for implementing these emerging new technologies without compromising patient safety.[29] Even though ideal patient selection criteria has not been established, the best candidate for this approach are average size (body mass index less than 30 kg/m^2) in a young patient who is concerned about having a visible neck scar or has a history of keloid or hypertrophic scar formation. Contraindications to this approach is similar for those patients that could be candidates for minimally invasive video assisted thyroid surgery (MIVAT). This includes: (1) a history of irradiation to the neck or previous neck surgery; (2) a malignancy with definite extrathyroidal tumor invasion, neck node metastases or distant metastasis; and (3) a lesion located in the thyroid dorsal area owing to possible injury to the trachea, esophagus or RLN.[33] Surgeons must also consider any problems with shoulder mobility and the presence of a rotator cuff injury if a transaxillary approach is considered. It is not recommended to operate on patients with Hashimoto's thyroiditis or Graves' disease during one's early experience (Table 7.1). These considerations may either make it difficult to position the patient safely for the procedure (especially for the transaxillary approach) or make dissection and exposure of the thyroid difficult with the robotic instrumentation. Recently, some authors have reported in their late experience the safety and feasibility of robotic surgery in patients with Graves' disease.[34,35]

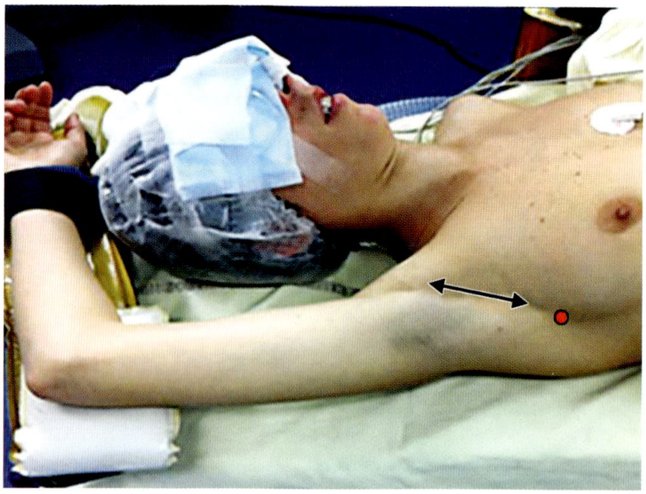

Fig. 7.5: The arm positioning for the transaxillary approach thyroidectomy.

Robotic Transaxillary Thyroidectomy

Modifications to the Asian robotic transaxillary thyroidectomy approach were necessary for US surgeons to be able to replicate the approach in the Western patient population without compromising safety and feasibility.[36] There have been concerns regarding the safety of the procedure when performed through a unilateral axillary incision in certain cases,[27] however, there is a significant learning curve for this approach. Kang et al. reported in their original series a significant decrease in the console time after 40-50 cases;[37] meanwhile, Kandil et al. reported a significant decrease in the console time after 45 cases.[27]

Surgical Technique

All patients undergo imaging studies prior to surgery that will help in the localization of the lesion. Patients are placed in the supine position and are usually intubated with the NIMS EMG endotracheal tube (neural integrity monitor electromyography) to allow intraoperative monitoring of the RLN function and to ensure its integrity. The arm ipsilateral to the lesion is positioned cephalad and flexed above the head as described by Ikeda et al. (Fig. 7.5).[38] This position optimizes the exposure to the axilla and shortens the distance from the axilla to the thyroid gland. Intraoperative ultrasound examination is routinely performed prior to the surgical incision to further aid the surgeon to the exact location of the lesion and to examine the relationship of the internal jugular vein to the thyroid gland in the anteroposterior plane. A 4 cm

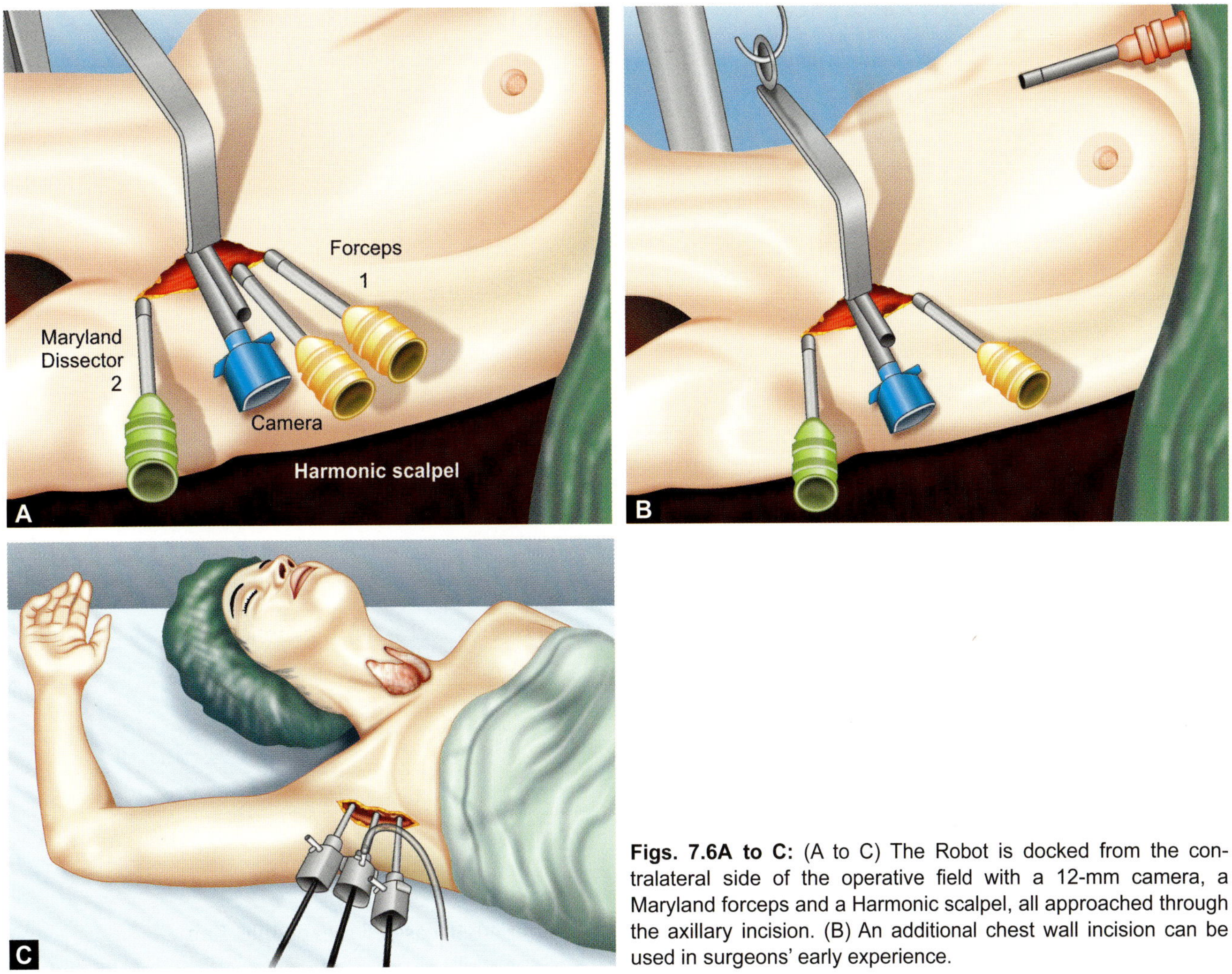

Figs. 7.6A to C: (A to C) The Robot is docked from the contralateral side of the operative field with a 12-mm camera, a Maryland forceps and a Harmonic scalpel, all approached through the axillary incision. (B) An additional chest wall incision can be used in surgeons' early experience.

axillary incision is then made along the lateral border of the pectoralis major muscle (Fig. 7.7).[33] A mycocutaneous flap is then raised in a subplatysmal plane in the direction of the thyroid until the sternal and clavicular heads of the sternocleidomastoid are visualized. A specially designed retractor is then secured to the table mount lift and placed under the sternal head of the sternocleidomastoid and the strap muscles, creating the working space superficial to the thyroid. The da Vinci S robot is then docked from the side of the bed contralateral to the operative field, with a 12-mm camera, a Maryland forceps and a Harmonic scalpel, approached through the axillary incision (Figs. 7.6A and B). An additional chest wall incision can be used in surgeons' early experience to assist in the manipulation and dissection of the thyroid gland (Fig. 7.6C). The dissection technique has been clearly described in Chapters 6 and 8 in this text.[25]

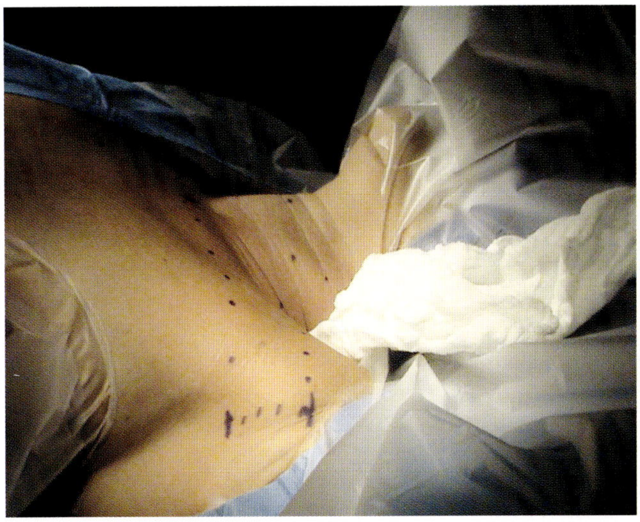

Fig. 7.7: The incision for the transaxillary approach is made in the postauricular crease and continued within the occipital hairline.

Robotic Facelift Thyroidectomy

In 2011, Terris et al. reported the feasibility of a novel robotic facelift approach for thyroidectomy. The idea for this approach originated when Terris et al. reported on the feasibility of a modified facelift incision for parotidectomy in 1994.[26] He also reported that a superior to inferior approach to the thyroid gland was optimal when compared to a series of transaxillary methods.[27] Lee et al. have built upon these concepts and employed a technique in which a postauricular portal is combined with the axillary approach using an insufflation technique to access the thyroid space.[29] Terris's hybrid technique combines the facelift parotidectomy,[26] the Chung gasless robotic thyroidectomy,[9] the Lee retroauricular insufflation technique[29] and the implementation of laryngeal nerve monitoring.[39]

This approach has a number of advantages including: (1) easier positioning of the patient and shorter distance to the thyroid gland as compared to the transaxillary approach, therefore reduced dissection that likely results in more rapid wound healing and less pain,[26] (2) the risk of brachial plexopathy is completely eliminated and (3) this approach is easier in slightly obese patients because of the ease of the flap creation as compared to the transaxillary approach.[36] In Western patients particularly in the US, the robotic facelift approach is the easiest to perform due to the larger BMI of patients. Some of the disadvantages of this approach are that it requires identification and protection of the greater auricular nerve as it is in the path of dissection and the inability to perform a total thyroidectomy via a unilateral incision.

Surgical Technique

Patients are positioned supine with the head turned slightly (30°) away from the side of the lesion. The patient is then intubated with a laryngeal EMG tube (NIMS-2, Medtronic Inc.) in order to monitor the laryngeal nerve intraoperatively. An incision is then made in the postauricular crease and continued within the occipital hairline. A musculocutaneous flap is then raised superficial to the greater auricular nerve and the external jugular vein and either deep[36] or superficial[28] to the platysmal muscle (Fig. 7.8). Terris described the dissection plan deep to platysma; however, we prefer in our experience to keep the dissection plane superficial to the platysma as described for neck lift operations to minimize any risk of injury to the greater auricular nerve. The triangle made up of the omohyoid muscle, the sternocleidomastoid muscle and the sternohyoid muscle is delineated and the omohyoid muscle is reflected ventrally to gain access to the superior pole of the thyroid gland. A customized retractor (Chung retractor) is then introduced to retract the strap muscles and to maintain the operative working space (Fig. 7.9A). An additional retractor (Greenberg retractor) can be used to retract the sternocleidomastoid muscle to maintain a wider operative field (Fig. 7.9B). The robotic surgical system is then docked using only three arms due to the limited space, which is in contrast to using four arms in the transaxillary approach. The camera arm is positioned 30° facing downward, parallel to the retractor, in the center of the surgical field, followed by a Maryland grasper placed in the nondominant arm and then the Harmonic CS14C device placed in the dominant arm (Fig. 7.10). Then the remainder of the procedure mimics that of the the transaxillary approach as described in Chapter 6 in this book.

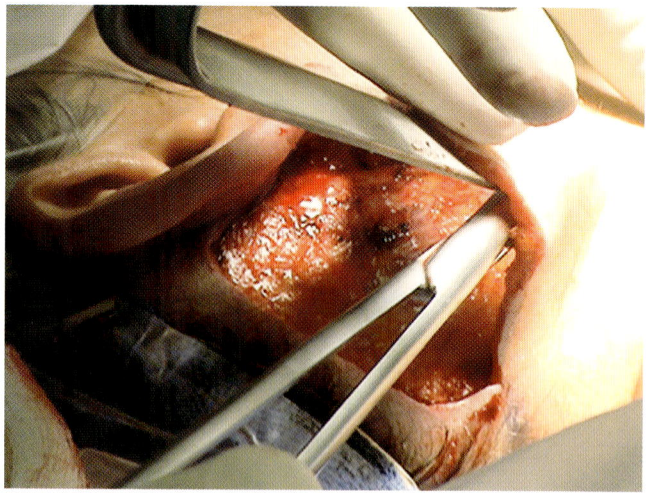

Fig. 7.8: A musculocutaneous flap is raised superficial to the greater auricular nerve and the external jugular vein and superficial to the platysmal muscle.

COMPLICATIONS

Conventional cervical thyroid surgery remains the gold standard for thyroidectomy with low morbidity and resulting in excellent outcomes. Therefore, it is essential to compare and evaluate these new technologies with the current standards. There are some complications that are not associated with the conventional thyroid surgery including muscle stiffness and prolonged paresthesia in the region of flap. Additionally, the arm positioning in the transaxillary approach can cause overtraction and lead to brachial plexus neuropraxia. This complication can be avoided by

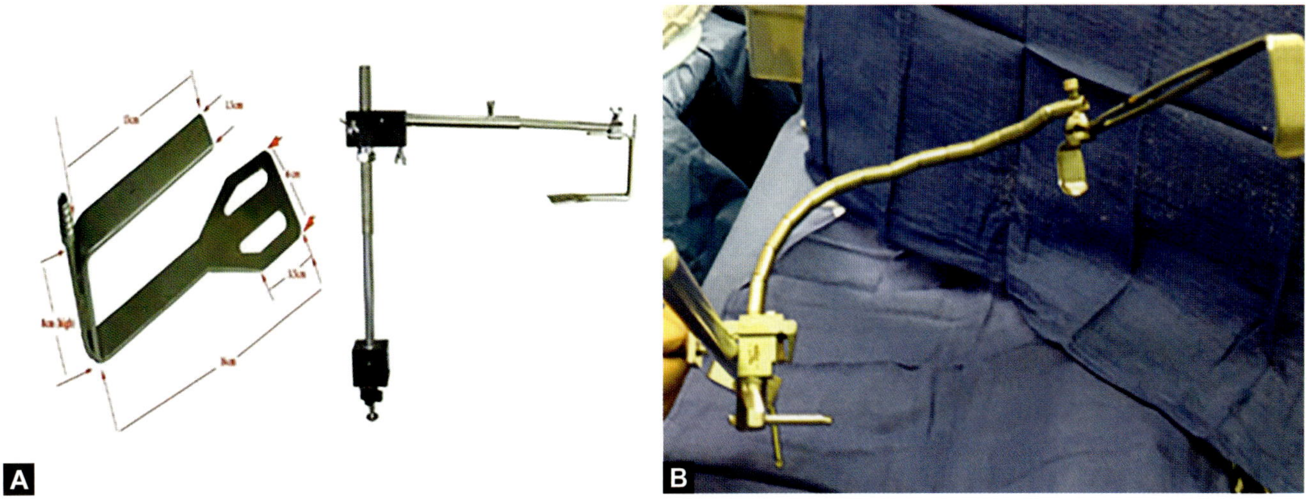

Figs. 7.9A and B: (A) The Chung retractor is used to retract the strap muscles and to maintain the operative pocket in the transaxillary and postauricular thyroidectomy approach. (B) An additional Greenberg retractor is used to retract the sternocleidomastoid muscle and keep a wider operative field in the postauricular approach.

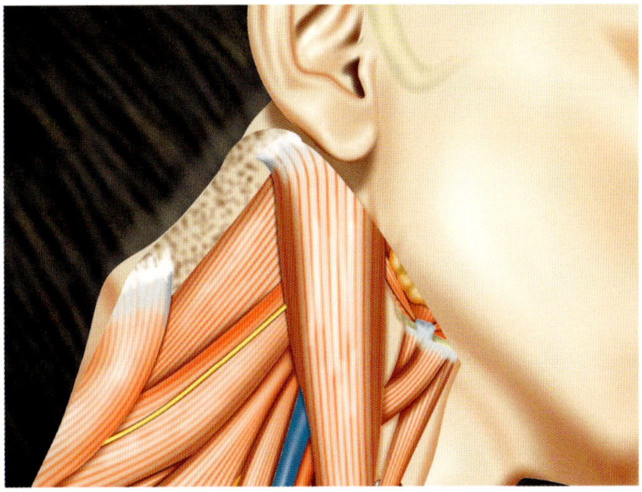

Fig. 7.10: The facelift incision approach is used to gain remote access to the thyroid space without having a visible cervical scar.

somatosensory evoked potential response nerve monitoring. All patients should be counseled regarding the possibility of conversion to an open procedure.

CONCLUSION

Robotic surgery has advanced the capabilities of surgeons in a very short period of time. Currently, uniform credentialing standards for surgeons do not yet exist and the training paradigms for these new technologies have not been validated. Efforts are currently under way to further outline these paths. It is essential to examine these new techniques and technologies responsibly as it is technically more complicated than the traditional approaches. Robotic thyroid surgery has a definite learning curve for both surgeons and operating room staff, and it is the surgeons' responsibility to ensure that they can perform the procedure without compromising patient safety. Additionally, the costs of these procedures must be weighed against the patients' psychological benefits of eliminating a visible neck scar, and the surgeons' benefit of enhanced visualization and instrumentation. A balanced investigation and a thorough data analysis are warranted to fully explore the advantages and the disadvantages of these new emerging technologies.

REFERENCES

1. Moran ME. Rossum's universal robots: not the machines. J Endourol. 2007;21:1399-402.
2. Gagner M. Endoscopic subtotal parathyroidectomy in patients with primary hyperparathyroidism. Br J Surg. 1996;83:875.
3. Huscher CS, Chiodini S, Napolitano C, et al. Endoscopic right thyroid lobectomy. Surg Endosc. 1997;11:877.
4. Kang SW, Jeong JJ, Yun JS, et al. Gasless endoscopic thyroidectomy using trans-axillary approach; surgical outcome of 581 patients. Endocr J. 2009;56:361-9.
5. Bellantone R, Lombardi CP, Rubino F, et al. Arterial PCO_2 and cardiovascular function during endoscopic neck surgery with carbon dioxide insufflation. Arch Surg. 2001;136:822-7.
6. Tanna N, Joshi AS, Glade RS, et al. Da Vinci robot-assisted endocrine surgery: novel applications in otolaryngology. Otolaryngol Head Neck Surg. 2006;135:633-5.
7. Miyano G, Lobe TE, Wright SK. Bilateral transaxillary endoscopic total thyroidectomy. J Pediatr Surg. 2008;43:299-303.

8. Kang SW, Lee SC, Lee SH, et al. Robotic thyroid surgery using a gasless, transaxillary approach and the da Vinci S system: the operative outcomes of 338 consecutive patients. Surgery. 2009;146:1048-55.
9. Lee KE, Rao J, Youn YK. Endoscopic thyroidectomy with the da Vinci robot system using the bilateral axillary breast approach (BABA) technique: our initial experience. Surg Laparosc Endosc Percutan Tech. 2009;19:e71-5.
10. Ballantyne GH. Telerobotic gastrointestinal surgery: phase 2—safety and efficacy. Surg Endosc. 2007;21:1054-62.
11. Anderson C, Ellenhorn J, Hellan M, et al. Pilot series of robot-assisted laparoscopic subtotal gastrectomy with extended lymphadenectomy for gastric cancer. Surg Endosc. 2007;21:1662-6.
12. Gutt CN, Oniu T, Mehrabi A, et al. Robot-assisted abdominal surgery. Br J Surg. 2004;91:1390-7.
13. Savitt MA, Gao G, Furnary AP, et al. Application of robotic-assisted techniques to the surgical evaluation and treatment of the anterior mediastinum. Ann Thorac Surg. 2005; 79:450-5; discussion 5.
14. Link RE, Bhayani SB, Kavoussi LR. A prospective comparison of robotic and laparoscopic pyeloplasty. Ann Surg. 2006;243:486-91.
15. Jacobsen G, Berger R, Horgan S. The role of robotic surgery in morbid obesity. J Laparoendosc Adv Surg Tech A. 2003;13:279-83.
16. Horgan S, Vanuno D, Sileri P, et al. Robotic-assisted laparoscopic donor nephrectomy for kidney transplantation. Transplantation. 2002;73:1474-9.
17. Cadiere GB, Himpens J, Vertruyen M, et al. Evaluation of telesurgical (robotic) NISSEN fundoplication. Surg Endosc. 2001;15:918-23.
18. Cadiere GB, Himpens J, Germay O, et al. Feasibility of robotic laparoscopic surgery: 146 cases. World J Surg. 2001; 25:1467-77.
19. Lee J, Kwon IS, Bae EH, et al. Comparative analysis of oncological outcomes and quality of life after robotic versus conventional open thyroidectomy with modified radical neck dissection in patients with papillary thyroid carcinoma and lateral neck node metastases. J Clin Endocrinol Metab. 2013;98:2701-8.
20. Ikeda Y, Takami H, Niimi M, et al. Endoscopic thyroidectomy by the axillary approach. Surg Endosc. 2001;15:1362-4.
21. Yoon JH, Park CH, Chung WY. Gasless endoscopic thyroidectomy via an axillary approach: experience of 30 cases. Surg Laparosc Endosc Percutan Tech. 2006;16:226-31.
22. Kang SW, Jeong JJ, Yun JS, et al. Robot-assisted endoscopic surgery for thyroid cancer: experience with the first 100 patients. Surg Endosc. 2009;23:2399-406.
23. Kang SW, Jeong JJ, Nam KH, et al. Robot-assisted endoscopic thyroidectomy for thyroid malignancies using a gasless transaxillary approach. J Am Coll Surg. 2009;209:e1-7.
24. Lee J, Yun JH, Nam KH, et al. The learning curve for robotic thyroidectomy: a multicenter study. Ann Surg Oncol. 2011;18:226-32.
25. Kuppersmith RB, Holsinger FC. Robotic thyroid surgery: an initial experience with North American patients. Laryngoscope. 2011;121:521-6.
26. Berber E, Siperstein A. Robotic transaxillary total thyroidectomy using a unilateral approach. Surg Laparosc Endosc Percutan Tech. 2011;21:207-10.
27. Landry CS, Grubbs EG, Perrier ND. Bilateral robotic-assisted transaxillary surgery. Arch Surg. 2010;145:717-20.
28. Kandil E, Winters R, Aslam R, et al. Transaxillary gasless robotic thyroid surgery with nerve monitoring: initial two experience in a North American center. Minim Invasive Ther Allied Technol. 2012;21:90-5.
29. Perrier ND, Randolph GW, Inabnet WB, et al. Robotic thyroidectomy: a framework for new technology assessment and safe implementation. Thyroid. 2010;20:1327-32.
30. Aliyev S, Taskin HE, Agcaoglu O, et al. Robotic transaxillary total thyroidectomy through a single axillary incision. Surgery. 2013;153:705-10.
31. Terris DJ, Singer MC, Seybt MW. Robotic facelift thyroidectomy: II. Clinical feasibility and safety. Laryngoscope. 2011;121:1636-41.
32. Terris DJ, Tuffo KM, Fee WE, Jr. Modified facelift incision for parotidectomy. J Laryngol Otol. 1994;108:574-8.
33. Kandil E, Abdelghani S, Noureldine SI, et al. Transaxillary gasless robotic thyroidectomy: a single surgeon's experience in North America. Arch Otolaryngol Head Neck Surg. 2012;138:113-7.
34. Kandil E, Noureldine S, Abdel Khalek M, et al. Initial experience using robot-assisted transaxillary thyroidectomy for Graves' disease. J Visc Surg. 2011;148:e447-51.
35. Kwon H, Koo dH, Choi JY, et al. Bilateral axillo-breast approach robotic thyroidectomy for Graves' disease: an initial experience in a single institute. World J Surg. 2013;37: 1576-81.
36. Kandil EH, Noureldine SI, Yao L, et al. Robotic transaxillary thyroidectomy: an examination of the first one hundred cases. J Am Coll Surg. 2012;214:558-64; discussion 64-6.
37. Katz L, Abdel Khalek M, Crawford B, et al. Robotic-assisted transaxillary parathyroidectomy of an atypical adenoma. Minim Invasive Ther Allied Technol. 2012;21:201-5.
38. Ikeda Y, Takami H, Niimi M, et al. Endoscopic thyroidectomy and parathyroidectomy by the axillary approach. A preliminary report. Surg Endosc. 2002;16:92-5.
39. Ikeda Y, Takami H, Sasaki Y, et al. Comparative study of thyroidectomies. Endoscopic surgery versus conventional open surgery. Surg Endosc. 2002;16:1741-5.

Chapter 8 Robotic Thyroidectomy—Facelift Approach

William S Duke, David J Terris

INTRODUCTION

The safety of thyroid surgery has improved significantly over the last century, and in experienced hands the modern thyroidectomy carries a low risk of complication. As the morbidity of the procedure decreased, increased attention has been given to the cosmetic consequences of the standard transverse cervical incision. Driven by patient interest and fueled by technological improvements, considerable advances have been made over the last 15 years in not only decreasing the size of the anterior cervical incision but also in removing the scar from the visible neck completely. These "remote access" procedures initially sought to improve postoperative cosmesis by transferring the incisions to the axilla, anterior chest or breast.[1,2] Attempts to extrapolate these approaches to North American patients have resulted in numerous complications, leading most surgeons to abandon these techniques.[3,4] Recently, however, a novel postauricular robotic-assisted facelift approach has been implemented to successfully manage surgical diseases of the thyroid.[5,6]

RATIONALE FOR PROCEDURE

The primary motivation for remote access thyroid procedures has been to completely remove the visible scar from the anterior neck. These techniques have largely evolved in Asian markets, where hypertrophic scarring is prevalent and there is significant social stigma associated with a neck scar.[7,8] A scar in the axilla, anterior chest or breast is considered more cosmetically favorable than a cervical scar in these societies.[8] Even if the scar can be removed from the neck, many Western patients would still consider a chest or breast scar equally unappealing. These social differences, as well as reports of significant complications from early experiences with remote access procedures in the United States,[3,9,10] prompted a search for alternative remote access approaches.

The robotic facelift thyroidectomy (RFT) was developed to offer both the patient and the surgeon several unique advantages over infraclavicular remote access approaches. One major advantage of the procedure is that there is no risk of brachial plexus injury and positioning neuropathies that may occur with axillary approaches. Additionally, the length of the dissection pocket is greatly reduced by placing the incision along the posterolateral neck, which results in less soft tissue trauma. This decreased dissection distance enables patients to have the procedure on an outpatient basis without the need for drains. The incision is placed behind the hairline, which is more cosmetically favorable than a scar on the anterior neck, axilla or breast. Finally, unlike other remote access approaches, the facelift approach involves anatomy that is more familiar to the head and neck surgeon.

APPLIED ANATOMY (FOR ROBOTIC SURGERY)

The anatomy relevant to successful RFT should be very familiar to most head and neck surgeons. The incision is placed in the postauricular sulcus and transitioned into the occipital hairline. The soft tissue flap is developed deep to the platysma along the lateral aspect of the sternocleidomastoid (SCM) muscle. Unlike other remote access approaches, patients with thicker skin and subcutaneous tissues benefit from a more robust flap with less chance of tissue necrosis or inadvertently creating a "button hole" through the skin during dissection. After the platysma, the first major landmark encountered is the great auricular nerve (GAN), which is generally identified 4 cm inferior to the apex of the incision. This nerve is preserved on the anterolateral aspect of the SCM. Dissection proceeds in an anteromedial vector and the external jugular vein is identified. This vessel may lie 2–3 cm anteromedial to the GAN and is preserved on the surface of the SCM. The anterior border of the SCM is then identified and dissected inferiorly to the clavicle.

Once the anterior border of the SCM is mobilized, the muscle is retracted posteriorly and laterally and the omohyoid muscle is identified. This muscle usually crosses under the SCM approximately 12 cm below the apex of the incision. The omohyoid is isolated and mobilized, then retracted ventrally to expose the sternohyoid and sternothyroid muscles. The superior vascular pedicle and superior aspect of the thyroid lobe is immediately deep to these muscles. The inferior constrictor muscle is medial to the superior aspect of the lobe and serves as a crucial land mark in thyroid surgery. The superior laryngeal nerve (SLN) may be identified descending along the inferior constrictor, and the recurrent laryngeal nerve (RLN) travels under the inferior aspect of the muscle to innervate the laryngeal muscles. The superior parathyroid gland lies dorsal to the coronal plane of the RLN, but due to ventral retraction of the thyroid may appear to reside anterior to the nerve. The middle thyroid vein crosses ventral to the RLN, and the inferior parathyroid gland and inferior vascular pedicle are encountered along the inferior aspect of the thyroid. The thyroid isthmus and medial aspect of the thyroid lobe are held to the trachea by the ligament of Berry.

INDICATIONS AND CONTRAINDICATIONS

Successful RFT depends on a host of patient and disease characteristics. Patients interested in RFT should be highly motivated to avoid a visible surgical scar, and they must be willing to accept an increased amount of dissection, increased surgical time and transient auricular hypesthesia to achieve their cosmetic goals. They should not be morbidly obese, but the presence of slightly thicker subcutaneous tissue may be advantageous to protect the soft tissue flap. Patients should be relatively healthy (American Society of Anesthesiologists class 1 or 2) and have no prior history of neck surgery or radiation.

The disease should preferentially be unilateral, though some patients may be candidates for staged bilateral RFT. The largest nodule should be <3 cm, and the patient should have no history of thyroiditis, which may lead to fibrosis around the gland. There should be no concerning associated lymphadenopathy and no concern for substernal or extrathyroidal extension (Table 8.1).

Table 8.1: Indications and contraindications for robotic facelift thyroidectomy

Indications	*Contraindications*
• Motivated patient willing to accept increased operative time, increased dissection and transient ear numbness in exchange for no visible scar	• Dominant nodule > 3 cm
• ASA class I or II	• Morbid obesity
• No prior neck surgery or radiation	• Thyroiditis
• Unilateral disease	• Associated lymphadenopathy
	• Substernal or extrathyroidal extension

PREOPERATIVE WORKUP

All patients undergoing surgery for thyroid disease should have a thyroid stimulating hormone (TSH) assay performed to evaluate for the presence of hypothyroidism due to autoimmune disease, which is a contraindication to RFT. An ultrasound should be performed to determine the size and location of the largest nodule. Patients with nodules larger than 3 cm may not be candidates for RFT at this time. Nodules larger than 1 cm should be evaluated with fine needle aspiration to assess for the presence of malignancy. While some patients with small well-differentiated papillary thyroid carcinoma (PTC) may be candidates for a unilateral RFT, patients with most malignancies would need bilateral RFT or a total thyroidectomy through an alternative approach. Further preoperative evaluation is at the discretion of the surgeon and contingent on the patient's medical comorbidities.

INSTRUMENTATION

Instrumentation for RFT can be divided into three groups, predicated upon the discrete segment of the operation: pocket creation, robotic dissection and wound closure.

Pocket Creation

- Surgical marker
- 15 blade
- Double-pronged skin hooks 2 (two)
- Terris long malleable suction (Medtronic, Jacksonville, FL)
- Electrosurgical handpiece with extension and Teflon-tipped guarded blade
- Terris thyroid retractors 2 (two) (Medtronic, Jacksonville, FL)
- Renal vein retractor
- Medium malleable retractor
- Long Debakey forceps
- 2-0 silk suture (Ethicon, Inc., Somerville, NJ).

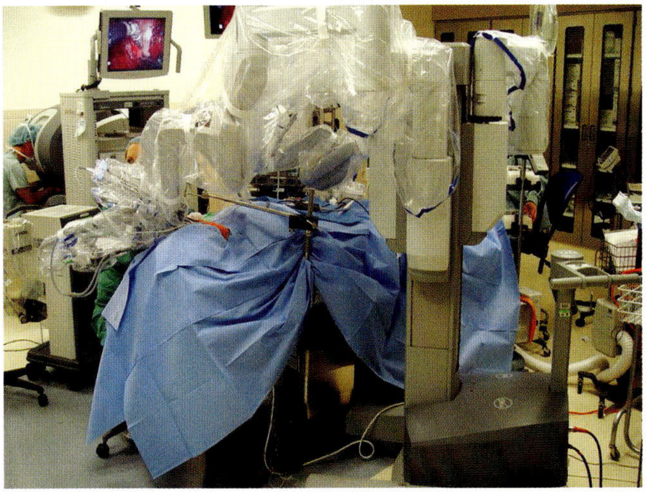

Fig. 8.1: The robotic console in position near the operating table opposite of the side being dissected, with the pedestal angled 30° away from the table.

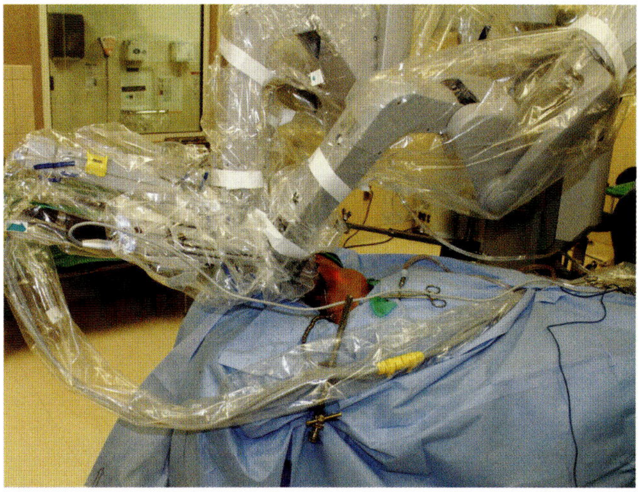

Fig. 8.2: Proper positioning of the robotic arms maximizes maneuverability during surgery.

Robot Dissection

- Da Vinci Si surgical robotic system (Intuitive Surgical Inc., Sunnyvale, CA) with the following three arms:
  - Camera arm with 30° down endoscope
  - Dominant arm: Harmonic device (Ethicon Endo-surgery Inc., Cincinnati, OH)
  - Nondominant arm: Maryland grasper
- Modified Chung retractor and fixed retractor system (Marina Medical, Sunrise, FL)
- Singer hook (Medtronic, Jacksonville, Florida) with adjustable Greenberg retractor arm (Codman & Shurtleff, Inc., Raynham, MA).

Wound Closure

- Surgicel (Ethicon, Inc., Somerville, NJ)
- 4-0 Vicryl (Ethicon, Inc., Somerville, NJ)
- Dermaflex tissue adhesive (Chemence Medical Products, Inc., Alpharetta, GA)
- ¼ inch Steri-Strips (3M Corporation, St. Paul, MN).

OPERATIVE SETUP WITH ROBOT

One of the most critical aspects of the procedure is correctly aligning and docking the robotic console with the patient. Unlike many robotic procedures in which docking ports are used to ensure correct placement, the open pocket technique used in RFT requires meticulous scrutiny to ensure that the camera and all arms are aligned to achieve maximum maneuverability and minimize operative interruptions to reposition the device.

The modified Chung retractor system (Marina Medical, Sunrise, FL) and the Singer hook SCM retractor (Medtronic, Jacksonville, FL) with the adjustable Greenberg retractor arm (Codman & Shurtleff, Inc., Raynham, MA) are used to maintain the dissection pocket. The robotic console is maneuvered into position near the operating table opposite of the side being dissected, with the pedestal angled 30° away from the table (Fig. 8.1). Fine adjustments in positioning are more easily accomplished by moving the table rather than by moving the robot console (8.1).

The camera arm with a 30° down facing endoscope is positioned first. The camera is advanced just beneath and parallel to the long axis of the modified Chung retractor. The camera may be angled upwards if necessary for improved visualization. The camera arm is nearly fully extended, so the elbow joints of the camera arm will not interfere with movement of the other arms. A Harmonic device (Ethicon Endosurgery Inc., Cincinnati, OH) is placed in the dominant arm and a Maryland grasper is used in the nondominant arm. These arms are brought into the operative field in such a manner that they will not cross or collide during dissection (Fig. 8.2).

OPERATIVE TECHNIQUE

Successful completion of the surgery begins in the preoperative holding area. With the patient sitting upright, a transverse anterior cervical incision is marked in case conversion to an open procedure is necessary. The facelift incision is then drawn beginning near the inferior extent of the earlobe just adjacent to the postauricular crease.

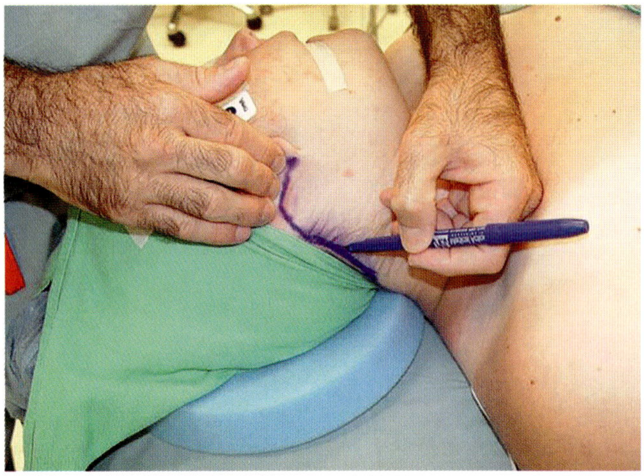

Fig. 8.3: The incision begins at the inferior extent of the earlobe adjacent to the postauricular crease, and is carried superiorly and posteriorly into the occipital hairline.
Source: From Terris D, Singer M, Seybt M. Robot facelift thyroidectomy: II. Clinical feasibility and safety. Laryngoscope. 2011;121: 1636-41.

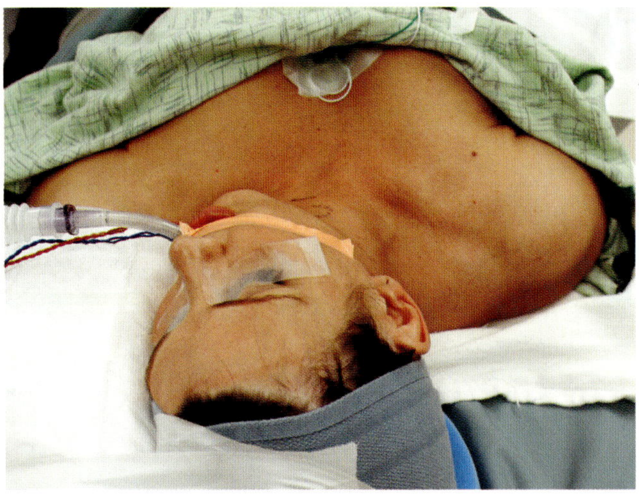

Fig. 8.5: The head is turned 20–30° away from the side of the surgery and the face is supported with soft towels to prevent excessive neck rotation.

The incision is carried superiorly and then posteriorly into the occipital hairline, which is shaved for a distance of 1 cm, in a gentle curve that will be obscured by the auricle. The incision is placed 1 cm within the hairline so that it is completely concealed once the hair re-grows. The incision is carried posteriorly and inferiorly as far as required to ensure adequate exposure (Fig. 8.3).

The patient is transferred to the operating room and transitioned to the OR: operating room table. The patient should lay just off-center of the middle of the table toward

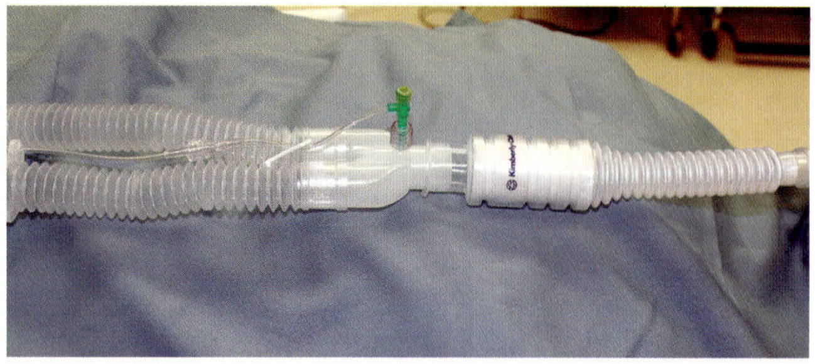

Fig. 8.4: A straight extension is placed on the anesthesia circuit and a three-way stopcock valve or right-angle connector is used to connect the CO_2 return tubing to the anesthesia circuit to prevent kinking of this tube.

the side to be operated on, with the top of the head almost at the top of the OR table. General anesthesia is induced using only a short-acting muscle relaxant if necessary. A propofol drip is used to maintain anesthesia. The patient is intubated with an electromyographic (EMG) endotracheal tube for continuous laryngeal nerve monitoring. A GlideScope (Verathon Inc, Bothell, WA) is used during intubation so that all members of the operative team can confirm adequate positioning of the EMG electrodes. A straight extension is placed on the anesthesia circuit and a three-way stopcock valve is used to connect the CO_2 return tubing to the anesthesia circuit to prevent kinking of this tube (Fig. 8.4). The bed is rotated 180° so that the patient's head is facing away from the anesthesiologist. The patient's arms are tucked at their sides and secured with wide silk tape. A formal safety strap that attaches to the table is not used to secure the arms in the tucked position because the strap interferes with placement of the retractor mechanisms. The head is turned 20°–30° away from the side of the surgery and the face is supported with soft towels to prevent excessive neck rotation (Fig. 8.5). The anesthesia circuit is taped to the operating table in such a manner that there is no excessive tension on the circuit that would cause the laryngeal EMG tube to twist or migrate (Fig. 8.6).

The planned incision line is infiltrated with 0.25% bupivacaine with 1:200,000 epinephrine and the patient is prepped and draped in sterile fashion. A 15 blade is used to incise the skin and the electrosurgical handpiece is used to elevate a subplatysmal flap until the fibers of the SCM muscle are identified. Dissection continues anteriorly and inferiorly along the SCM until the GAN is identified. Continued dissection along the same vector in a plane superficial to the GAN reveals the external jugular vein and subsequently the anterior border of the SCM (Fig. 8.7). The external jugular vein is preserved and reflected dorsally, though it may be ligated and divided if necessary to

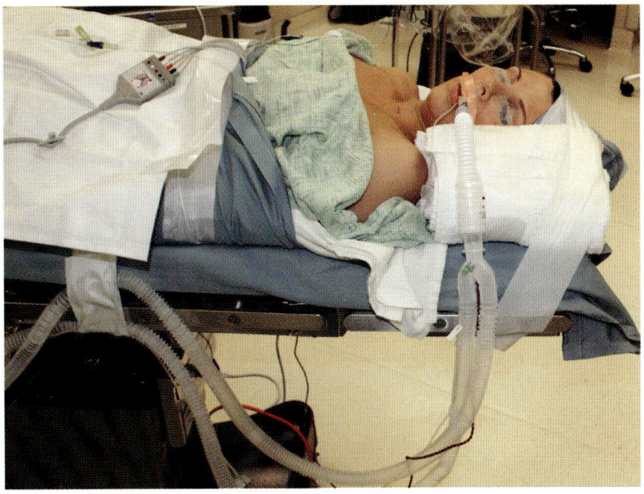

Fig. 8.6: The anesthesia circuit is taped to the operating table in such a manner that there is not excessive tension on the circuit that would cause the laryngeal electromyographic tube to twist or migrate.

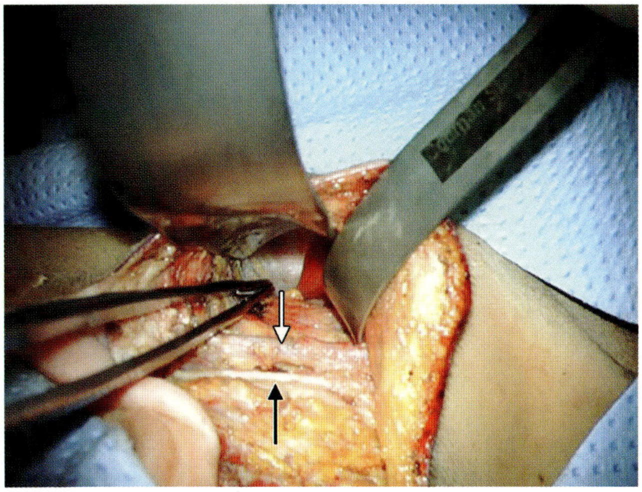

Fig. 8.7: The great auricular nerve (black arrow) and external jugular vein (white arrow) are identified on the surface of the sternocleidomastoid muscle.

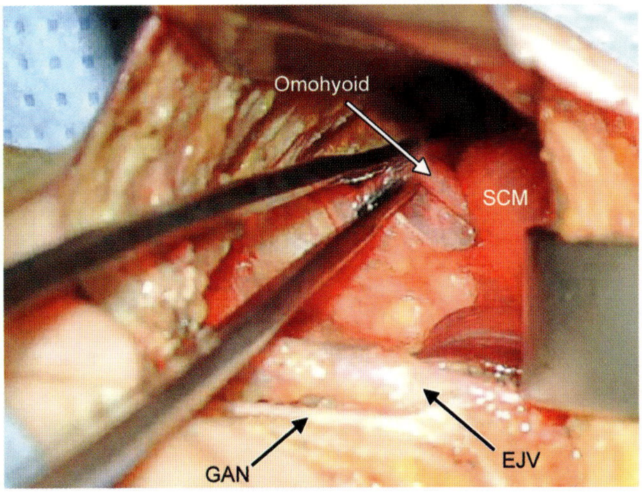

Fig. 8.8: A muscular triangle bordered by the anterior border of the sternocleidomastoid (SCM) the superior border of the omohyoid and the posterior border of the sternohyoid is defined. The great auricular nerve (GAN) and external jugular vein (EJV) are preserved.

Source: From Terris D, Singer M, Seybt M. Robot facelift thyroidectomy: II. Clinical feasibility and safety. Laryngoscope. 2011;121: 1636-41.

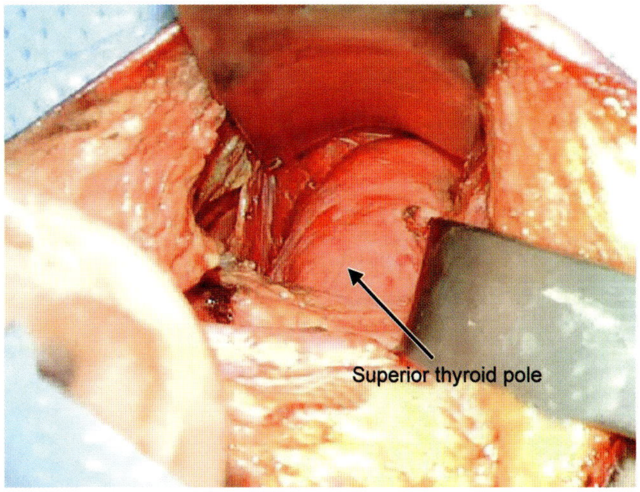

Fig. 8.9: The omohyoid, sternohyoid and sternothyroid muscles are retracted ventrally, exposing the superior pole of the thyroid gland.

Source: From Terris D, Singer M, Seybt M. Robot facelift thyroidectomy: II. Clinical feasibility and safety. Laryngoscope. 2011;121: 1636-41.

improve exposure. The anteromedial border of the SCM is freed down to the clavicle. A series of progressively deeper retractors are utilized to facilitate the dissection. The malleable retractor is used to reflect the SCM dorsally and laterally during dissection. The surgeon should be seated during this dissection, and the operating table is placed in reverse Trendelenburg and rotated away from the surgeon to facilitate visualization of the surgical field (8.1).

A muscular triangle bounded by the anterior border of the SCM, the superior border of the omohyoid and the posterior border of the sternohyoid is then defined (Fig. 8.8). The omohyoid, sternohyoid and sternothyroid muscles are retracted ventrally, exposing the superior pole of the thyroid gland (Fig. 8.9). The strap muscles are elevated off of the thyroid gland. The thyroid itself is mobilized as much as possible during this phase, which

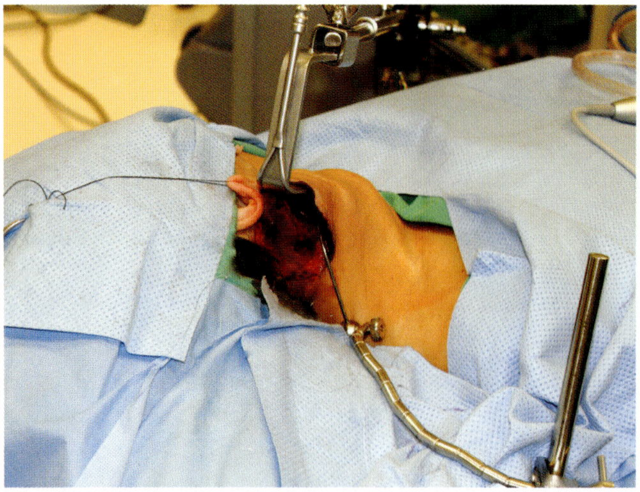

Fig. 8.10: The operative pocket with retractors in place.

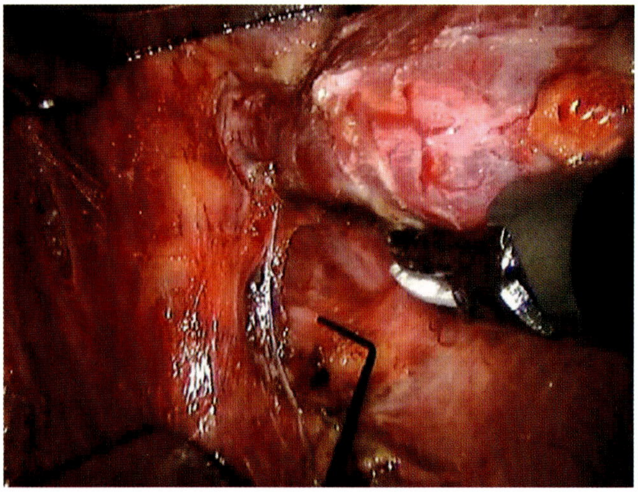

Fig. 8.12: The recurrent laryngeal nerve, at the tip of the nerve stimulator, is identified just inferior to the inferior constrictor.

Source: From Terris D, Singer M, Seybt M. Robot facelift thyroidectomy: II. Clinical feasibility and safety. Laryngoscope. 2011;121: 1636-41.

facilitates the robotic dissection, including isolation of the superior pedicle and identification of the superior parathyroid gland. The modified Chung retractor (Marina Medical, Sunrise, FL) is placed under the omohyoid and other strap muscles to retract them ventrally. The retractor system is anchored to the frame of the operating table on the side opposite the lobe being resected. A Singer hook (Medtronic, Jacksonville FL) with adjustable retractor arm is secured to the ipsilateral side of the table and used to retract the SCM laterally and dorsally, thereby securing the open surgical pocket (Fig. 8.10). The robotic cart is then deployed as described above.

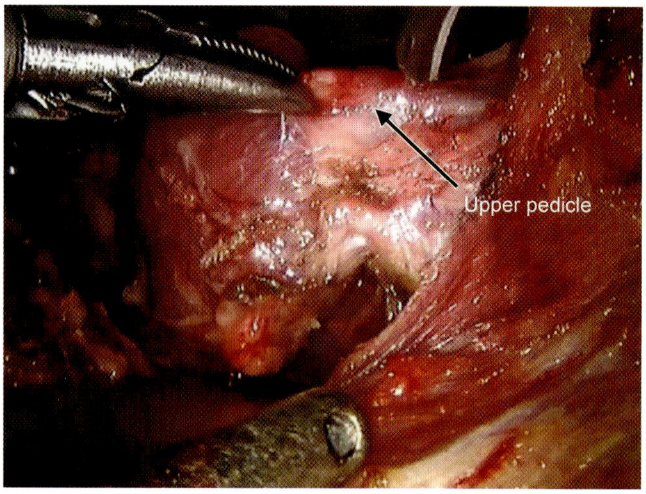

Fig. 8.11: The superior vascular pedicle is defined and transected with the Harmonic device.

Source: From Terris D, Singer M, Seybt M. Robot facelift thyroidectomy: II. Clinical feasibility and safety. Laryngoscope. 2011;121: 1636-41.

The robotic portion of the procedure involves sequential identification and dissection of a series of landmarks. First, the superior vascular pedicle is transected with the Harmonic device (Ethicon Endosurgery Inc., Cincinnati, OH) (Fig. 8.11 and 8.1). The superior thyroid pole is retracted inferiorly and ventrally, exposing the inferior constrictor muscle. This muscle is followed inferiorly until its lower border is identified. Care should be taken to avoid injuring the SLN, which usually travels along the surface of the muscle. If it has not already been dissected, the superior parathyroid gland is identified on the posterior aspect of the thyroid and reflected posteriorly and superiorly away from the thyroid. The RLN is then identified laterally as it courses under the inferior constrictor. The nerve is followed inferiorly, exposing the ligament of Berry (Fig. 8.12). With the nerve under direct vision, the ligament is transected with the Harmonic device and then the isthmus is divided. The middle thyroid vein is divided. The inferior parathyroid gland is dissected inferiorly away from the thyroid, and the inferior vascular pedicle is isolated and transected with the Harmonic device. Any remaining attachments between the gland and the surrounding soft tissue or trachea are divided and the specimen is removed.[6,11]

Hemostasis is assured, and the robot is removed. The surgical field is irrigated and Surgicel (Ethicon, Inc., Somerville, NJ) is placed into the thyroid bed. The wound edges are approximated using buried interrupted deep

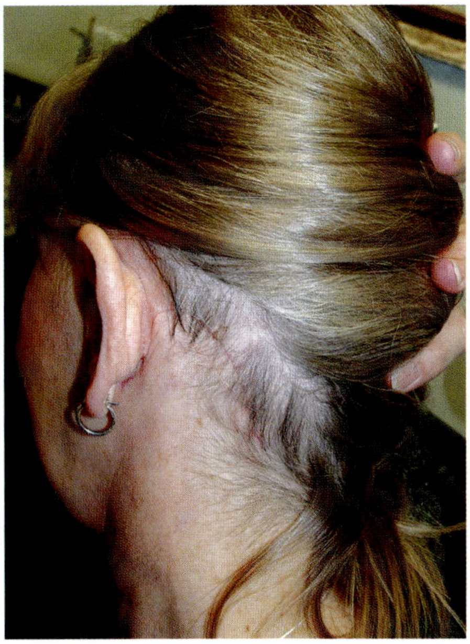

Fig. 8.13: The healed incision is concealed within the hairline.

dermal 4-0 Vicryl sutures (Ethicon, Inc., Somerville, NJ). The skin edges are sealed with Dermaflex tissue adhesive (Chemence Medical Products, Inc., Alpharetta, GA) and ¼ inch Steri-Strips (3M Corporation, St. Paul, MN) placed horizontally along the incision. No drains are utilized. The patient is extubated deeply to minimize coughing or straining on emergence from anesthesia. The healed incision is concealed within the hairline (Fig. 8.13).

COMPLICATIONS AND THEIR MANAGEMENT

During any thyroid operation, meticulous surgical technique and identification and preservation of the RLN and parathyroid glands are required to minimize the risk of iatrogenic morbidity. While most potential complications of RFT are inherent to any thyroid procedure, there are several that are unique to this approach.

As suggested earlier, operative success begins with proper patient selection and preparation. Since the main advantage of this approach is cosmetic in nature, patients should be properly counseled that this procedure is not "minimally invasive" and in fact requires more dissection than an anterior cervical approach. Appropriate management of patient expectations will prepare them for the postoperative discomfort and potential neck swelling that, while mild, may be more prominent than that associated with an anterior cervical operation. It is possible that conversion to an anterior approach may be needed (although this has not been necessary in our experience), and patients should be aware of this possibility. Patients should also be counseled to expect several months of decreased auricular sensation related to dissection of the GAN.

Due to the increased extent of dissection required compared with anterior cervical approaches, patients undergoing RFT may experience lateral neck swelling or seroma. Unless the seroma is causing significant pain or functional limitation, conservative management that allows natural absorption of the fluid rather than aspiration is preferred, as this may introduce bacteria into the neck and precipitate a postoperative infection.

FOLLOW-UP

Patients are discharged from the hospital on the day of surgery, unless there is a specific medical contraindication or immediate postoperative complication. Patients who live within 2 hours of the hospital are allowed to return home, while those who travel longer distances are encouraged to remain overnight in a local hotel. Patients are discharged with narcotic pain medication, an antiemetic and a stool softener. Those patients undergoing completion thyroidectomy are also placed on levothyroxine 100 mcg daily and given supplemental calcium and vitamin D. The standard supplementation regimen consists of 1 gram of Os-Cal D (GlaxoSmithKline) taken three times daily for 1 week, twice daily for 1 week then once daily for 1 week. Patients are thoroughly counseled about the signs and symptoms of hypocalcemia, and in the event that the symptoms occur are instructed to take two additional calcium pills every 30 minutes until they subside. If they fail to resolve, patients are instructed to call their surgeon.

The patients resume a regular diet the day after surgery. They are instructed to avoid any strenuous activity or heavy lifting for at least 2 weeks. They may shower the day after surgery, but should avoid scrubbing the incision to prevent inadvertent removal of the Steri-Strips (3M Corporation, St. Paul, MN). The Steri-Strips (3M Corporation, St. Paul, MN) are left in place for 3 weeks, after which time they may be removed by the patient. Most of the skin glue comes off with the Steri-Strips (3M Corporation, St. Paul, MN); any residual glue can be removed with baby oil.

Approximately 4-6 weeks after surgery, the patients follow up with their referring physicians to have their TSH level evaluated to determine if any postoperative levothyroxine treatment is required. Patients who live within 2 hours of the hospital return for a postoperative visit with the surgeon 4-6 weeks after surgery. Those who travel longer distances are not required to physically return if they are doing well.

RESULTS

Robotic facelift thyroidectomy was pioneered at our institution, and while other institutions are pursuing this procedure none of these groups has yet published on their outcomes. We have performed 57 procedures on 50 patients since implementing the technique in June, 2010. Seven patients had bilateral procedures due to the diagnosis of malignancy on final pathology after the initial thyroid lobe was removed. The first patient was managed with a drain and was kept overnight in the hospital for observation. All subsequent patients have been discharged on the day of surgery without a drain. A unilateral RFT initially took a mean time of 157 minutes to complete, though with increased experience the operative time is <2 hours for most patients.[11,12] All attempted RFT procedures were successfully completed with no conversions to an open procedure. This compares favorably with the robot transaxillary approach, which has a reported conversion rate of up to 2% and usually requires an inpatient stay.[10,13,14] The RFT procedure has been used successfully for small PTCs and in patients as young as 12 years old.[12]

Complications associated with the RFT technique in our series include one seroma (1.8%), one transient case of accessory nerve weakness (1.8%) and three cases of transient vocal cord paresis (5.3%). These rates also compare favorably with those seen in robotic transaxillary thyroidectomy.[9,10,13-15]

FUTURE DIRECTIONS

As with any new surgical procedure, the long-term efficacy of RFT remains to be determined. Robotic facelift thyroidectomy typically takes longer to perform than an anterior cervical thyroidectomy, but is reimbursed in the United States at the same rate as standard thyroid surgery. This differs from Korea, where robotic-assisted thyroid surgery is reimbursed at four times more than a conventional thyroidectomy.[8] The procedure also requires specialized capital resources that may not be available in every hospital, and one or two additional assistants to assist with retraction. These resource and reimbursement constraints may limit the ease with which the procedure could be adopted outside of major medical or academic centers. However, the viability and safety of RFT in the hands of an experienced, well-trained thyroid and robotic surgeon have been well-established, and patients wary of any anterior neck incision continue to travel great distances to benefit from the superior cosmetic and functional outcome of the procedure.

As the robotic technology inevitably improves along with other instrumentation, it seems likely that remote access thyroid procedures will become easier to perform, and that indications will expand. Technology developed for single-incision laparoscopic surgery seems particularly likely to have applicability in transoral surgery and remote access thyroid surgery.

VIDEO LEGEND

Video 8.1: Robotic Thyroidectomy—Facelift Approach.

REFERENCES

1. Ohgami M, Ishii S, Arisawa Y, et al. Scarless endoscopic thyroidectomy: breast approach for better cosmesis. Surg Laparosc Percutan Tech. 2000;10(1):1-4.
2. Ikeda Y, Takami H, Sasaki Y, et al. Clinical benefits in endoscopic thyroidectomy by the axillary approach. J Am Coll Surg. 2003;196(2):189-95.
3. Kuppersmith R, Holsinger F. Robotic thyroid surgery: an initial experience with North American patients. Laryngoscope. 2011;121:521-6.
4. Perrier N. Why I have abandoned robot-assisted transaxillary thyroid surgery. Surgery. 2012;152:1025-6.
5. Singer M, Seybt M, Terris D. Robot facelift thyroidectomy: I. Preclinical simulation and morphometric assessment. Laryngoscope 2011;121:1631-5.
6. Terris D, Singer M, Seybt M. Robotic facelift thyroidectomy: patient selection and technical considerations. Surg Laparosc Percutan Tech. 2011;21(4):237-42.
7. McCurdy J. Considerations in Asian cosmetic surgery. Facial Plast Surg Clin North Am. 2007;15:387-97.
8. Duh Q. Robot-assisted endoscopic thyroidectomy: has the time come to abandon neck incisions? Ann Surg. 2011; 253(6):1067-8.
9. Landry C, Grubbs E, Warneke C, et al. Robot-assisted transaxillary thyroid surgery in the United States: is it comparable to open thyroid lobectomy? Ann Surg Oncol. 2012;19:1269-74.
10. Kandil E, Noureldine S, Yao L, et al. Robotic transaxillary thyroidectomy: an examination of the first one hundred cases. J Am Coll Surg. 2012;214:558-66.

11. Terris D, Singer M, Seybt M. Robot facelift thyroidectomy: II. Clinical feasibility and safety. Laryngoscope. 2011;121: 1636-41.
12. Terris D, Singer M. Qualitative and quantitative differences between 2 robotic thyroidectomy techniques. Otolaryngol Head Neck Surg. 2012;147(1):20-5.
13. Lee J, Lee JH, Nah K, et al. Comparison of endoscopic and robotic thyroidectomy. Ann Surg Oncol. 2011;18:1439-46.
14. Lin H, Folbe A, Carron M, et al. Single-incision transaxillary robotic thyroidectomy: challenges and limitations in a North American population. Otolaryngol Head Neck Surg. 2012;147(6):1041-6.
15. Lee S, Ryu H, Park J, et al. Excellence in robotic thyroid surgery: a comparative study of robot-assisted versus conventional endoscopic thyroidectomy in papillary thyroid microcarcinoma patients. Ann Surg. 2011;253:1060-6.

Section 3

Head and Neck Reconstruction

Chapter Outline

Chapter 9 Transoral Robotic Surgery in Head and Neck Reconstruction

Anya Joyce Miller, Tamer Abdel-Halim Ghanem

INTRODUCTION

The field of robotic-assisted surgery is rapidly expanding especially in the field of otolaryngology. Robotic approaches to the clivus, and base of tongue, have led to the development of new applications in the field of neurosurgery and sleep medicine, respectively. For head and neck cancer in particular, the robot has allowed otolaryngologists to offer cancer patients a less morbid surgery as an alternative to chemoradiation in treating oropharyngeal cancer. Since primary cancer resection via the transoral robotic surgery (TORS) route has been proven to be safe and effective,[1] this has naturally extended to using robotic techniques for reconstruction as well. Many of the principles of microvascular surgery remain the same with the adjunctive use of the robot to assist in flap insetting.

In this chapter, we will describe a newer application of robotics in oropharyngeal reconstruction after larger resections for more advanced disease. It is important to note that current federal drug administration (FDA) approval for oropharyngeal cancer is limited to T1 and T2 stages, and its use in T3 and T4 stages is an off-label use.

RATIONALE FOR PROCEDURE

Large base of tongue/oropharyngeal defects are difficult to access with traditional transoral surgical instruments. The space is narrow, deep and often not accessible or visible with straight instrumentation. The robot allows "around the corner" access to these areas with angled telescopes and small jointed instruments negating the need for a morbid open procedure such as a transmandibular approach.

Reconstruction after ablative procedures in the oropharynx is necessary to accomplish a number of goals such as:[2]

1. Prevention of fistula communication from the oropharynx to the neck
2. Protection of the great vessels of the neck

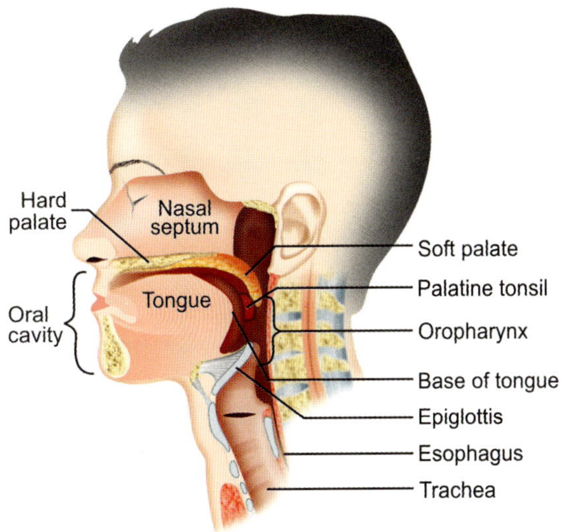

Fig. 9.1: Anatomy of the upper airway.
Source: Reprinted with permission from http://www.cancer.net/multimedia/medical-illustrations-gallery?mitid=248.

3. Improving swallow function by:
   a. Restoring tongue bulk for bolus propulsion
   b. Restoring natural apposition of sphincters
   c. Preserving velopalatal competence
4. Building velopharyngeal competence to help with clarity of speech
5. Restoring sensation (if possible)

APPLIED ANATOMY

Robotic surgical anatomy is the same as that for any open or endoscopic laryngeal and oropharyngeal surgery. (Fig. 9.1).

INDICATIONS

Indications for robotic-assisted flap reconstruction are as follows (Table 9.1):

- Class III defects
- Class IV defects

Table 9.1: Defect classification

Class I	Involves one subsite of the oropharynx without any complicating features
Class II	Involves more than one subsite without any complicating factors
Class III	Involves one subsite with complicating features
Class IV	Involves more than one subsite with complicating features • Carotid artery exposure • Pharyngocervical communication • Extensive palatal defect (>50%)

CONTRAINDICATIONS

Contraindications for robotic-assisted flap reconstruction are as follows:

- Class I defect may be allowed to remucosalize
- Class II defect may be left to heal secondarily

In regard to the goals of reconstructive surgery in the oropharyngeal region, protection of the neck from contents within the aerodigestive tract is paramount, i.e. saliva. Carotid artery exposure is a key indication for reconstruction, where the parapharyngeal fat that normally protects the carotid artery is removed during cancer resection of deep tonsillar cancers. This can usually be predicted by preoperative computed tomography (CT) or magnetic resonance imaging scan, but in some cases it is not known until time of surgery, such as when there is a positive deep margin on the superior constrictor muscle. Another important indication for pharyngeal reconstruction is the creation of a pharyngocervical communication after cancer resection. This often happens if the ipsilateral level I neck nodes are addressed during the neck dissection. For a defect involving >50% of the palate, flap reconstruction for adequate swallow and speech function postoperatively is an indication but not a necessity. A palatal obturator is also an adequate option for swallow and speech rehabilitation and may be offered to the patient.

For defects without complicating features but involving more than one subsite (Class II defects), a flap for reconstruction is not always necessary. Of course this should ultimately be left to the surgeon at the time of the surgery along with the patient's wishes. Examples where a flap might be useful would be a deep resection of the base of tongue where bolus propulsion during swallowing might be difficult without bulk in that area. An extensive tonsillar resection may warrant a flap for closure even if there is no communication with vessels of the neck. In this scenario, a free flap may not be indicated, but a mucosal flap from the buccal mucosa may instead be adequate. While the list of possible scenarios is large, the outlined classification scheme should provide surgeons with general guidelines for management of defects in this area.

Besides the above indications, when TORS is performed in the setting of salvage surgery, the threshold to use microvascular free tissue transfer should be lowered. Many times, these wounds are very slow to heal, and risk of carotid blowout is higher.

PREOPERATIVE WORKUP

Preoperative workup should be no different from the standard evaluation of any cancer patient about to undergo a major surgery. The patient should have a thorough physical examination of the head and neck. All medical problems, medications and prior surgery and radiation treatments should be reviewed. If necessary, the patient should be medically optimized by their primary care physician and other necessary specialists such as a cardiologist, pulmonologist or nutritionist. We recommend that all aspirin and plavix products be stopped at least 7 days prior to surgery and that all anticoagulation be stopped prior to surgery. In some instances, especially patients with peripheral vascular disease and those with cardiac and non-cardiac stents, we keep the patients on their home dose of anticoagulation before and after surgery. The patient's internist should make recommendations about anticoagulation in the perioperative period in regard to the patient's thromboembolic risk. A CT scan of the head and neck for operative planning and cancer staging is recommended.

The type of flap to be utilized is at the discretion of the surgeon. Factors to consider include the surface area to be covered, the amount of bulk needed and the location of the defect. The donor limb should also be assessed for skin pliability, thickness of the subcutaneous fat layer and patency of the vessels. The ideal donor site harvest for oropharyngeal reconstruction is the radial forearm flap. It has a long pedicle, consistent anatomy and provides thin and pliable skin. Prior to harvesting the radial forearm flap, the patient should not have any blood draws or intravenous lines started in the donor limb. Typically the patient's nondominant side is utilized. Another option in patients with thin subcutaneous fat tissue is an anterolateral thigh flap, but the skin is not as thin and pliable as the forearm skin. The patient should be warned that any hair bearing skin that is transferred will continue to grow hair after the surgery as well.

Limitations that may hinder the use of TORS include limited neck extension and limited mouth opening or temporomandibular joint problems. These issues may preclude adequate exposure with the retractor and may make it difficult or impossible for the camera and robot arms to fit inside the oral cavity with enough degrees of freedom to work freely. Sometimes with muscle relaxant, mouth opening may be increased but occasionally the trismus is so severe that adequate exposure cannot be obtained. The patient should be forewarned that the procedure may have to be aborted and another route may have to be used such as a mandibulotomy or visor approach. We recommend that the patient be consented for an alternative approach in these instances.

As with any surgery, preoperative counseling should include the risks associated with the surgery and in this case, risks specific to use of transoral technique. Due to prolonged time in suspension with tongue compression, some patients develop transient tongue swelling, altered taste sensation and tongue numbness after surgery. The risk of damage to the lips, teeth, tongue and gums must be discussed with the patient as well. Also, as with any transoral approach utilizing laser or electrocautery, there is a potential risk for airway fire. The possibility of flap failure must also be discussed.

INSTRUMENTATION

The basic instruments necessary for any robotic resection and flap reconstruction are as follows (Table 9.2).

OPERATIVE SETUP WITH ROBOT

General anesthesia should be initiated and the patient intubated with a small 6.5 mm or 7.0 mm tube. While orotracheal intubation can be performed especially in tonsillar cancers, nasotracheal intubation is our preferred choice for base of tongue cancers as it moves the tube out of the way. The table should be turned 90° or 180° away from anesthesia depending on the setup of the room. There should be adequate space for an assistant to sit at the head of the bed and for the robot to be docked next to the patient bed (Fig. 9.2).

Table 9.2: Instruments for transoral robotic surgery

Instrument name	*Model number*	*Manufacturer*	*Number needed*
Before beginning			
Da Vinci S-Robot	S	Intuitive Surgical, Inc.	1
Opti-Gard eye protector	D28300CE	Dupaco	1
Suspension			
Feyh-Kastenbauer Basic frame retractor	640001	Gyrus	1
Attachment for connection of frame to chest support	640003	Gyrus	1
Tongue blade curved 22 cm	640013	Gyrus	1
Tongue blade curved to right, 22 cm	640016	Gyrus	1
Tongue blade curved to left, 22 cm	640017	Gyrus	1
Cheek retractor, flexible, 22.5 cm	640011	Gyrus	2
Wollenberg laryngeal blade, concave, 17 cm	640019	Gyrus	1
Wollenberg diverticuloscope blade, concave, 22 cm	640050	Gyrus	1
Simon mandible blade, 14 cm	640020	Gyrus	1
Robotic surgery			
Maryland dissector	400143/420143	Intuitive Surgical, Inc.	1
Monopolar spatula cautery	400160/420142	Intuitive Surgical, Inc.	1
Needle driver	400117/420117	Intuitive Surgical, Inc.	2

Notes: Intuitive Surgical, Inc., Sunnyvale, CA
Dupaco Oceanside, CA
Gyrus ENT, L.L.C., Bartlett, TN

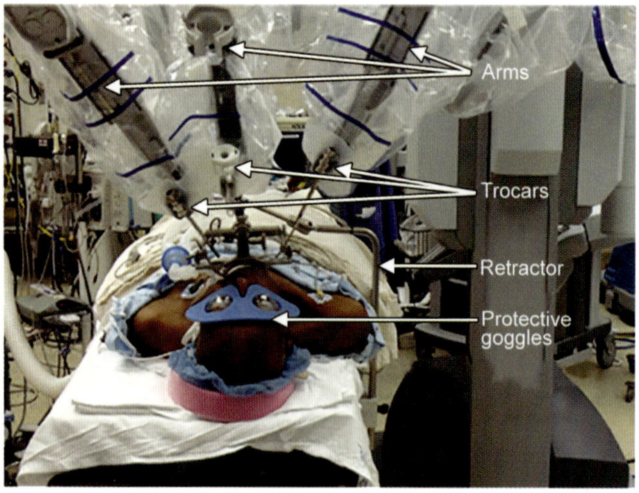

Fig. 9.2: Operative setup with the robot. The robot is positioned parallel to the bed, the patient turned 180° away from anesthesia. The patient is in suspension with the FK retractor and is wearing eye goggles.

The patient's teeth should be protected with a tooth guard. If the patient is edentulous, a wet Raytec may be used to protect the gums. The eyes should be protected with eye shields, not eye pads. We prefer the Dupaco Opti-Gard eye protector (Oceanside, CA).

A single silk suture is placed in the midline of the tongue to help with placement of the retractor. The Feyh-Kastenbauer (FK) retractor (Gyrus ENT, LLC, Bartlett, TN) is optimal as it allows both the jaws to open, the tongue to be pulled forward and the cheeks to be retracted. A Crow-Davis or Dingman mouth gag may be adequate for tonsil lesions, but the different types of tongue retractors available in the FK retractor set allow for easy base of tongue and supraglottic access. Once the mouth gag has been positioned for adequate operative visibility, the mouth gag is then secured to the bed either by suspension or with the FK-frame/chest support connection.

Once the patient is placed into suspension, the robot is brought into the field. It is positioned parallel to the bed with the base at approximately the level of the patient's waist. Trocars are inserted and the endoscope and instruments are then inserted through the trocars. The telescope is first inserted into the patient's mouth. The 0° telescope is typically used for more posterior pharyngeal or tonsillar lesions while the 30° endoscope is typically used for deeper base of tongue, vallecula or supraglottic lesions. We prefer the 12.5 mm scope because it provides better optical resolution than the 8 mm scope but if a patient has a particularly small mouth, the 8 mm scope may be preferred.

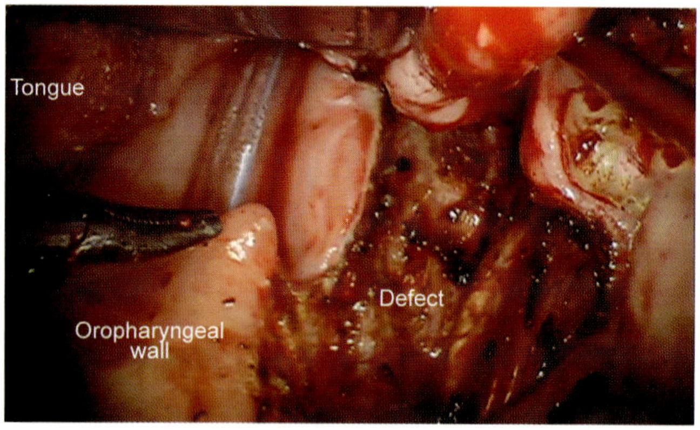

Fig. 9.3: Postablation prior to flap inset.

The instrument arms are then brought into the oral cavity. They should be positioned at approximately a 20° angle to the endoscope. The arms should be at 45° to an axial and coronal plane with the patient to allow for insertion into the narrow field (Fig. 9.2). We use 5 mm trocars with 5 mm EndoWrist instruments. The most commonly used instruments are the Maryland Dissector, the monopolar spatula cautery and a needle driver.

One video monitor should be placed on the side opposite the robot for the assistant sitting at the head of the bed to visualize. The assistant's instruments should include a velvet eye suction, baby Yankauer suction, long forceps, long scissors, long needle driver, spatula, tonsil sponges, epinephrine soaked pledgets, curved hemostats, ligature clips and a suction Bovey. Their main job will be to help the surgeon with retraction.

OPERATIVE TECHNIQUE

All reconstructed patients should have a tracheostomy placed at least temporarily until the swelling from the flap is decreased. While the tracheostomy may be performed at any time, if done before the robotic portion of the surgery, removal of the endotracheal tube from the oral cavity may help facilitate use of the robot. The ablative procedure is then performed with the robot. If neck dissections are to be done, they should be done at this time as well. The neck is then explored and vessels are preserved for microvascular anastomosis. The flap is harvested (radial forearm, anterolateral thigh etc.) according to standard flap harvest techniques. This should be done following the ablation (Fig. 9.3) the size and location of the defect can be assessed relative to the skin paddle to be harvested.

For flap inset, two needle drivers are placed on either arm. Initially, the flap is tacked with silk suture. This allows for the surgeon to assess the size match, establish

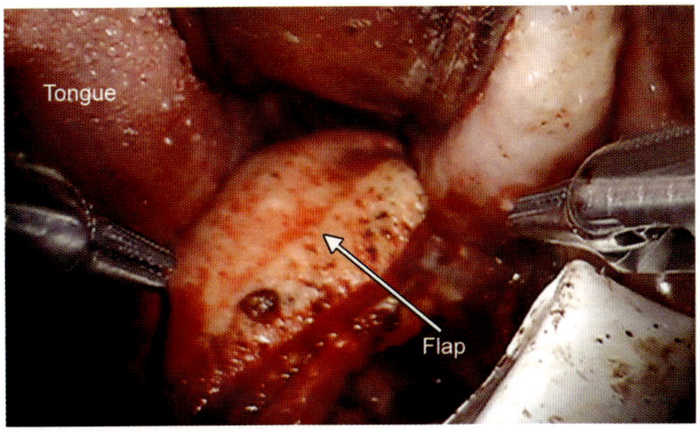

Fig. 9.4: Flap placed intraorally to assess orientation prior to inset and microvascular anastomosis.

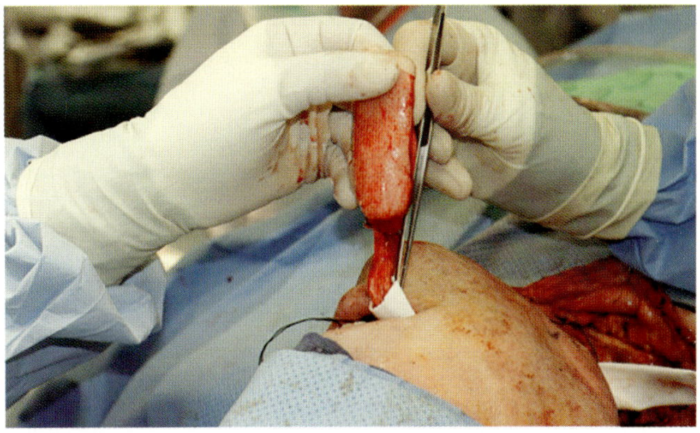

Fig. 9.5: Flap after microvascular anastomosis, prior to inset with the robot.

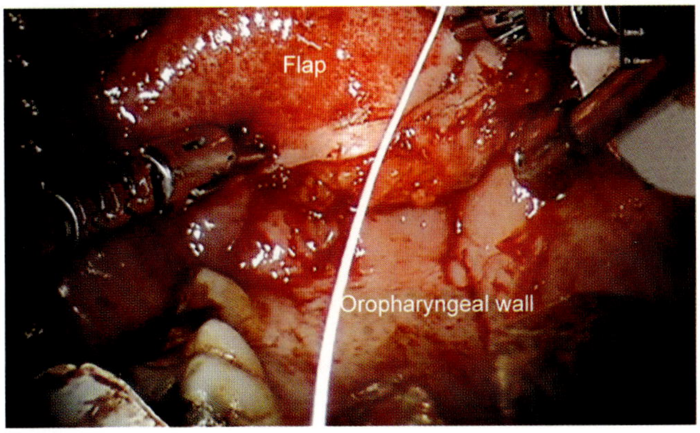

Fig. 9.6: Sewing the flap in.

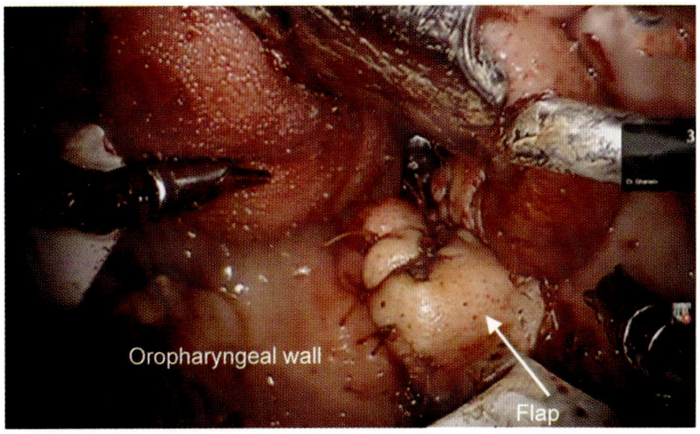

Fig. 9.7: Flap after inset.

the orientation, assess vessel length and prevent kinking or twisting of the vessel (Fig. 9.4).[3] If a pedicled flap is being used, the surgeon may proceed with insetting of the flap. If a free flap is being used, after tacking the flap, the microvascular anastomosis can begin (🎥 9.1).

The microvascular portion can be done either using loupe magnification, the operating microscope or with microvascular instrumentation with the robot.[4,5] For microvascular anastomosis with the robot, Black Diamond Micro Forceps (Intuitive surgical 400033/420033) should be placed in the arms and 8-0 or 9-0 nylon suture may be used for microvascular anastomosis with the robot. The arms should be placed nearly horizontal with the bed and a third arm should be attached to hold the vessels in position.[5] The surgeon should perform the microvascular anastomosis with whatever method he or she is most comfortable with (Fig. 9.5).

Vicryl suture (2-0 or 3-0) (Ethicon, Somerville, NJ) is then used to secure the flap with interrupted horizontal mattress or Connell sutures (Fig. 9.6). However, in some instances, due to geometrical constraints, simple interrupted suture is the only option. These should be loaded on an RB-1 needle as the curvature of the needle allows it to be easily handled in the limited working field.[3] We prefer suturing with two needle holders loaded, so either arm can throw the suture. The mucosal surfaces should be everted into the oropharynx. The sutures are cut to a shorter length (~10–12 cm) before loading them on to the needle drivers. The short length is more manageable with the narrower operative field and requires less suture be pulled through the tissue. During this time, the assistant should be aiding the surgeon with retraction, cutting the suture and loading the suture. Occasionally, if the space is tight, the assistant may need to help by repositioning the arms at a severe angle or tying down the suture by hand after it has been thrown.[5]

Once insetting of the flap is complete (Fig. 9.7), a watertight seal must be ensured. Copious amounts of saline should be poured into the oral cavity and evidence of a leak should be observed. The flap should be pricked with an 18 gauge needle to ensure appropriate perfusion.

Once the surgery has been terminated, the robot is removed from the field, the patient is taken out of suspension and the table is turned back to anesthesia. The decision to wean the patient off ventilatory support should be left to the anesthesiologist and surgeon.

COMPLICATIONS AND THEIR MANAGEMENT

Pearls and Pitfalls

- Starting with good exposure of the operative field is the key to make the rest of the operation run smoothly. Spend time adjusting the retractor and position the camera and robot arms exactly where you want them to save time later.
- A good assistant can make the surgery run much smoother if they provide good retraction and visibility of the surgical field. Suction is the key and the spatula can be a very useful instrument.
- The view with the robotic endoscope can sometimes be akin to tunnel vision. It is important that the assistant should be aware of where the arms of the patient are at all times to prevent the arms from knocking into the patient or each other.
- Sometimes a combination of the robot plus traditional surgical approaches can complement each other. Do not stick to just one modality if you are struggling.
- In cases of salvage surgery, the threshold for a flap should be lowered.

FOLLOW-UP

Standard postoperative flap care is utilized after TORS reconstructive surgery. Decisions regarding flap checks, blood pressure, anticoagulation, antibiotic coverage and diet are generally left up to the microvascular surgeon. Our flap monitoring protocol consists of utilizing an implantable Doppler, which allows for intensive care unit nurses to perform Q1 hour Doppler checks for the first 48 hours, then Q4 hour Doppler checks once the patient is moved to the general floor. Flaps are pricked as needed to ensure appropriate perfusion.

We do not typically use anticoagulation postoperatively other than subcutaneous heparin for deep vein thrombosis prophylaxis. Broad spectrum antibiotic coverage is used for 7 days due to the clean-contaminated nature of the wound. Patients are kept nil per os (NPO) for at least 7 days. Nutrition is initiated via percutaneous endoscopic gastrostomy (PEG) or nasogastric (NG) tube during that time. The patient is not allowed to have any oral care except for very gentle suctioning with soft tipped catheters for the first few days and then mouth washes with Peridex are initiated. We also do not allow anything around the neck, such as tracheostomy ties, for the first few days to prevent compression over the anastomosis.

Patients are made to ambulate on postoperative day 1. Depending on the location of the flap, decannulation takes places either as an outpatient or inpatient. In general, our patients are discharged on postoperative day 7–10 with oral feeding initiated as an outpatient with the aid of speech pathologists.

RESULTS

At our institution we have published the results of four TORS ablations with free flap reconstructions.[6] There were no flap failures and complications were minor: a small dehiscence in the tonsillar pillar that healed secondarily and a neck infection that resolved with antibiotics. Since publication, over 10 TORS ablations with free flap reconstructions have been performed with no flap failures, revisions or fistulas to date. Publication of this data is in progress but we will report preliminarily on the results of our first 10 robotic-assisted flaps (Table 9.3).

Bonawitz and Duvvuri had similar results in his case series of four as well.[4] He reported no flap failures, no returns to the operating room and all patients were free of disease at the time of submission. Garfein et al. reported one patient whose base of tongue was reconstructed with a free flap who had good swallow function following the surgery without complications.[6] Mukhija et al. described two cases of transoral robotic insetting of free flaps.[7] While long-term outcomes were not reported, both patients had good flap success and tolerated oral diets. Selber had the largest case series with five robotically assisted free flaps inset with no major complications.[5] Both Selber and Bonawitz performed one case where the microvascular anastomosis was performed robotically without leak or flap failure.[4,5]

FUTURE DIRECTIONS

Transoral robotic surgery has increased in popularity for ablative procedures for head and neck cancer. Robotic assistance with the reconstruction of these defects is also now taking a foothold. However, most surgeons are still performing their microvascular anastomosis with an operating microscope or with loupe magnification. In a

Table 9.3: First 10 robotic-assisted flap reconstructions by Dr Tamer Ghanem

Patient	*Salvage*	*Ablation*	*Flap*	*Flap failure*	*Complication*
1	No	Tongue	Radial forearm	No	Urinary retention
2	No	Pharynx	Radial forearm	No	Flap dehiscence
3	No	Tongue, floor of mouth	Radial forearm	No	Infection
4	No	Tonsil	Anterolateral thigh	No	Urinary retention
5	No	Tonsil	Radial forearm	No	None
6	Yes	Tonsil	Radial forearm	No	Urinary retention
7	No	Tonsil, pharynx, soft palate	Radial forearm	No	None
8	Yes	Tonsil, soft palate, tongue	Radial forearm	No	None
9	No	Tongue, tonsil, base of tongue	Radial forearm	No	None
10	No	Base of tongue	Radial forearm	No	None

search of the literature, only Bonawitz and Selber describe using the robot for the microvascular anastomosis.[4,5] While traditional methods of microsurgical technique can be used, the robot often needs to be brought into and out of the field, which adds to surgical time. This technique may be particularly useful when there is already a large communication between the neck and oral cavity, so access is facilitated.

Further studies also need to be done in cases of salvage surgery. In our first 10 patients, two were for salvage after radiation with/without chemotherapy. While there were no complications associated with any of those cases, further studies should be performed to ascertain the efficacy and safety of the robot in salvage cases. We hope that as robotic surgery continues to gain acceptance in medical treatment, its indications for use will continue to expand.

VIDEO LEGEND

Video 9.1: Transoral robotic surgery free flap.

REFERENCES

1. Weinstein GS, O'Malley BW, Jr, Magnuson JS, et al. Transoral robotic surgery: a multicenter study to assess feasibility, safety, and surgical margins. Laryngoscope. 2012;122:1701-7.
2. de Almeida JR, Genden EM. Robotic assisted reconstruction of the oropharynx. Curr Opin Otolaryngol Head Neck Surg. 2012;20:237-45.
3. Ghanem TA. Transoral robotic-assisted microvascular reconstruction of the oropharynx. Laryngoscope. 2011;121:580-2.
4. Bonawitz SC, Duvvuri U. Robot-assisted oropharyngeal reconstruction with free tissue transfer. J Reconstr Microsurg. 2012;28:485-90.
5. Selber JC. Transoral robotic reconstruction of oropharyngeal defects: a case series. Plast Reconstr Surg. 2010;126:1978-87.
6. Garfein ES, Greaney PJ, Jr, Easterlin B, et al. Transoral robotic reconstructive surgery reconstruction of a tongue base defect with a radial forearm flap. Plast Reconstr Surg. 2011;127:2352-4.
7. Mukhija VK, Sung CK, Desai SC, et al. Transoral robotic assisted free flap reconstruction. Otolaryngol Head Neck Surg. 2009;140:124-5.

Section 4

Robotic Procedures in Evolution

Chapter Outline

Chapter 10 Robot-Assisted Neck Dissection via a Modified Facelift or Retroauricular Approach

Yoon Woo Koh, Eun Chang Choi

INTRODUCTION

Cervical lymph node metastasis is the single most adverse prognosticator in head and neck cancer except for distant metastasis. Selective neck dissection (SND) of level I-III/II-IV and modified radical neck dissection (MRND) are frequent surgical procedures conducted by head and neck surgeons. Although there are still some controversies regarding the optimal management for clinical N0 neck of head and neck cancers, several reports demonstrated that SND level I-III/II-IV improved regional control and disease specific survival. The MRND is the treatment of choice for clinically obvious neck metastasis and the accumulated data show quite favorable treatment outcomes especially when combined with adjuvant therapies. Currently, transoral robotic surgery (TORS) is actively being investigated as a minimally invasive surgery for the treatment of laryngopharyngeal cancer. This operation allows the cancer to be excised en bloc through the oral cavity without an external incision. Accordingly, the procedure has some advantages in the aspect of postoperative recovery and functional preservation compared to conventional open surgery. The surgical technique of SND or MRND is standardized in most centers and may be performed without significant surgical morbidity such as injury of neurovascular structures. However, a external scar of the neck is unavoidable and despite the efforts to minimize scarring, some patients may suffer from disfiguring hypertrophic scar or keloid formation, which can affect patient's quality of life adversely. The lymphedema is also one of the frequent complaints that the patient can have after the MRND. The long transverse incision in the neck can disrupt normal lymphatic drainage from head and face to neck area and consequently, this disruption causes facial or neck edema. We attempted the incisional shift that can avoid the downside of the conventional neck dissection (ND). Owing to the recent development of robotic surgical systems, the ND with remote incisions became possible. With the accumulation of robot-assisted neck dissection (RAND) via various incisions, we realized that the retroauricular (RA) or the modified facelift (MFL) incisions are more suitable for the management of neck metastasis in head and neck cancer. In this chapter, our novel surgical technique of RAND via an RA or MFL incisions is introduced in detail.

RATIONALE FOR PROCEDURE

Previously, RAND via a transaxillary approach was reported for the management of thyroid carcinoma with cervical lymph node metastasis. However, it is difficult to visualize levels I, IIB and VA in patients with prominent clavicles because the dissection proceeds in the inferior-to-superior direction. Then, our group modified and reported the technique and performed RAND via the transaxillary and retroauricular (TARA) approach for the ND in patients with head and neck squamous cell carcinoma (HNSCC). After the initial report of RAND via TARA, we tried to dissect the upper neck levels I-III through RAND via an MFL approach, avoiding an axillary incision to reduce the extent of dissection. We reported on the feasibility and excellent cosmetic benefits of robot-assisted SND levels I-III via an MFL approach in patients with oral cavity cancer. Because it was performed through an RA or MFL incision, the postoperative scar was hidden behind the hairline, and the patients were extremely satisfied with their cosmetic results. Recently, after having accumulated additional experience with RAND, we are trying to perform level IV and V as well as level I-III dissections via an RA or MFL incision without an axillary incision.

APPLIED ANATOMY

Firstly, the surgeon should be well-acquainted with the surgical anatomy required for conventional ND. The sound understanding of regional anatomy can guarantee the successful operation without complications. The surgical anatomy for the RAND is similar to the conventional ND. Here, we will discuss some aspects specific for the RAND. Robot-assisted neck dissection requires wider skin flap elevation from the RA incision site to the midline of the neck. Therefore, the surgeon should become familiar with subplatysmal flap elevation. Using the greater auricular nerve (GAN) and external jugular vein (EJV) as a landmark of the skin flap and identifying the platysma muscle above them will be the first gateway of this surgery. In conventional ND, the platysma muscle is a guiding light in flap elevation. However, with the RA or MFL approach, the platysma muscle can be encountered only after the flap elevation process is well under way. The surgeons who want to take advantage of the RA or MFL incision should understand the superficial musculoaponeurotic system (SMAS) fascia. The SMAS is a fibromuscular extension of the platysma muscle fascia. This is connected inferiorly to the platysma muscle and superiorly to the superficial temporal muscle. The sub-SMAS flap elevation secures the parotidomasseteric fascia that covers the parotid gland which consequently helps preserve and protect the marginal mandibular branch of the facial nerve (MMN). The anatomy of the facial artery from the proximal to the distal portion located deep to the marginal branch of the facial nerve should be considered during level I dissection to preserve the nerve and ligate the vessel without troublesome bleeding. It goes without saying that experience of conventional ND is necessary to conduct RAND. The surgeon should be fully aware of the location of MMN, hypoglossal nerve, lingual nerve, spinal accessory nerve (SAN), vagus nerve, GAN, phrenic nerve and brachial plexus, which should be preserved during the surgery. The SAN has some variations. The SAN can have branches to the sternocleidomastoid (SCM) muscle without passing through it. However, in some other cases, the SAN passes through the SCM muscle with branching into the SCM muscle. Since, this difference can have a large impact on the dissection procedure of type III MRND, each variation of the SAN course should be kept in mind. Since the procedure of robotic SND levels I-III proceeds in a posterior to anterior direction (i.e. from the anterior border of the SCM muscle to the lateral border of the strap muscles), it may be helpful to accumulate surgical experience of conventional ND in the same manner.

The thoracic duct is the lymphatic vessel that drains into the left brachiocephalic vein. Since the identification failure or inadvertent ligation of the thoracic duct results in the chyle leakage, particular care should be taken to the dissection procedure of the level IV region near the thoracic duct.

INDICATIONS

Robot-assisted SND levels I-III or II-IV

1. Oral cavity cancer with clinical N0 neck indicated for elective SND
2. Parotid cancer with clinical N0 neck indicated for elective SND (*see* Fig. 10.27A)
3. Laryngopharyngeal cancer with clinical N0 neck indicated for elective SND
4. Patients in whom the primary lesion can be removed through transoral resection or TORS without an external incision
5. Patients with no previous history of treatment for head and neck cancer

Robot-assisted MRND levels I–V/II–V (*see* Fig. 10.27B)

1. Patients with biopsy proven lymph node metastasis of the head and neck cancer
2. Patients with no previous history of treatment for head and neck cancer
3. Lymph node metastasis without severe extracapsular spread (ECS) on imaging studies [computed tomography (CT), magnetic resonance imaging (MRI)].

CONTRAINDICATIONS

1. Past history of neck surgery of any kind
2. Patients with previous history of chemoradiation as primary treatment (relatively contraindicated)
3. Unresectable lymph node metastasis (e.g. carotid artery encasement)
4. Recurrent primary tumor
5. Patients who require cervical incisions to remove the primary tumor
6. Patients who require cervical incisions for microvascular flap reconstruction (relatively contraindicated)
7. Patients with distant metastasis at the time of initial presentation.

PREOPERATIVE WORKUP

Choice of Surgical Approach

The body mass index (BMI) (kg/m^2), length and circumference of the neck should be considered since they may affect the difficulty and operation time of the procedure. There is no absolute contraindication regarding the body habitus or BMI. With over 100 cases of RAND experiences, we could successfully accomplish the planned procedures without conversion to the conventional ND regardless of

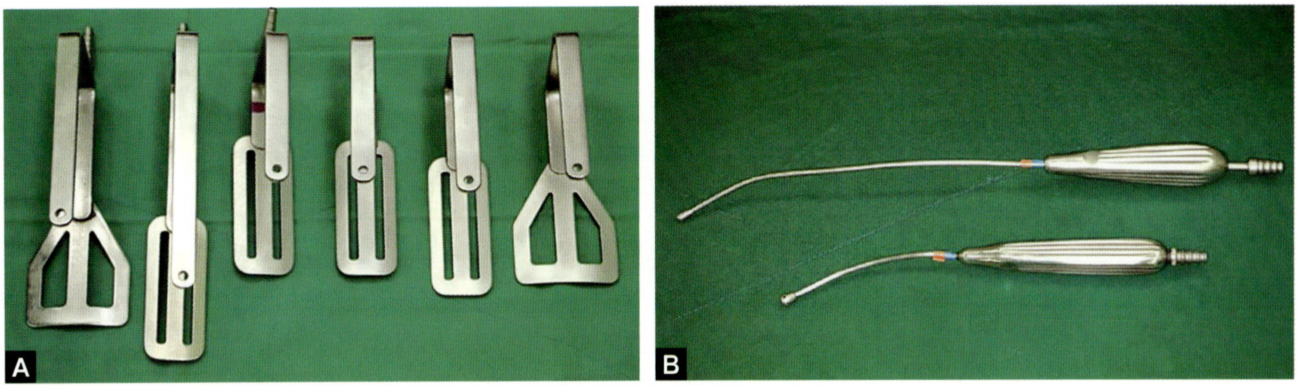

Figs. 10.1A and B: Self-retaining retractor and Yankauer suction. (A) The left two retractors are Chung's retractor used for endoscopic or robotic thyroidectomy and the other four on the right are self-developed retractors for neck dissection via retroauricular approach or modified facelift incision. (B) New self-developed Yankauer suction with longer or shorter length.

BMI. Obese patients are not an absolute contraindication to surgery; however, the possible prolonged operative time should be explained to the patient. Since RAND requires more time to perform compared to the conventional technique, elderly patients or those with significant comorbidities should be carefully selected.

All patients should be counseled about the advantages and disadvantages of RAND as well as alternative options including conventional ND, definitive chemoradiation as well as the possibility of conversion to a conventional ND.

Preoperative Imaging

Radiologic studies such as CT, MRI and positron emission tomography PET-CT may be useful to identify metastatic cervical lymph nodes. Lymph nodes that are suspicious for metastasis should undergo fine needle aspiration biopsy. Ultrasonography may be useful to target the lymph nodes during the biopsy procedure. CT and MRI are the most useful imaging studies and can reveal the size, number, location and extent of cervical lymph node metastasis. It can also detect the presence of extracapsular extension of a suspicious metastatic lymph node. The SCM muscle, internal jugular vein (IJV) or SAN invasions are not an absolute contraindication of this procedure and the type of MRND can be determined preoperatively based on the imaging studies.

Precautions for Anesthesia

For the flap elevation and upper ND under direct vision, the operator should be seated near the head of the patient looking cephalo-caudally. The endotracheal tube should be directed to the contralateral side and connected to the ventilator that is located near the patient's feet. For tracheotomized patients, the tracheotomy tube should be secured with sutures to avoid inadvertent dislodgement. Risks of any other anesthesia-related complications or difficulties for intubation and anesthesia are not specifically increased with this procedure. The airway is not naturally compromised or disturbed in any way through this procedure.

INSTRUMENTATIONS

Retractors for skin flap elevation:

- Skin hook
- Army-Navy retractor
- Right-angle "breast" retractor
- Self-retaining retractor (L & C BIO, Gyeonggi-do, Korea) (Fig. 10.1A).

Instruments for dissection under direct vision:

- Monopolar cautery tips with variable length (spatula tip is preferred)
- Harmonic Curved Shears (Harmonic Ace 23E; Johnson & Johnson Medical, Cincinnati, OH)
- Debakey forceps or Russian forceps
- Yankauer suction (Fig. 10.1B).

Robotic instrument (da Vinci Robotic System—Intuitive Surgical, Inc., Sunnyvale, CA):

- 12-mm, 30° facedown endoscope (Intuitive Surgical, Inc., Sunnyvale, CA)
- 5-mm, Maryland forceps (Intuitive Surgical, Inc., Sunnyvale, CA)
- 5-mm, Harmonic Curved Shears (Intuitive Surgical, Inc., Sunnyvale, CA)

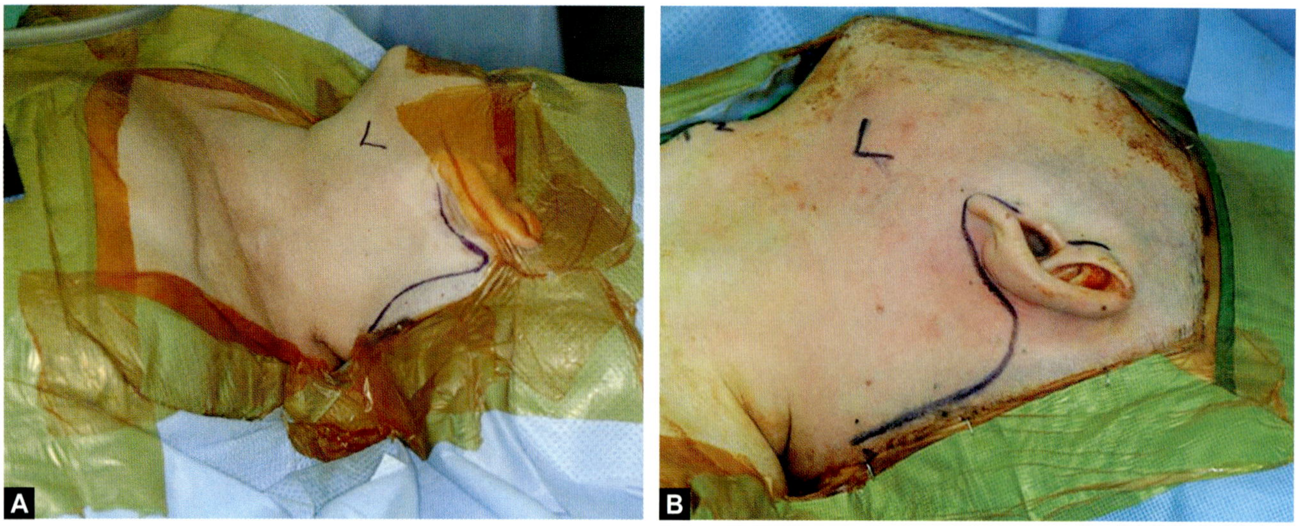

Figs. 10.2A and B: Position of the patient and design of the skin incision. (A) Retroauricular incision. (B) A modified facelift incision.

- 8-mm, ProGrasp forceps (Intuitive Surgical, Inc., Sunnyvale, CA): Installed at left or right arm depending on the side of ND. It could be substituted by an endoscopic alligator forceps manipulated by a patient-side assistant.

Vessel ligation system:

- Hem-o-lok Ligation System (Teleflex, Inc., Research Triangle Park, NC)

OPERATIVE TECHNIQUES

Step 1 Positioning of the Patient

The patient is set in supine position with the neck slightly extended by inserting a soft pillow under the shoulder and head rotated towards the contralateral side (Figs. 10.2A and B). Sometimes, the neck may be relaxed in its natural position and not extended.

Step 2 Skin Incision Design

An MFL or RA incision is designed. The RA incision is made behind the auricle starting from the lower end of the RA sulcus and moves upward to the midpoint of the sulcus, and then smoothly angulated downward 0.5 cm inside the hairline (Fig. 10.2A). Modified facelift incision is extended from the RA incision to the natural preauricular fold and continued behind the tragus (Fig. 10.2B). Care should be taken not to make the RA skin flap too narrow or too long, so that skin flap necrosis may be prevented. Initially, the MFL approach was preferred because it provided a wider working space for the robotic instrument arms than the RA approach. As our experience with RAND increased, we realized that the RA approach allowed sufficient working space for the robotic arms without the preauricular incision. Subsequently, the RA approach is mainly used for RAND.

Step 3 Skin Flap Elevation

Subplatysmal skin flap is elevated using a monopolar coagulator. Surgeon needs a surgical headlight to visualize the surgical field. The assistant can use the skin hook, Army-Navy retractor or Right-angle "breast" retractor to facilitate the procedure as the dissection proceeds towards the midline of the neck. GAN and EJV should be preserved superficial to the SCM muscle (Fig. 10.3). To prevent postoperative deformity or adhesion of neck, the fascia of the SCM muscle should also be preserved. Skin flap elevation below the mandible should be conducted with care not to give thermal injury to the marginal branch of the facial nerve (MMN). After identifying the contour of the submandibular gland (SMG), lateral border of the strap muscles should be identified medially and superior belly of the omohyoid muscle should be identified inferiorly. For MRND, the dissection is continued medially to the opposite anterior belly of the digastric muscle, inferiorly to the clavicular prominence and laterally to the anterior border of the trapezius muscle. When sufficient working space is acquired, a self-retaining retractor is applied.

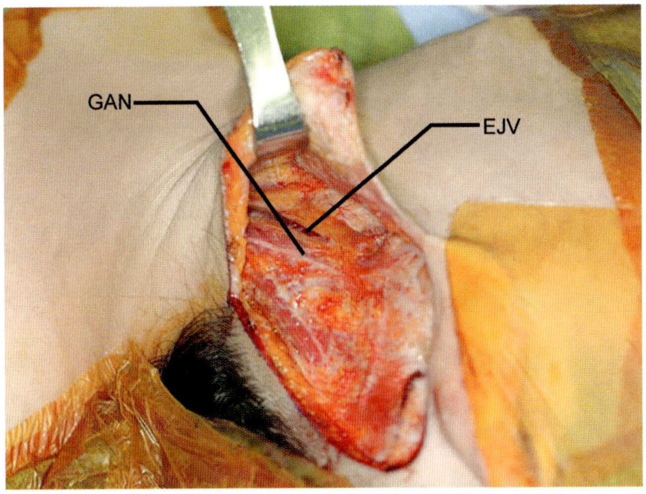

Fig. 10.3: Skin flap elevation and acquirement of working space. The greater auricular nerve (GAN) and external jugular vein (EJV) should be preserved superficial to the sternocleidomastoid (SCM) muscle.

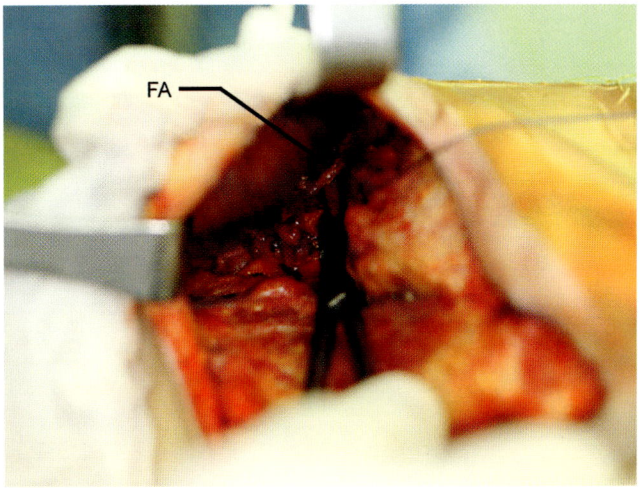

Fig. 10.4: Distal facial artery (FA) and marginal mandibular branch of the facial nerve (MMN). The MMN should be identified. The distal FA located deep to the nerve may be a good landmark.

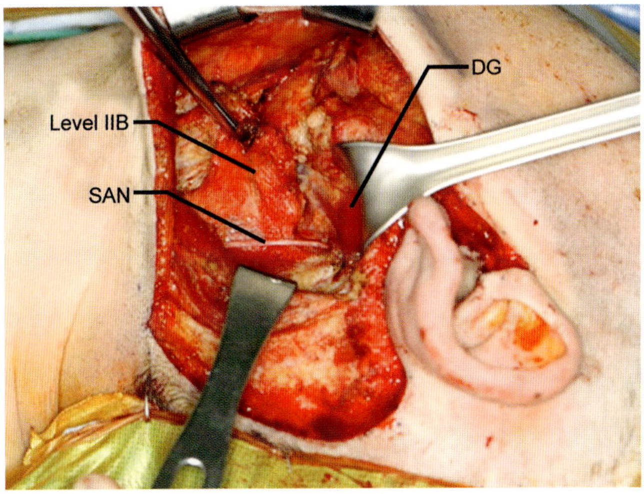

Fig. 10.5: Identifying the spinal accessory nerve (SAN) and level IIB dissection. The lymphofatty tissues are dissected from the medial border of the SCM muscle and the SAN is traced in the inferior direction (DG: Posterior belly of digastric muscle).

Step 4 Upper ND Under Direct Vision

Selective neck dissection levels I-III: Upper part of level IB including the SMG, level IIB and fibrofatty tissues of levels IIA and III lateral to the carotid sheath can be dissected under direct vision using conventional instruments. First of all, the marginal branch of the facial nerve (MMN) is identified so that perifacial lymph nodes can be removed safely. The distal facial artery and vein, which is located deep to the nerve, may be a good landmark (Fig. 10.4). After identifying the nerve, the vessels are ligated with the Harmonic Curved Shears (Harmonic Ace 23E; Johnson & Johnson Medical, Cincinnati, OH) and the surrounding fibroadipose tissues can be separated from the inferior border of the mandible. The lymphofatty tissues inferior to the parotid tail are dissected using monopolar coagulator. Dissection of the inferior border of SMG leads to identification of the posterior belly of the digastric muscle. Fibroadipose tissues are dissected from the anterior surface of the SCM muscle using monopolar coagulator. Dissection between the inferior border of digastric muscle and anterior border of SCM leads to exposure of the IJV. The transverse process of the atlas can be palpated at this area where the SAN usually crosses the IJV. After identifying the SAN and dissecting it, level IIB can be dissected (Fig. 10.5). While preserving the cervical plexus, the fibroadipose tissues of level IIB and III can be dissected towards the carotid sheath using a monopolar cautery.

Modified radical neck dissection levels I–V or II–V: When level I is omitted, there is no need to elevate the skin flap as high up as the inferior border of the mandible and that the working space must cover far below to the clavicle in order to address levels IV and V. Therefore, the skin flap must be elevated more laterally based on the posterior border of the SCM so that the lymph nodes of level V are sufficiently included. Here, it is helpful if the operator positions himself at above the patient's head.

In case of type III MRND that preserves the SCM muscle, the lymphofatty tissues are dissected from the medial border of the SCM muscle and the SAN is traced in

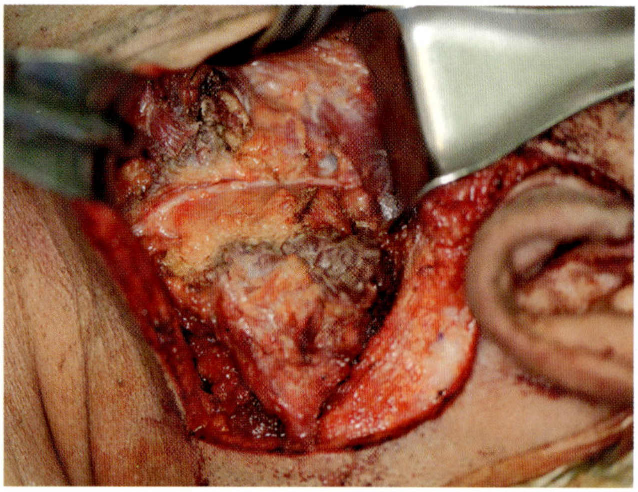

Fig. 10.6: The spinal accessory nerve (SAN) tracing (type II MRND). The SAN is identified near the transverse process of the second cervical spine and traced to the insertion to the trapezius muscle.

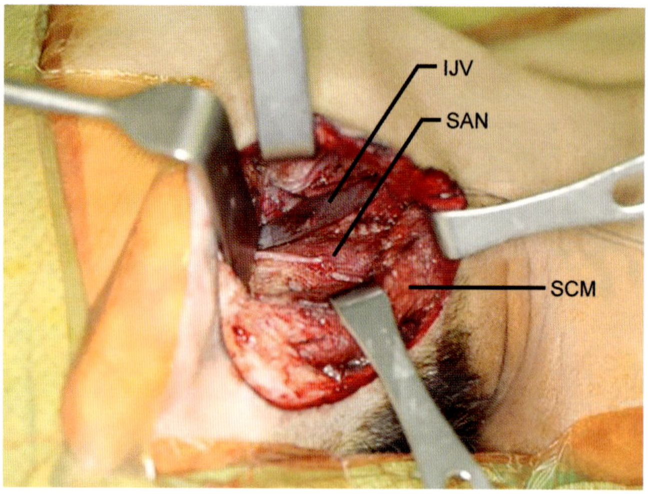

Fig. 10.7: The surgical view of robot-assisted selective neck dissection (levels II–V). Surgical field after lateral traction of the sternocleidomastoid muscle (IJV: Internal jugular vein; SCM: Sternocleidomastoid muscle; SAN: Spinal accessory nerve).

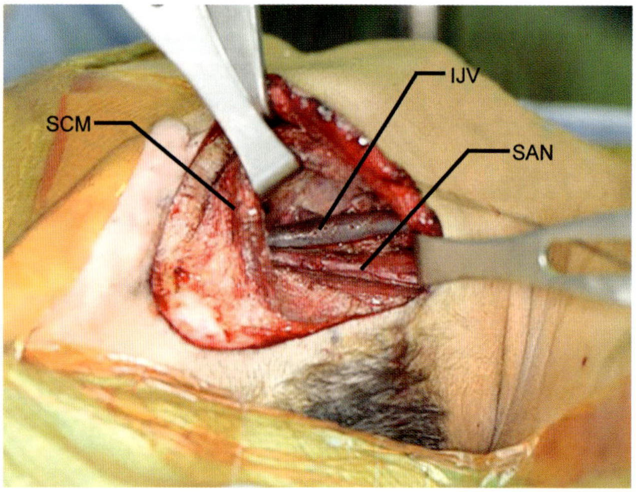

Fig. 10.8: The surgical view of robot-assisted selective neck dissection (level II-V). Surgical field after superior traction of the sternocleidomastoid muscle (IJV: Internal jugular vein; SCM: Sternocleidomastoid muscle; SAN: Spinal accessory nerve).

the inferior direction (Fig. 10.5). In case of type II MRND that sacrifices the SCM muscle, the SCM muscle branch of the SAN may be cut. The SAN is identified at the lateral border of the SCM muscle (Fig. 10.6). The fascia of the SCM is opened at the anterior border of the SCM and continued as far below as possible to level IV. The SAN is traced and skeletonized as it is followed toward the trapezius muscle. The SAN is located at Erb's point on the posterior border of the SCM (Fig. 10.7). The entire SAN from the skull base to the trapezius muscle is identified and skeletonized. Next, the surgeon opens the fascia along the whole posterior border of the SCM, and the fibrofatty tissue is dissected from the medial side of the SCM by elevating it upward using an Army-Navy retractor (Fig. 10.8). All fibroadipose tissues are dissected off the SCM during this procedure, and care must be taken not to damage the SAN running to the trapezius at this point (Fig. 10.8). With lifting up the skeletonized SCM muscle, levels IIB, VA and the lateral aspect to the carotid sheath of IIA, and upper III are dissected under direct vision (Fig. 10.9). Following the accumulation of surgical experiences, most of the upper ND including levels IIA and III medial to the carotid sheath can be accomplished under direct vision. A self-retaining retractor (L&C BIO, Gyeonggi-do, Korea) is then inserted through the working space and the SCM muscle is elevated upwards and now it is ready to introduce the robotic arms. Describing the sequence of the operation in general, before docking of the robotic arms, levels IIB and VA must be dissected first at the lateral portion of the SAN and after elevating the SCM muscle, some portion of levels IIA and III located lateral to the carotid sheath should be dissected under direct vision (Fig. 10.9).

Step 5 Robot-assisted Neck Dissection Technique

Selective neck dissection levels I-III: A facedown 30° endoscope is used for visualization of the surgical field and two robotic instrument arms, equipped at either side of the endoscopic arm with 5-mm Maryland forceps and

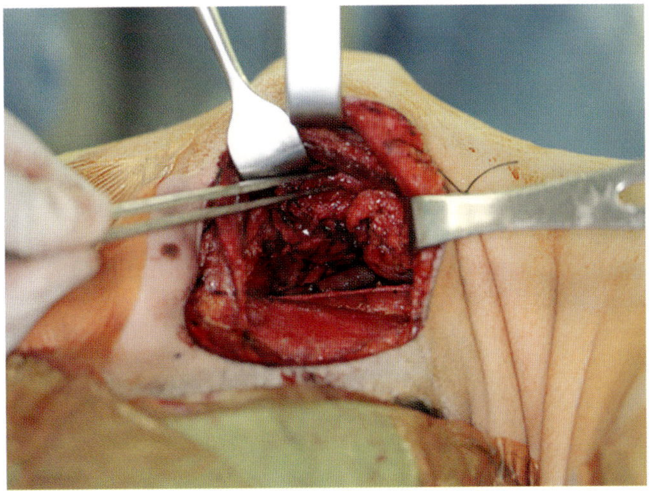

Fig. 10.9: Levels IIB, VA, IIA and upper III dissections. With the upward retraction of the skeletonized sternocleidomastoid muscle (SCM), levels IIB, VA and the lateral aspect to the carotid sheath of IIA, and upper III are dissected under direct vision.

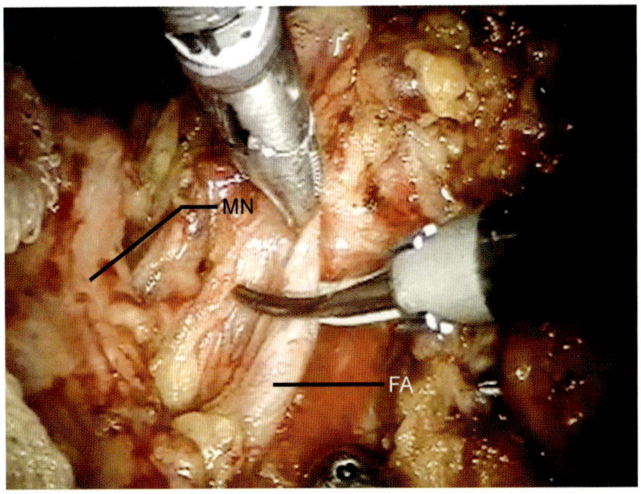

Fig. 10.10: Ligation of proximal facial artery (MN: Marginal branch of facial nerve; FA: Facial artery).

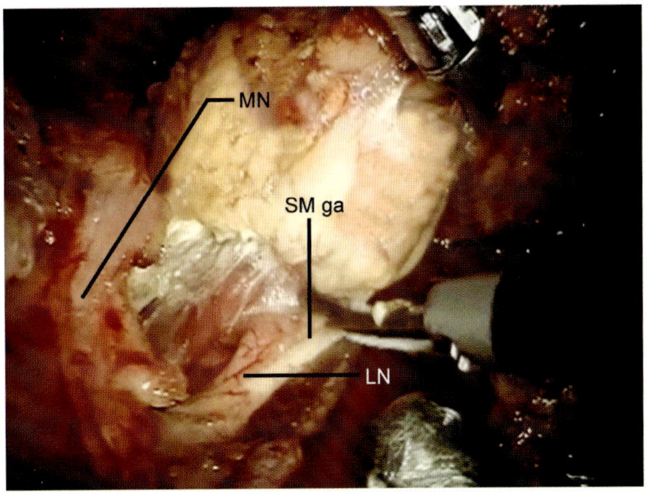

Fig. 10.11: Lingual nerve and submandibular ganglion (LN: Lingual nerve; MN: Marginal branch of facial nerve; SM ga: Submandibular ganglion).

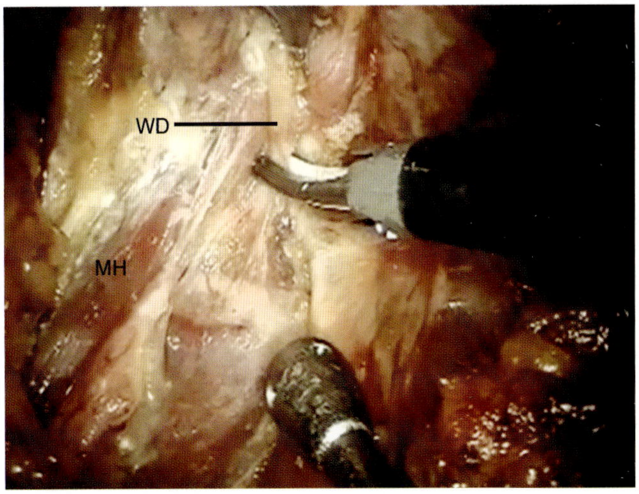

Fig. 10.12: Wharton's duct (WD). The duct is ligated deep to the mylohyoid muscle (MH).

5-mm Harmonic Curved Shears respectively, are utilized throughout the operation. A patient-side assistant can facilitate the robotic dissection by exposing the surgical field using an Army-Navy retractor or a Yankauer suction. The robotic dissection begins from level I. Dissection of level I is conducted as lateral to medial direction. The posterior belly of the digastric muscle is first identified, and then the proximal facial artery is sealed with Harmonic Curved Shears or double ligated with Hem-o-lok Ligation System (Teleflex, Inc., Research Triangle Park, NC) performed by the assistant (Fig. 10.10). While pulling the fibroadipose tissues with the Maryland dissector, level I is dissected from the surrounding muscles. The MMN, lingual nerve (LN) and hypoglossal nerve should be safely preserved during the dissection of the SMG. After identification of the mylohyoid muscle, the SMG ganglion and the Wharton duct are sealed, with preservation of the hypoglossal and lingual nerve (Figs. 10.11 and 10.12). Submental artery is sealed with Harmonic Curved Shears. The fibrofatty tissues between both anterior bellies of digastric muscle (level IA) are detached using Harmonic Curved Shears. After completing level I dissection (Fig. 10.13), the

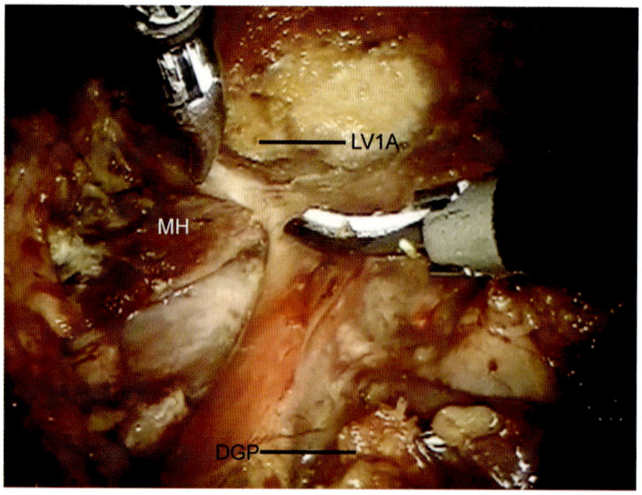

Fig. 10.13: Completion of level I dissection. Fibroadipose tissues of level IA and level IB above the posterior belly of digastric muscle are removed (LV1A, level IA; MH: Mylohyoid muscle; DGP: Posterior belly of digastric muscle).

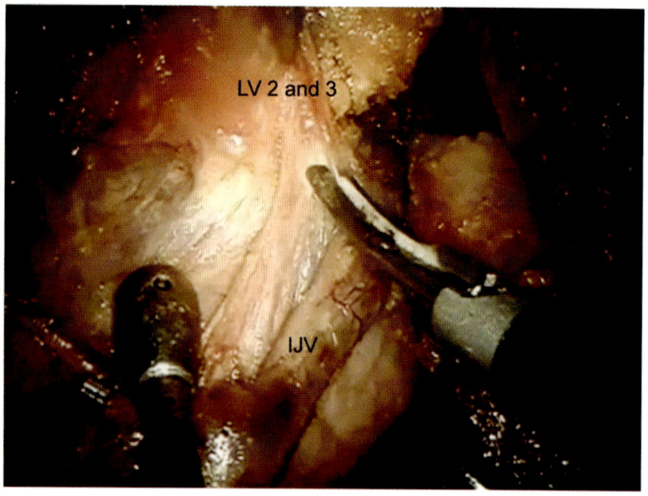

Fig. 10.14: Lymph node dissection from the carotid sheath and the internal jugular vein. Fibroadipose tissues of levels II and III (LV 2&3) are dissected.

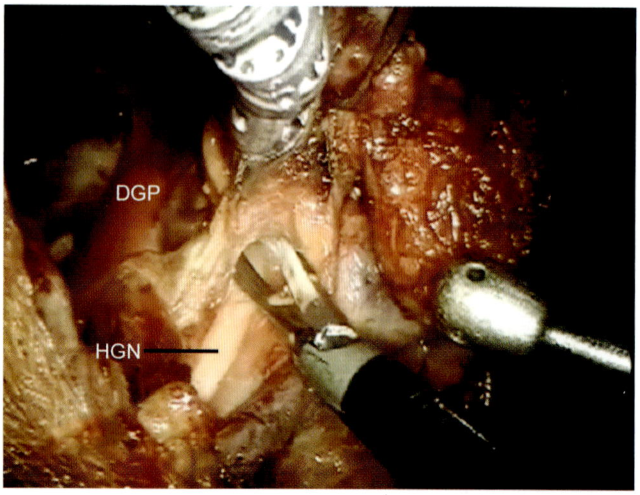

Fig. 10.15: Hypoglossal nerve (HGN). The nerve is easily identified deep to the posterior belly of digastric muscle (DGP).

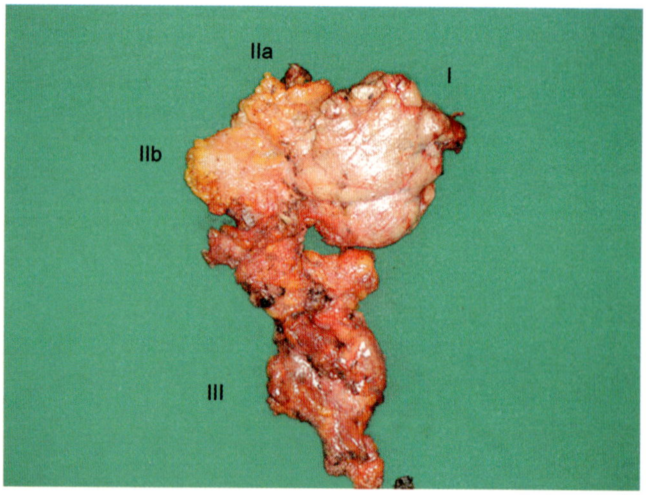

Fig. 10.16: Surgical specimen.

fibroadipose tissues of levels II and III dissected under direct vision are pulled medially using the Maryland dissector and dissected from the carotid sheath and the IJV (Fig. 10.14). During the level IIA dissection, the hypoglossal nerve can be easily identified and preserved (Fig. 10.15). Dissection is conducted inferiorly to the superior belly of the omohyoid muscle and medially to the lateral border of the strap muscles. Superior thyroid artery and ansa cervicalis can be easily identified through the magnified view and preserved. After completing the dissection, the specimen is removed (Fig. 10.16). The specimen should be mapped according to each level and sent for biopsy.

Modified radical neck dissection levels I–V/II–V: The main difference with regard to SND levels I-III is that in this procedure, dissection of levels IV and V is required. Therefore, the robotic arms must be inserted so that they are addressed towards levels IV and V. Retracting the previously dissected specimen of level IIB superiorly and medially, level IIA dissection is started in a superior to inferior manner. The hypoglossal nerve is identified and preserved near the carotid bifurcation area. During the level IIA dissection, the superior thyroid and lingual artery are identified and preserved. Next, level III is dissected using the robotic system, again from superior to inferior

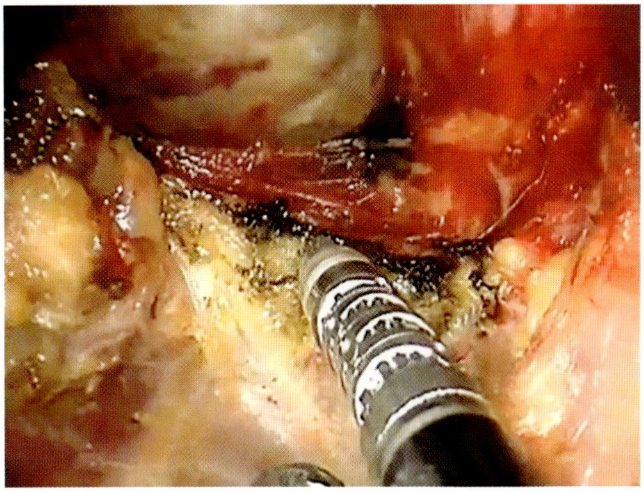

Fig. 10.17: Level VB dissection. The fibrofatty tissues in level VB are dissected in a lateromedial direction.

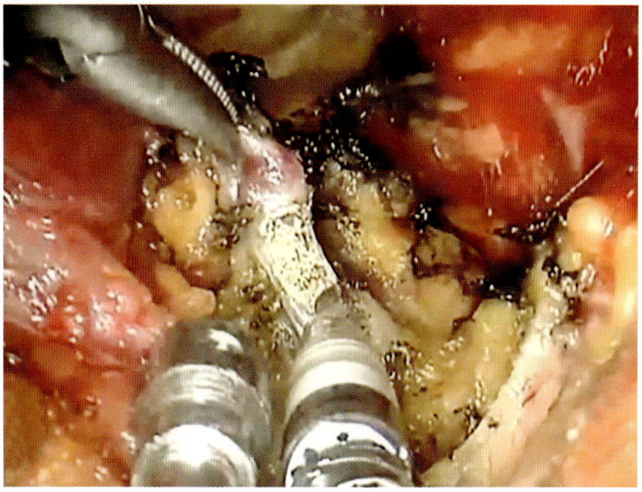

Fig. 10.18: Resection of the omohyoid muscle. The omohyoid muscle is identified and cut using Harmonic Curved Shears.

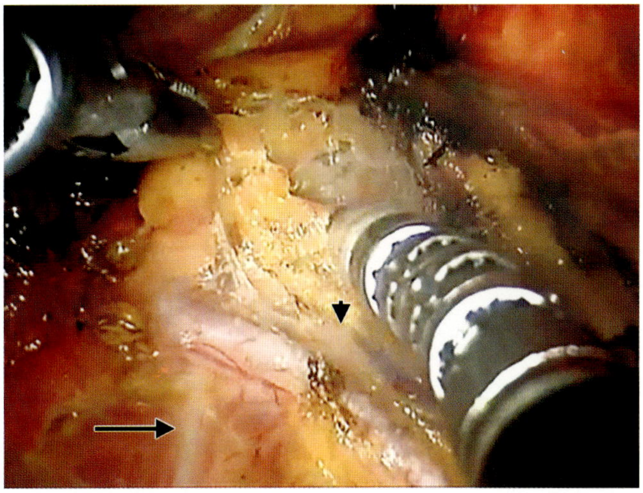

Fig. 10.19: Identification and preservation of the transverse cervical artery. The transverse cervical artery and vein (arrowhead) are verified and the phrenic nerve (arrow) is identified beneath the transverse cervical vessels.

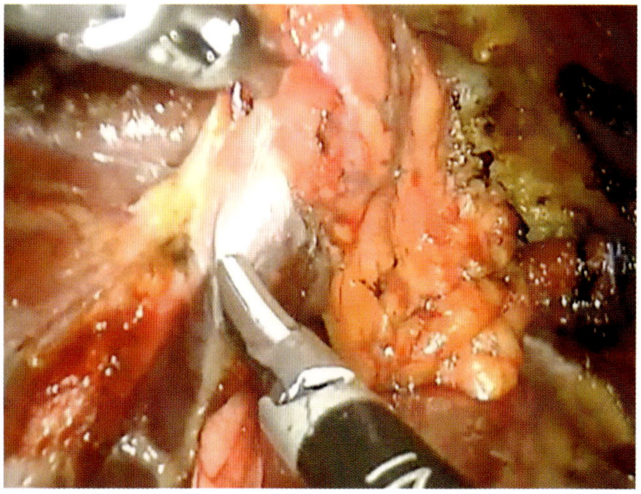

Fig. 10.20: Carotid sheath dissection. The fibrofatty tissues near carotid space in level IV are dissected using Harmonic Curved Shears.

direction. Fibroadipose tissue is carefully dissected from the IJV using Harmonic Curved Shears equipped with robotic arms. Since the skin flap and SCM muscle are already elevated, it is not difficult to dissect level V (posterior to anterior) in cases in which level V dissection is required. In a lateromedial direction, the fibrofatty tissues in level VB are dissected (Fig. 10.17). The omohyoid muscle is identified and cut using Harmonic Curved Shears (Fig. 10.18). The transverse cervical artery and vein are verified on the floor of level V and the phrenic nerve is identified beneath the transverse cervical vessels (Fig. 10.19). The specimen is then retracted superiorly and medially, and level IV dissection is performed. The fibrofatty tissues near carotid space in level IV are dissected using Harmonic Curved Shears. The vagus nerve, carotid artery and jugular vein are identified and preserved by carefully opening the carotid sheath (Fig. 10.20). During the dissection of level IV, the lymphatic or thoracic duct should be ligated using hemoclips or Hem-o-lok Ligation System to prevent a chyle leakage (Fig. 10.21). The branches of IJV are ligated with Harmonic Curved Shears or Hem-o-lok Ligation System (Fig. 10.22). In case of type II MRND, the sternal and clavicular heads of the SCM are cut with Harmonic Curved Shears (Fig. 10.23). After the ND is complete, the neck

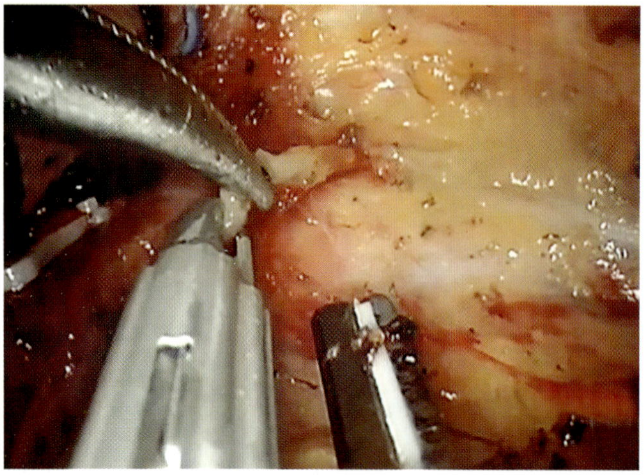

Fig. 10.21: Ligation of the lymphatic duct. The lymphatic duct is sealed with Hem-o-lok to prevent a chyle leakage

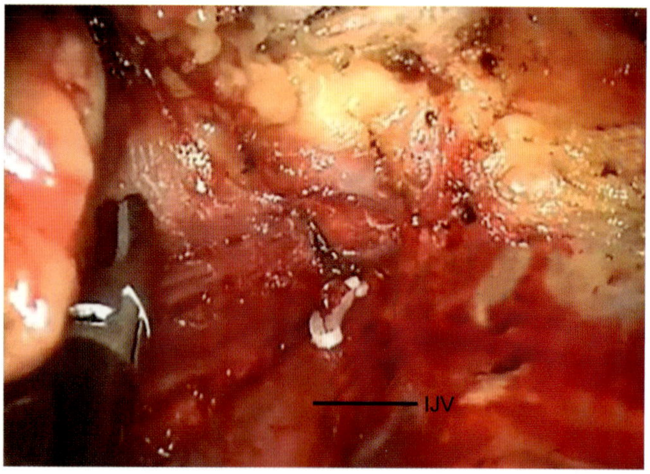

Fig. 10.22: Ligation of the branch of internal jugular vein with Hem-o-lok Ligation System. (IJV: Internal jugular vein).

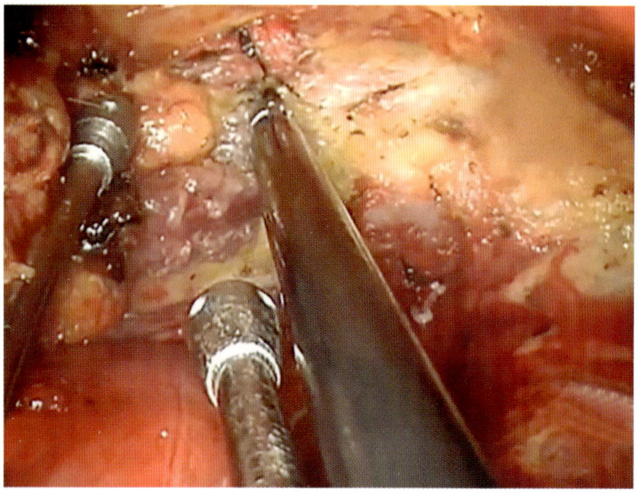

Fig. 10.23: Resection of sternocleidomastoid muscle (SCM). The sternal and clavicular heads of the SCM are cut with Harmonic Curved Shears.

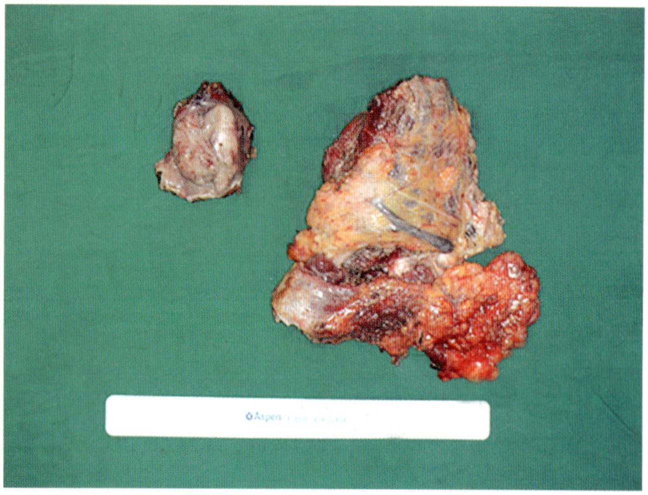

Fig. 10.24: Surgical specimens of primary tumor and neck. The specimen is removed through the retroauricular or modified facelift incision. The specimen can be separately removed with level-by-level strategy.

specimens are removed through the MFL or RA incision (Fig. 10.24). During the operation, one assistant is situated near the incision port while the three robotic arms are inserted; the assistant should actively provide suction and aspiration of irrigation from the surgical field and engage in ligating vessels or lymphatic ducts using a hemoclip or Hem-o-lok Ligation System.

Step 6 Finishing the Operation

The surgical bed is irrigated with warm saline and bleeding control under both endoscopic view and direct vision should be performed (Figs. 10.25 and 10.26). A closed suction drain is placed in the wound and the incision is closed with 4-0 Vicryl and 5-0 Nylon sutures.

COMPLICATIONS AND THEIR MANAGEMENT

Some possible postoperative complications are listed below. In uncomplicated situations, the RA or MFL skin incisions heal well without any wound disruptions. Massive hemorrhage or hematoma can rarely occur from rupture or loosening of the previously ligated or clipped vessels or the nearby carotid artery. Minor, trivial bleeding or hematoma can be managed locally with compression but in such uncontrollable or massive bleeding situations, do not hesitate to open the wound in the operating room.

Possible Postoperative Complications from Therapeutic RAND

- Nerve-related injury
  - Lingual nerve injury
  - Marginal mandibular branch of facial nerve injury (Mouth corner deviation)
  - Glossopharyngeal nerve injury
  - Vagus nerve injury (vocal cord palsy)
  - Spinal accessory nerve injury (SAN syndrome)
  - Hypoglossal nerve injury
  - Phrenic nerve injury
  - Sympathetic nerve injury (Horner's syndrome)

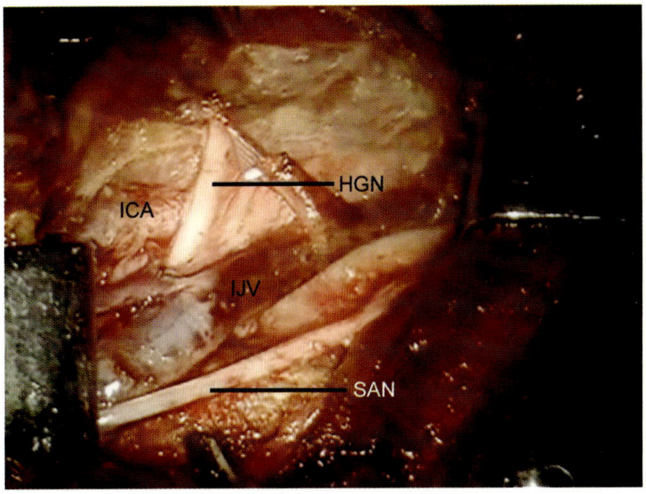

Fig. 10.25: Surgical field after selective neck dissection levels I-III (SAN: Spinal accessory nerve; IJV: Internal jugular vein; ICA: Internal carotid artery; HGN: Hypoglossal nerve).

- Hematoma/hemorrhage
- Seroma
- Chyle leakage
- Wound infection, dehiscence
- Discoloration or necrosis of skin flap.

1. *Hemorrhage or hematoma*: Minor bleeding from the skin flap or muscles that may lead to postoperative hematoma may be resolved with conservative management. However, major bleeding possibly from ligated or clipped vessels may present as abrupt swelling of the neck. Surgical exploration under general anesthesia should be conducted in such cases. However, significant postoperative hemorrhage after RAND is rare, based on our experience. We have experienced several cases of postoperative bleeding from the EJV stump and skin flap. The harmonic scalpel is effective in vessel sealing in most cases, but careful examination must be done before ending the operation.
2. *Neurologic deficit*: The marginal branch of the facial nerve can be injured by excessive thermal insult and retraction or mechanical trauma. We have experienced several cases of temporary paralysis of the marginal branch of facial nerve that recovered within 2–3 months. Therefore, both the surgeon and the assistant should take care to prevent such injury at the inferior border of mandible. In addition, greater auricular nerve, hypoglossal nerve, lingual nerve, SAN, vagus nerve and sympathetic nerve injury may occur. To prevent these various nerve injuries, comprehensive understanding of the anatomy of the neurovascular

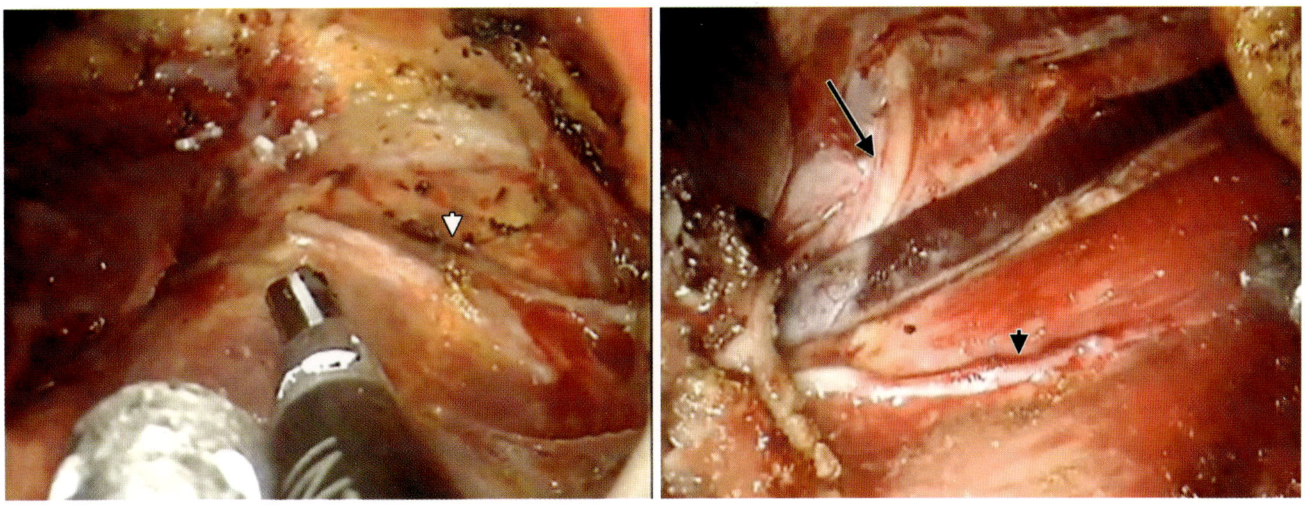

Fig. 10.26: Surgical field after modified radical neck dissection. The transverse cervical vessels (white arrowhead) can be identified intact in level IV. The hypoglossal nerve (black arrow) and the spinal accessory nerve (black arrowhead) can be identified and preserved.

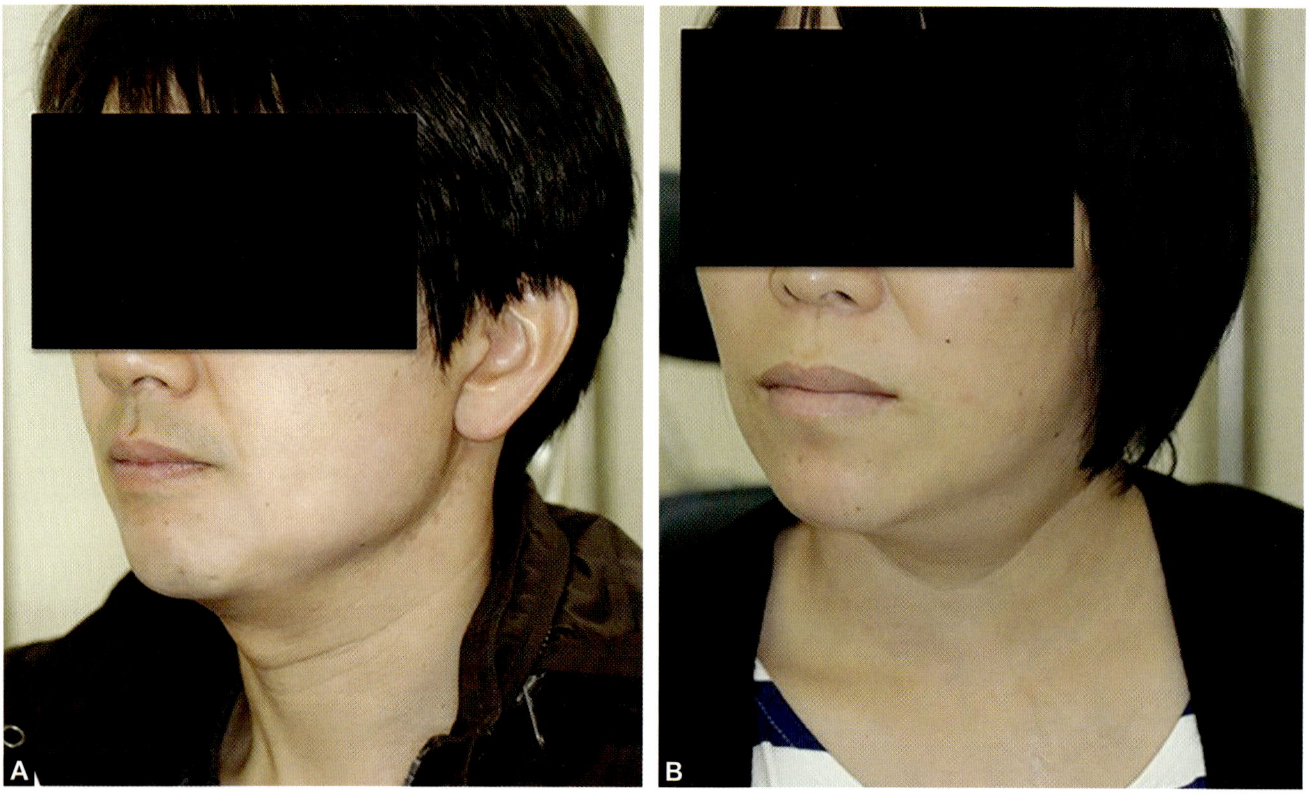

Figs. 10.27A and B: Postoperative photograph. (A) Robot-assisted selective neck dissection levels I-III for parotid cancer. (B) Robot-assisted modified radical neck dissection for primary unknown cancer. Postoperative scar is hidden by the auricle and hair without any significant lymphedema or fibrotic change of the dissected area.

structures is essential. Temporary or permanent numbness of ear lobe due to injury of the greater auricular nerve may occur due to thermal injury to the nerve. Injury of the hypoglossal nerve, lingual nerve, SAN and vagus nerve is extremely rare with thorough anatomical understandings of the structures and magnified visualization. However, these nerves may be more vulnerable to dissection with harmonic scalpel during RAND rather than during conventional ND. So, surgeons should be familiar with the use of the harmonic scalpel even in the conventional neck surgery.

3. *Chyle leakage*: The lymphatic duct or thoracic duct are also very thin-walled structures even though the pressure is not high, so great care must be given when ligating the thoracic or lymphatic duct exclusively with the harmonic scalpel. After removal of the ND specimen, level IV should be inspected for any chyle leak. If chylous leakage is suspected, hemoclip or Hem-o-lok Ligation System should be applied. We routinely check for any chylous leakage with the Valsalva maneuver before finishing the operation.
4. *Discoloration or necrosis of skin flap*: Such complications may occur at the tip of the RA skin flap due to insufficient blood supply. We have not experienced serious skin necrosis but discoloration (ischemic change) but care must be taken so that the skin flap does not become too thin. The platysma muscle should be always identified as you proceed for the skin flap elevation. Otherwise it may lead to thinning of the skin flap that could result in postoperative skin necrosis, discoloration, depression or even penetration of the skin.
5. *Hypertrophic scar or keloid formation*: Meticulous handling of the skin flap and minimizing tissue injury during the surgery may be helpful to prevent such complications. Skin closure should be conducted with minimal skin tension after proper suture of the subcutaneous tissue.
6. *Hair loss along the skin incision*: Occasionally, hair loss along the skin incision within the hairline could occur. In order to prevent such situations, beveling the skin incision or designing the incision in front of the hairline might be useful.

FOLLOW-UP

Postoperative management is no different to conventional ND. The neck should be closely monitored for any signs of hemorrhage, hematoma or infection. According to our experience, an average amount of blood loss during uncomplicated endoscopic ND is <100 mL. A closed Hemovac suction drain can be removed if the drainage amount falls to <20 mL/day. Generally, Hemovac can be removed in no more than a week. The patient can be discharged in about a week, 1 day after the suction drain has been removed. Second, any change of skin color or signs of skin flap necrosis should be detected. Third, the possibility of orocervical fistula should be borne in mind when RAND is followed by TORS.

RESULTS

Robot-assisted neck dissection is a feasible and safe technique as an elective or therapeutic neck treatment in cN0 and cN + head and neck squamous cell carcinoma patients. Terris et al. developed the technique of MFL incision for parotidectomy, and the feasibility of robotic thyroidectomy via MFL was recently reported by the same group. Based on that, we added MFL or RA to the transaxillary approach, and we named this hybrid approach TARA. With increasing experience with the RAND via the TARA approach, we realized that omitting the transaxillary approach for ND was feasible, and we now complete ND via the RA or MFL alone. We previously reported the feasibility of robot-assisted supraomohyoid ND for clinically node negative oral tongue cancer and documented the satisfactory operative parameters obtained. These findings were the foundation of the rationale for the MRND via the RA or MFL approaches. The hindrance caused by clavicular prominence during the levels IV and V dissection can be bypassed because a superior-to-inferior dissection is performed in an RA or MFL approach. Moreover, an abbreviated transaxillary incision allowed for shorter operating times better results in terms of cosmesis and invasiveness.

This RAND technique via an RA or MFL approach may be successfully applied to selected cases by an experienced surgeon. It may be especially helpful in patients who have undergone TORS to remove a primary lesion because it does not leave an apparent scar around the neck. In this era of minimally invasive surgery, transoral surgery with or without robotic system for head and neck cancer is on the increase. Moreover, several reports presented worldwide show an increase of oral cavity or oropharynx cancer in young patients. These patients may have more demands for better postoperative cosmetic outcomes. In addition, we expect that there are benefits of RAND compared with conventional ND in functional aspects such as subcutaneous induration/fibrosis, lymphedema, incision site sensory disturbance and objective range of neck motion. Based on the normal anatomic subcutaneous lymphatic channel of the head and the neck, the transverse incision in the anterior neck can significantly disrupt lymphatic drainage, which is generally prevented by the use of RA or MFL incisions. We confirmed a decreased rate of postoperative lymphedema in the RAND group (data are not shown), and plan to examine the postoperative lymphedema results in a follow-up study. Despite all these advantages of RAND, improving cosmetic result is a secondary issue in ND and should never compromise oncologic safety. Retrieval of lymph nodes in the RAND group was not significantly different from that in the conventional ND group. Satisfaction with the resulting scar was significantly higher in the RAND group than in the conventional ND group.

Moreover, the procedure should be conducted with minimal complications or morbidities. Therefore, RAND should be conducted after sufficient acquisition of surgical anatomy and experience of conventional ND. Since the robotic procedure is conducted from lateral to medial direction, experiencing conventional ND in the same manner may be helpful to shorten the learning curve. Long-term results on oncologic safety and functional outcomes are required to establish the validity of RAND. This operative procedure, however, has a disadvantage of relatively longer operation times. Another important disadvantage of this operation is that it requires a considerable experience for the surgeon before he/she feels comfortable and is familiar with it. It is recommended that for optimal treatment outcomes, careful selection of clinically node negative patients must be carried out.

FUTURE DIRECTIONS

Our experience of performing comprehensive ND using the RA or MFL incision has shown that this approach is feasible in almost all cases of nodal metastases as long as there is no severe ECS. Nowadays, nearly all cases of ND can be performed by RA incision alone and the MFL incisions are seldom applied. Also, in cases of thyroid cancer with lymph node metastasis, ND as well as total thyroidectomy are being attempted by the RA approach only and without the axillary incision. It is expected that reports on its feasibility will be possible before long. If a single port or single arm technique is to be introduced with the advancement of the robotic system in the near future, great progress in the selective or comprehensive ND through the RA approach would be expected.

SUGGESTED READING

1. Byeon HK, Ban MJ, Lee JM, et al. Robot-assisted Sistrunk's operation, total thyroidectomy, and neck dissection via a transaxillary and retroauricular (TARA) approach in papillary carcinoma arising in thyroglossal duct cyst and thyroid gland. Ann Surg Oncol. 2012;19(13):4259-61.
2. Byeon HK, Holsinger FC, Kim DH, et al. Feasibility of robot-assisted neck dissection followed by transoral robotic surgery. Br J Oral Maxillofac Surg. 2015;53(1):68-73.
3. Byeon HK, Holsinger FC, Koh YW, et al. Endoscopic supraomohyoid neck dissection via a retroauricular or modified facelift approach: preliminary results. Head Neck. 2014;36(3):425-30.
4. Byeon HK, Holsinger FC, Tufano RP, et al. Robotic total thyroidectomy with modified radical neck dissection via unilateral retroauricular approach. Ann Surg Oncol. 2014;21(12):3872-5.
5. Kim CH, Byeon HK, Shin YS, et al. Robot-assisted sistrunk's operation via a retroauricular approach for thyroglossal duct cyst. Head Neck. 2014;36(3):456-8.
6. Kim CH, Chang JW, Choi EC, et al. Robotically assisted selective neck dissection in parotid gland cancer: preliminary report. Laryngoscope. 2013;123(3):646-50.
7. Kim CH, Koh YW, Kim D, et al. Robotic-assisted neck dissection in submandibular gland cancer: preliminary report. J Oral Maxillofac Surg. 2013;71(8):1450-7.
8. Kim WS, Ban MJ, Chang JW, et al. Learning curve for robot-assisted neck dissection in head and neck cancer: a 3-year prospective case study and analysis. JAMA Otolaryngol Head Neck Surg. 2014;140(12):1191-7. Erratum in: JAMA Otolaryngol Head Neck Surg. 2015;141(1):83.
9. Kim WS, Byeon HK, Park YM, et al. Therapeutic robot-assisted neck dissection via a retroauricular or modified facelift approach in head and neck cancer: a comparative study with conventional transcervical neck dissection. Head Neck. 2015;37(2):249-54.
10. Kim WS, Koh YW, Byeon HK, et al. Robot-assisted neck dissection via a transaxillary and retroauricular approach versus a conventional transcervical approach in papillary thyroid cancer with cervical lymph node metastases. J Laparoendosc Adv Surg Tech A. 2014;24(6):367-72.
11. Kim WS, Lee HS, Kang SM, et al. Feasibility of robot-assisted neck dissections via a transaxillary and retroauricular ("TARA") approach in head and neck cancer: preliminary results. Ann Surg Oncol. 2012;19(3):1009-17.
12. Koh YW, Choi EC. Robotic approaches to the neck. Otolaryngol Clin North Am. 2014;47(3):433-54.
13. Koh YW, Chung WY, Hong HJ, et al. Robot-assisted selective neck dissection via modified face-lift approach for early oral tongue cancer: a video demonstration. Ann Surg Oncol. 2012;19(4):1334-5.
14. Lee HS, Kim J, Lee HJ, et al. Transoral robotic surgery for neurogenic tumors of the prestyloid parapharyngeal space. Auris Nasus Larynx. 2012;39(4):434-7.
15. Lee HS, Kim WS, Hong HJ, et al. Robot-assisted supraomohyoid neck dissection via a modified face-lift or retroauricular approach in early-stage cN0 squamous cell carcinoma of the oral cavity: a comparative study with conventional technique. Ann Surg Oncol. 2012;19(12):3871-8.
16. Lee HS, Lee D, Koo YC, et al. Endoscopic resection of upper neck masses via retroauricular approach is feasible with excellent cosmetic outcomes. J Oral Maxillofac Surg. 2013;71(3):520-7.
17. Lee HS, Park do Y, Hwang CS, et al. Feasibility of robot-assisted submandibular gland resection via retroauricular approach: preliminary results. Laryngoscope. 2013;123(2): 369-73.
18. Park YM, Holsinger FC, Kim WS, et al. Robot-assisted selective neck dissection of levels II to V via a modified facelift or retroauricular approach. Otolaryngol Head Neck Surg. 2013;148(5):778-85.
19. Park YM, Lee WJ, Yun IS, et al. Free flap reconstruction after robot-assisted neck dissection via a modified face-lift or retroauricular approach. Ann Surg Oncol. 2013;20(3): 891-8.
20. Shin YS, Choi EC, Kim CH, et al. Robot-assisted selective neck dissection combined with facelift parotidectomy in parotid cancer. Head Neck. 2013.
21. Shin YS, Hong HJ, Koh YW, et al. Gasless transaxillary robot-assisted neck dissection: a preclinical feasibility study in four cadavers. Yonsei Med J. 2012;53(1):193-7.
22. Singer MC, Seybt MW, Terris DJ. Robotic facelift thyroidectomy: I. Preclinical simulation and morphometric assessment. Laryngoscope. 2011;121(8):1631-5.
23. Singer MC, Terris DJ. Robotic facelift thyroidectomy. Otolaryngol Clin North Am. 2014;47(3):425-31.
24. Terris DJ, Tuffo KM, Fee WE Jr. Modified facelift incision for parotidectomy. J Laryngol Otol. 1994;108(7):574-8.

Chapter 11 Robotic-Assisted Skull Base Surgery

Michael E Kupferman, Ehab Hanna

INTRODUCTION

In the past several years, transnasal endoscopic approaches have been increasingly used for surgical access and treatment of neoplastic and benign lesions of the anterior and central skull base. Endoscopic surgery is used with increasing frequency for surgical resection of tumors of the sinonasal tract such as inverted papilloma, angiofibroma, osteomas and other benign fibro-osseous lesions, and in selected patients with malignant sinonasal tumors.[1-5] Endoscopic approaches are also becoming popular for trans-sphenoidal access to the sella turcica, and are considered by many centers as the preferred surgical approach for treatment of pituitary adenomas.[6-9] More recently, there has been an emerging trend to expand the use of transnasal endoscopic approaches in the surgical treatment of suprasellar, petroclival, infratemporal and other intracranial skull base tumors.[10-14]

The increasing popularity of these endoscopic skull base approaches may be attributed to a larger trend towards more "minimally invasive" techniques across all surgical disciplines. The main advantage of transnasal endoscopic skull base approaches is providing more direct access to the anterior and central skull base while avoiding craniofacial incisions and extensive bone removal commonly used in open surgical approaches. Also, the wider angle of vision and angled lenses increases the range of the endoscopic visual surgical field compared with the "line of sight" visual field gained by surgical loupes or microscopes.

One major disadvantage of transnasal endoscopic approaches is the inability to provide watertight dural closure and reconstruction, which limits its safety and widespread adoption in surgery for intradural skull base tumors. Current techniques of endoscopic skull base reconstruction, such as tissue grafts, mucosal flaps and tissue sealants, provide adequate reconstruction of limited skull base defects such as a posttraumatic cerebrospinal fluid leak.[15,16] However, for larger dural defects, these endoscopic techniques have higher cerebrospinal fluid leak rates compared with traditional reconstructive techniques used in open surgery such as the vascularized pericranial flap.[10]

While the application of robotic technology to surgery has rapidly expanded over the last 5 years, one of the least studied but fertile areas for application of surgical robotics in the head and neck is for minimally invasive skull base surgery. Certain advantages that these novel systems offer are the ability to perform bimanual surgery in confined cavities with instrumentation that exceeds the capabilities of the human hand, providing the surgeon with a three-dimensional (3D) view of the surgical field. Significant advances in surgical robotics have been made,[17] although a role for robotic-based applications in skull base surgery has not been completely defined.

TECHNIQUES

Approach to the Anterior Cranial Fossa

The feasibility of using the surgical robot to access the anterior and central skull base was demonstrated by the authors in a cadaver model.[18] Caldwell-Luc incisions and wide anterior maxillary antrostomies, followed by wide middle meatal antrostomies are the entry points for the surgical arms (Fig. 11.1A). Sufficient access can be obtained without compromising the infraorbital nerves (Fig. 11.1B), and a posterior septectomy provides a common bilateral surgical field. The robotic endoscope is then placed into the patient's nare and the right and left surgical arms introduced through the respective maxillary sinus (Fig. 11.1C). Anterior and posterior ethmoidectomies are performed, and sphenoidotomies provide exposure to the planum sphenoidale, sella turcica and parasellar regions (Figs. 11.2A and B). Finally, access to the anterior cranial fossa is provided by sharp dissection of the anterior skull base and incision of the dura (Figs. 11.3A to C). The dual robotic arms can be used for primary repair of the dura.[19]

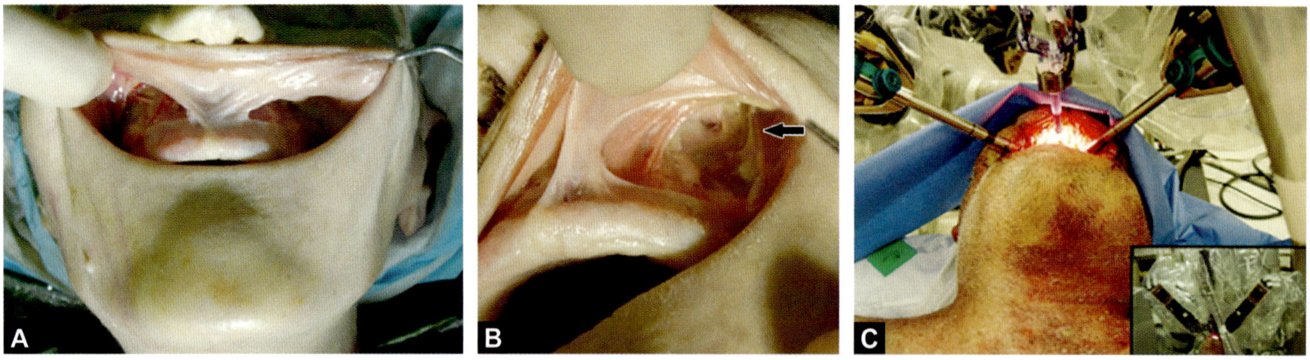

Figs. 11.1A to C: (A) Sublabial incisions with bilateral exposure of the face of the maxilla. (B) Identification and preservation of the infraorbital nerve (arrow). (C) Docking of the camera (C) and the robotic arms via maxillary antrostomies.

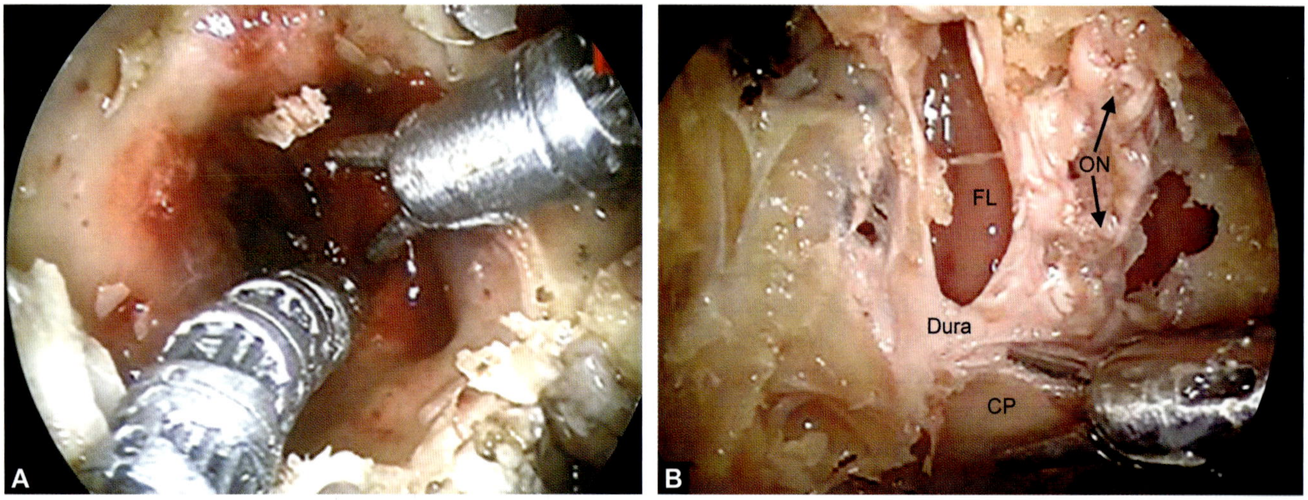

Figs. 11.2A and B: (A) Dissection of the posterior wall of the sphenoid sinus. (B) The cribriform plate (CP) is removed bilaterally, and the cut edges of the olfactory nerves (ON) are shown; the dura is incised or resected to expose the inferior surface of the frontal lobes (FL) intracranially.

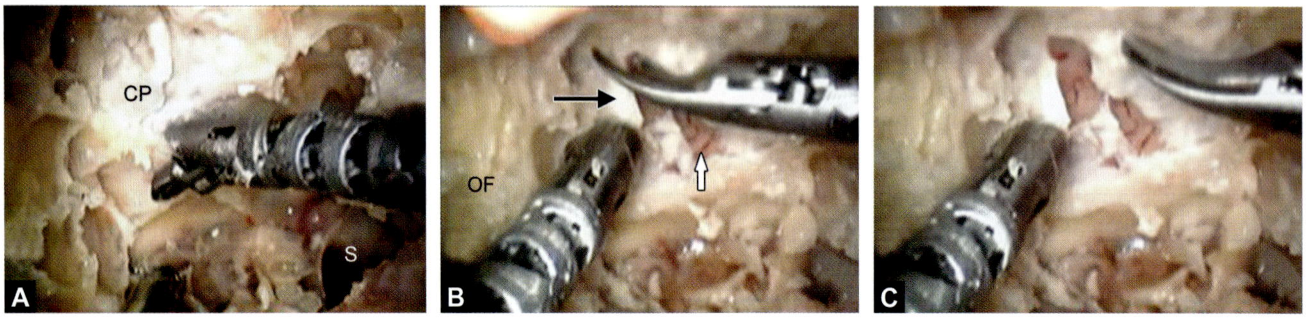

Figs. 11.3A to C: (A) Resection of the cribriform plate (CP) and (B and C) incision of the dura (black arrow) with the robotic instrumentation after complete exposure of medial orbital walls (OF-orbital fat) and sphenoid sinus (S). The frontal lobe is visible (white arrow).

This approach provides excellent access to the anterior and central skull base including the cribriform plate, fovea ethmoidalis, medial orbits, planum sphenoidale, nasopharynx, pterygopalatine fossa and clivus. The most significant advantage of this approach is the ability to perform two-handed tremor-free endoscopic closure of dural defects. To date, this approach remains investigational in nature.

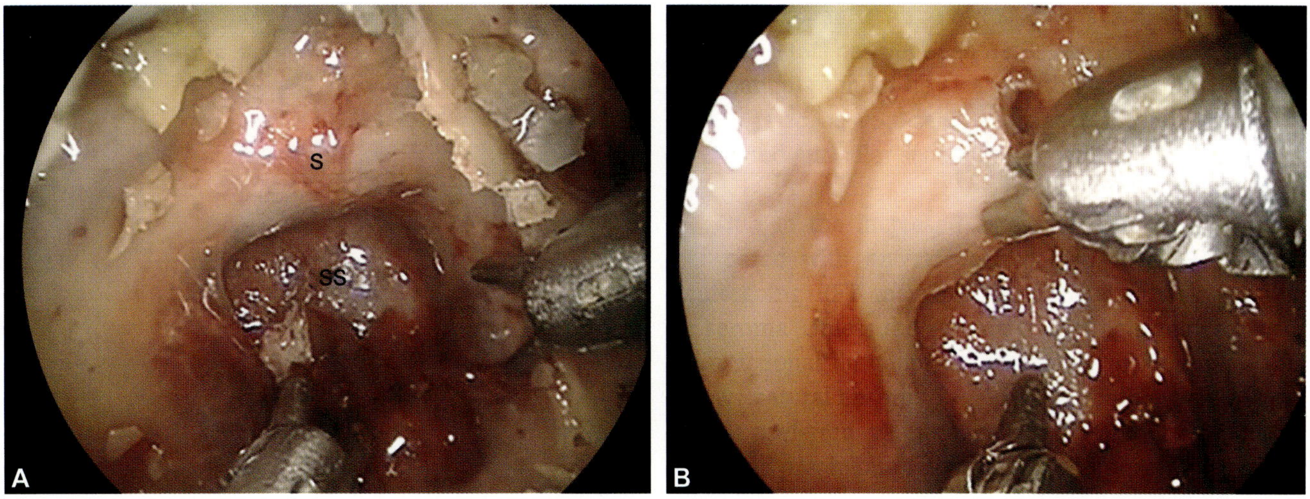

Figs. 11.4A and B: (A) Exposure of the anterior face of the sella (*S*-sella, *SS*-sphenoid sinus). (B) Entry into the pituitary fossa.

Approach to the Pituitary Fossa

While the transnasal endoscopic approach to the pituitary fossa has become a widely utilized technique for surgical resection,[20,21] robotic surgery in this anatomic location may provide unique advantages over the four-handed technique. The feasibility of a robotic approach to the pituitary fossa has been described by the authors, and remains investigational.[22]

Similar to the approach to the anterior cranial fossa, access involves creating bilateral maxillary antrostomies and docking the robotic arms and camera, as described above. An anterior sphenoidotomy is then performed, and the sellar floor removed to expose the dura of the pituitary fossa (Figs. 11.4A and B). The dura is opened sharply with the robotic scissors to allow for exploration of the pituitary gland (Fig. 11.5A). Blunt and sharp dissection may then be performed to excise the pituitary gland after the optic chiasm and hypothalamus are exposed (Fig. 11.5B). Dissection of the lateral wall of the sphenoid sinus may also be performed with high-speed drills and fine rongeurs to access the cavernous sinus. Using this technique access to the central skull base, including the planum sphenoidale, the pituitary gland, cavernous carotid, mammillary bodies and optic chiasm can be achieved (Fig. 11.5C).

The transcervical approach to the skull base in canine and cadaver models has been previously described. Access to the sphenoid, clivus, sella and suprasellar anterior fossa is achieved by placing a 30° robotic endoscope transorally and placing the right and left robotic arms through the lateral pharyngeal walls via a transcervical technique, posterior to the submandibular gland.[23]

Approach to the Nasopharynx

Robotic surgery of the nasopharynx is perhaps the only anatomic site of the skull base that is most amenable to surgical dissection with current iterations of surgical robotics. The feasibility of robotic resection of nasopharyngeal lesions in a cadaver was first described in 2008,[24] and subsequent case reports of surgical management of nasopharyngeal cancers have been published in the literature.[25]

A Dingman retractor is utilized to expose the oral cavity, and the soft palate is divided under direct visualization—lateral retraction of the divided palate is achieved with Vicryl suture (Fig. 11.6A). The da Vinci robot is then docked at the head of the bed, and the robotic arms are positioned into the oral cavity. Typically a 30° endoscope providing a superiorly oriented view of the oropharynx and nasopharynx is utilized. Using the grasper and the spatula cautery, the nasopharynx soft tissue may then be progressively degloved (Fig. 11.6B) between the carotid arteries and Eustachian tubes (Fig. 11.6C) laterally and the skull base and prevertebral musculature posteriorly. Once the tumor is resected, the palate is closed in three layers with absorbable suture. The advantage of this technique is that it allows for en bloc excision of nasopharyngeal lesions, and may offer the advantage of decreased morbidity compared to either reirradiation or open surgical approaches for recurrent nasopharyngeal carcinoma. Further study is necessary to delineate the optimal surgical indications.

Approach to the Infratemporal Fossa

Both preclinical studies and case reports addressing the infratemporal fossa and parapharyngeal space via robotic

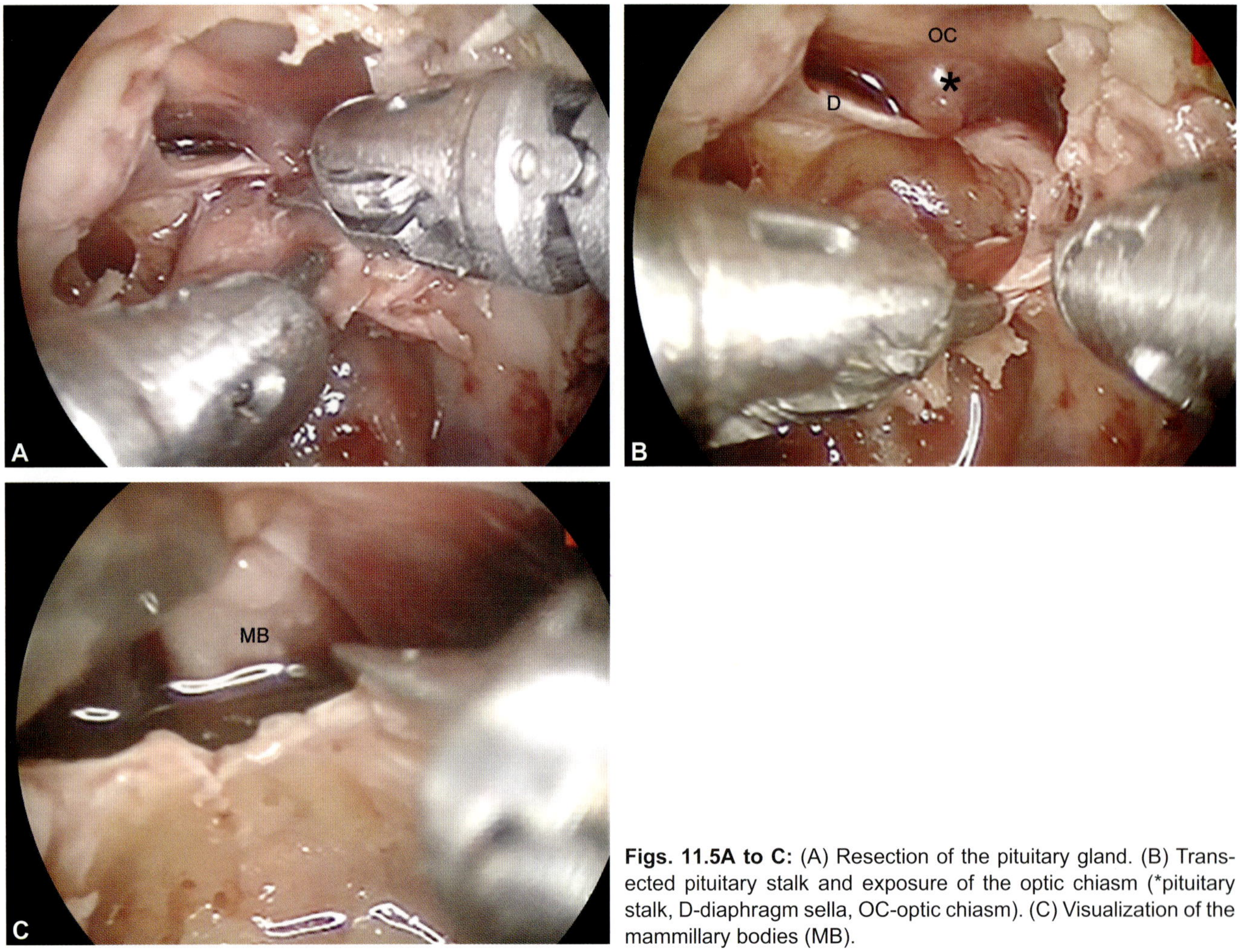

Figs. 11.5A to C: (A) Resection of the pituitary gland. (B) Transected pituitary stalk and exposure of the optic chiasm (*pituitary stalk, D-diaphragm sella, OC-optic chiasm). (C) Visualization of the mammillary bodies (MB).

approaches have been described.[26,27] Dissection is performed through the lateral pharyngeal wall to access the parapharyngeal space. Using the 30° endoscope directed superiorly, the parapharyngeal space can be carefully explored to identify the neurovascular contents—jugular vein, internal carotid and cranial nerve (CN) IX, X, XI and XII. To gain exposure superiorly and laterally (to the infratemporal fossa) the styloid musculature can be resected and pterygoid muscles partially released. This approach may be best suited for well-circumscribed benign lesions.

SKULL BASE RECONSTRUCTION

Perhaps the most significant limitation of current transnasal endoscopic techniques is the inability to reconstruct dural defects with a sutured watertight dural closure. Options for repair of the skull base include free mucosal grafts, fascia lata grafts, pedicled mucosal grafts and biological materials.[15,16,28-30] While each has advantages and disadvantages, only the pedicled mucoperiosteal grafts are vascularized,[31] a necessary component of any reconstruction in patients undergoing postoperative irradiation, or in previously irradiated patients. One of the major drawbacks of the endoscopic approach is the inability to perform a suture-based reconstruction of the dura using currently available technology, an approach that is easily undertaken with a pericranial flap through the transcranial approach. We previously reported the feasibility of an endonasal robotic surgical dural reconstruction to address this problem in skull base surgery.

Repair of the skull base defect can be performed robotically with two distinct techniques. First, repair of the dura may be primarily reconstructed with both continuous and interrupted suture techniques (Fig. 11.7A). Additionally, harvested sinonasal mucoperiosteal graft can be sutured

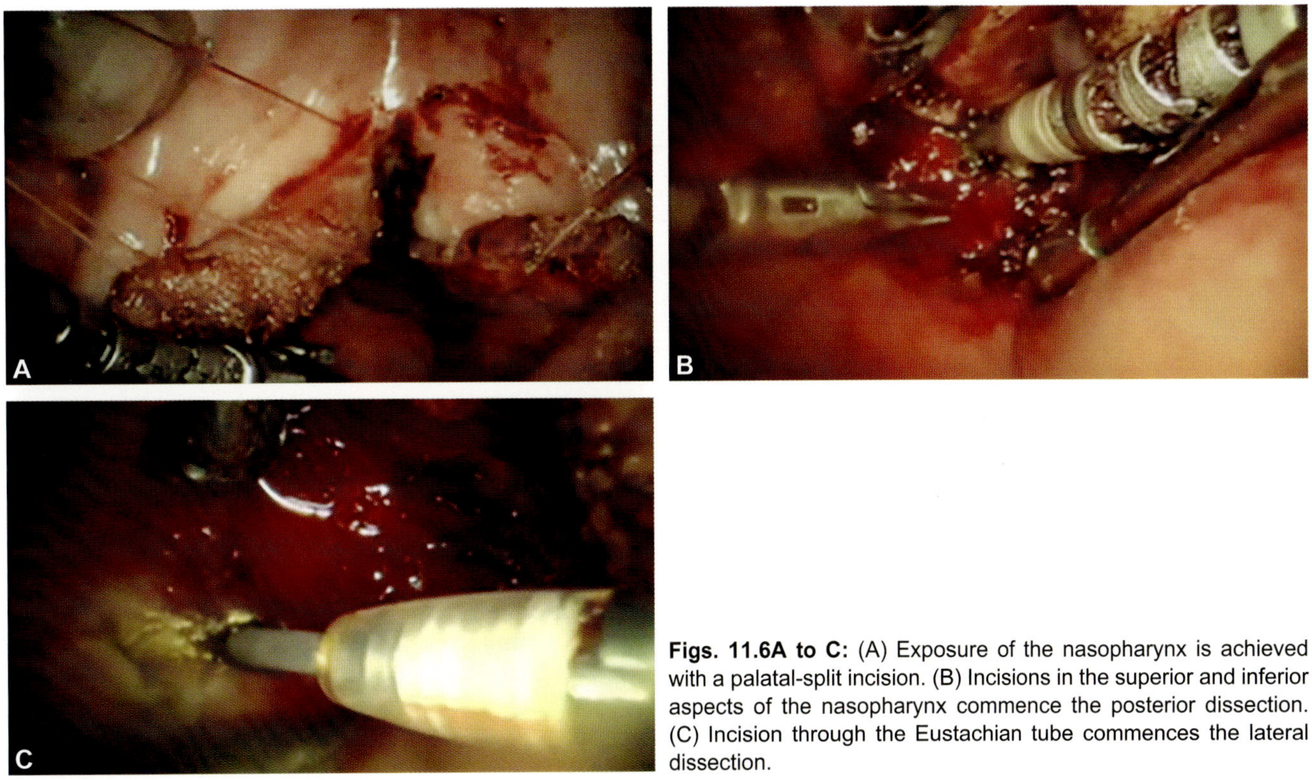

Figs. 11.6A to C: (A) Exposure of the nasopharynx is achieved with a palatal-split incision. (B) Incisions in the superior and inferior aspects of the nasopharynx commence the posterior dissection. (C) Incision through the Eustachian tube commences the lateral dissection.

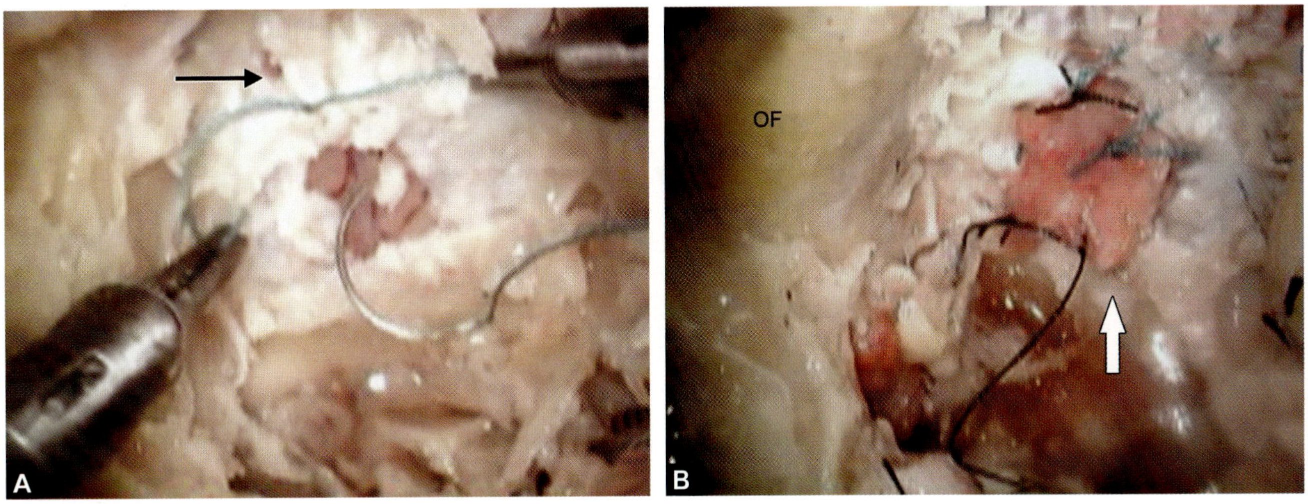

Figs. 11.7A and B: (A) Primary repair of a dural defect (arrow) with polyglactin suture (Ethicon). (B) Repair of a large dural defect with a mucosal graft (white arrow).

into dural defects with both running and interrupted suture techniques (Fig. 11.7B). While these techniques have been demonstrated in cadaver models, their application in human use has yet to be realized.

A balanced analysis of where robotic surgery may lie on the spectrum of surgical modalities suggests that robotic assisted skull base surgery offers unique advantages that are lacking in either microscopic or transnasal endoscopic techniques. These can be divided in four major areas: optical, ergonomic, dissection and reconstructive. The following is a discussion of how endoscopic robotic surgery can overcome some of the limitations of these other techniques, and where robotic surgery has limitations.

OPTICAL LIMITATIONS

The two-dimensional visualization provided by single channel optical systems in current endoscopes lacks the depth perception of 3D vision provided by the binocular optical systems used in standard microsurgery. During endoscopic surgery, depth perception relies more on tactile than on visual cues. Visual depth perception is particularly important when operating on critical intracranial neurovascular structures, especially when working in a deep and limited space. The 5-mm robotic endoscope has a dual channel optical system coupled with a dual charge-coupled device, which allows for 3D visualization of the surgical field at the surgeon's console. This "binocular endoscope" allows the surgeon to have the combined benefit of a wider angle of vision and the depth perception of 3D visualization.

ERGONOMIC LIMITATIONS

Current endoscopic techniques have several ergonomic limitations. Bimanual surgery is only feasible if the endoscope is held by an assistant or a mechanical holder. A surgical assistant is preferred because of the constant need to adjust the position (depth and angle) of the endoscope during endoscopic surgery. This not only limits the direct control of the endoscope by the primary surgeon but also requires the assistance of a relatively experienced endoscopic surgeon who can seamlessly follow the primary surgeon in every step of the operation.

Also, both surgeons have to work within the confined space provided by the nostrils, which in some cases limits ergonomic freedom. In addition, as the surgical field gets deeper, longer instruments are needed and, with lack of proper arm support, precision may be limited by fine tremor, especially when using fine instrumentation for delicate dissection of critical neurovascular structures. The robotic system has four arms, all of which are controlled by the primary surgeon sitting at the console. One arm, the camera port, holds the endoscope; two arms hold right and left hand instruments; and a fourth "spare" arm may be dedicated for retraction or a third instrument. This allows the primary surgeon simultaneous direct control of the endoscope and the instrumentation, an advantage not feasible with nonrobotic endoscopic techniques. Another advantage of the "endowrist" technology used in the da Vinci robotic instrumentation is its ability to provide movement at the instrument tip with 7° of freedom and 90° of articulation and motion scaling. This allows the surgeon, who sits comfortably at the console with an adjustable arm, support to perform precise tremor-free movement in a deep and confined space, with working angles usually not achievable with nonrobotic instruments.

DISSECTION LIMITATIONS

In its current iteration, the da Vinci robotic system is designed exclusively for soft tissue surgery, while the paranasal sinuses and skull base are bony anatomic structures. Access to tumors in these domains requires bone-cutting instrumentation, including rongeurs, osteotomes and drills. The exquisitely tuned internal pulley system within the robotic arms is not engineered for the stress forces that bony dissection requires. In our experience, use of the robotic dissecting instruments led to rapid deterioration in the functionality and life span of the equipment (unpublished data). Further optimization of the robotic arms will be required before skull-base surgery can be effectively performed with the novel technology.

RECONSTRUCTIVE LIMITATIONS

The most significant limitation of current transnasal endoscopic techniques is the inability to suture and provide watertight dural closure or reconstruction of dural defects. Endoscopic repair of dural defects relies on nonvascularized fat, mucosal, or allogeneic grafts, or vascularized septal or nasal rotational mucosal flaps. These reconstructions are then covered with fibrin sealants and supported by either absorbable or nonabsorbable packing. While these methods may provide adequate reconstruction of minor dural tears or defects, their ability to provide safe and reliable reconstruction of larger dural defects remains to be seen. Preliminary results suggest that these methods have a higher cerebrospinal fluid leak rate compared with the more standard dural reconstruction using pedicled (axial) flaps, such as the pericranial flap or microvascular free flaps. Adequate and reliable dural reconstruction is critical in minimizing the morbidity of skull base resections, particularly in patients who received or will undergo high-dose radiation therapy. As described above, robotic-assisted surgery allows for successful and precise endoscopic suturing of the dura. This may drastically impact the utility and safety of endoscopic surgery of intracranial intradural lesions of the skull base.

CONCLUSION

While still in the developmental stages, robotic applications to skull base surgery are forthcoming. Transantral robotic surgery provides stereoscopic endoscopic access to the anterior skull base and pituitary fossa, and allows for two-handed endoscopic manipulation and reconstruction. Traditional suture and reconstructive techniques can be implemented in this confined surgical site with the use of robotic technology. These advantages may expand the indications of minimally invasive endoscopic approaches to the skull base. Future development and refinement of endonasal robotic instrumentation is critical before applying these techniques in the clinical setting.

REFERENCES

1. Hanna E, DeMonte F, Ibrahim S, et al. Endoscopic resection of sinonasal cancers with and without craniotomy: oncologic results. Arch Otolaryngol Head Neck Surg. 2009; 135(12):1219-24.
2. Lund V, Howard DJ, Wei WI. Endoscopic resection of malignant tumors of the nose and sinuses. Am J Rhinol. 2007;21(1):89-94.
3. Nicolai P, Battaglia P, Bignami M, et al. Endoscopic surgery for malignant tumors of the sinonasal tract and adjacent skull base: a 10-year experience. Am J Rhinol. 2008; 22(3):308-16.
4. Suriano M, De Vincentiis M, Colli A, et al. Endoscopic treatment of esthesioneuroblastoma: a minimally invasive approach combined with radiation therapy. Otolaryngol Head Neck Surg. 2007;136(1):104-7.
5. Shipchandler TZ, Batra PS, Citardi MJ, et al. Outcomes for endoscopic resection of sinonasal squamous cell carcinoma. Laryngoscope. 2005;115(11):1983-7.
6. Anand VK, Schwartz TH, Hiltzik DH, et al. Endoscopic transphenoidal pituitary surgery with real-time intraoperative magnetic resonance imaging. Am J Rhinol. 2006;20(4): 401-5.
7. Schwartz TH, Stieg PE, Anand VK. Endoscopic transsphenoidal pituitary surgery with intraoperative magnetic resonance imaging. Neurosurgery. 2006;58(1 Suppl):ONS44-51; discussion ONS44-51.
8. Sethi DS, Leong JL. Endoscopic pituitary surgery. Otolaryngol Clin North Am. 2006;39(3):563-83, x.
9. Teo C. Application of endoscopy to the surgical management of craniopharyngiomas. Childs Nerv Syst. 2005;21 (8-9):696-700.
10. Kassam A, Carrau RL, Snyderman CH, et al. Evolution of reconstructive techniques following endoscopic expanded endonasal approaches. Neurosurg Focus. 2005;19(1):E8.
11. Kassam A, Snyderman CH, Mintz A, et al. Expanded endonasal approach: the rostrocaudal axis. Part I. Crista galli to the sella turcica. Neurosurg Focus. 2005;19(1):E3.
12. Kassam AB, Gardner P, Snyderman C, et al. Expanded endonasal approach: fully endoscopic, completely transnasal approach to the middle third of the clivus, petrous bone, middle cranial fossa, and infratemporal fossa. Neurosurg Focus. 2005;19(1):E6.
13. Kassam AB, Snyderman C, Gardner P, et al. The expanded endonasal approach: a fully endoscopic transnasal approach and resection of the odontoid process: technical case report. Neurosurgery. 2005;57(1 Suppl):E213; discussion E213.
14. Solari D, Magro F, Cappabianca P, et al. Anatomical study of the pterygopalatine fossa using an endoscopic endonasal approach: spatial relations and distances between surgical landmarks. J Neurosurg. 2007;106(1):157-63.
15. Basu D, Haughey BH, Hartman JM. Determinants of success in endoscopic cerebrospinal fluid leak repair. Otolaryngol Head Neck Surg. 2006;135(5):769-73.
16. Locatelli D, Rampa F, Acchiardi I, et al. Endoscopic endonasal approaches for repair of cerebrospinal fluid leaks: nine-year experience. Neurosurgery. 2006;58(4 Suppl 2):ONS-246-256; discussiom ONS-256-247.
17. Weinstein GS, O'Malley BW, Jr, Snyder W, et al. Transoral robotic surgery: supraglottic partial laryngectomy. Ann Otol Rhinol Laryngol. 2007;116(1):19-23.
18. Hanna EY, Holsinger C, DeMonte F, et al. Robotic endoscopic surgery of the skull base: a novel surgical approach. Arch Otolaryngol Head Neck Surg. 2007;133(12):1209-14.
19. Kupferman ME, Demonte F, Levine N, et al. Feasibility of a robotic surgical approach to reconstruct the skull base. Skull base. 2011;21(2):79-82.
20. Cappabianca P, Cavallo LM, de Divitiis O, et al. Endoscopic pituitary surgery. Pituitary. 2008;11(4):385-90.
21. Liu JK, Weiss MH, Couldwell WT. Surgical approaches to pituitary tumors. Neurosurg Clin N Am. 2003;14(1):93-107.
22. Kupferman M, Demonte F, Holsinger FC, et al. Transantral robotic access to the pituitary gland. Otolaryngol Head Neck Surg. 2009;141(3):413-5.
23. O'Malley BW, Jr, Weinstein GS. Robotic anterior and midline skull base surgery: preclinical investigations. Int J Radiat Oncol Biol Phys. 2007;69(2 Suppl):S125-8.
24. Ozer E, Waltonen J. Transoral robotic nasopharyngectomy: a novel approach for nasopharyngeal lesions. Laryngoscope. 2008;118(9):1613-6.
25. Wei WI, Ho WK. Transoral robotic resection of recurrent nasopharyngeal carcinoma. Laryngoscope. 2010;120(10): 2011-4.
26. McCool RR, Warren FM, Wiggins RH, 3rd, et al. Robotic surgery of the infratemporal fossa utilizing novel suprahyoid port. Laryngoscope. 2010;120(9):1738-43.
27. O'Malley BW, Jr, Weinstein GS. Robotic skull base surgery: preclinical investigations to human clinical application. Arch Otolaryngol Head Neck Surg. 2007;133(12):1215-9.

28. Hadad G, Bassagasteguy L, Carrau RL, et al. A novel reconstructive technique after endoscopic expanded endonasal approaches: vascular pedicle nasoseptal flap. Laryngoscope. 2006;116(10):1882-6.
29. Leong JL, Citardi MJ, Batra PS. Reconstruction of skull base defects after minimally invasive endoscopic resection of anterior skull base neoplasms. Am J Rhinol. 2006;20(5):476-82.
30. Mehta RP, Cueva RA, Brown JD, et al. What's new in skull base medicine and surgery? Skull Base Committee Report. Otolaryngol Head Neck Surg. 2006;135(4):620-30.
31. Kassam AB, Thomas A, Carrau RL, et al. Endoscopic reconstruction of the cranial base using a pedicled nasoseptal flap. Neurosurgery. 2008;63(1 Suppl 1):ONS44-ONS53.

Chapter 12 Robotic-Assisted Surgery for Nasopharyngeal Tumors

Raymond K Tsang, William I Wei

INTRODUCTION

The nasopharynx has traditionally been considered a difficult place for surgical access. The nasopharynx is situated in the center of the skull and bounded by bony structures on all sides except the inferior aspect where it connects to the oropharynx. Multiple surgical approaches to the nasopharynx have been devised, including the inferior approach with palatal split[1] with or without mandibular split:[2] an anterior approach with a midfacial degloving operation, an anterolateral approach with the maxillary swing[3] and a lateral approach with the infratemporal fossa approach.[4] All these approaches require a facial incision and osteotomy of the facial skeleton, with their associated morbidities.

The advent of endoscopic sinus surgery allowed minimally invasive operations to be performed in the paranasal sinuses and subsequently within the nasopharynx. Endoscopic operations in the nasopharynx, however, are not without difficulties. The nasal cavity and the nasopharynx are confined spaces, making manipulation of instruments for en bloc resection of lesions difficult. Moreover, triangulation of instruments for traction and countertraction can be very awkward, as the bony walls allow minimal lateral movements of the instruments. There are reports of endoscopic nasopharyngectomy for resection of nasopharyngeal carcinomas (NPCs) in the literature, but these have been for small tumors located in the nasopharynx with minimal lateral extension.[5] The pterygoid plates that form the lateral boundaries of the anterior nasopharynx can block the view and limit instrument movements in endoscopic nasopharyngectomy. In order to circumvent these obstacles, an endoscopic transpterygoid approach for nasopharyngectomy has been devised.[6] This approach removed the pterygoid plates and medial maxillary wall to allow visualization and instrumentation of the lateral nasopharyngeal wall. This operation has not been popular, as it requires a significant amount of bone work by a team of skillful endoscopic sinus surgeons before gaining full access to the nasopharynx.

The surgical robot has two distinct advantages in performing minimally invasive surgery. First, the surgical robot has a three-dimensional (3D) magnified view that allows the surgeon to visualize the anatomy and pathology with unprecedented clarity. Second, the wristed instrument arms of the robot can allow complex maneuvers in multiple planes to be performed in a very tight space. These two distinct advantages are especially useful in operations within a confined space such as the nasopharynx.

RATIONALE FOR PROCEDURE

Cancers of the nasopharynx are primarily treated with external beam radiation with or without concurrent chemotherapy. The endemic type of NPC in Southern China is especially sensitive to radiation. Local failure after primary radiotherapy for NPC has been shown to be low as noted in one large-scale review that demonstrated a local failure rate of 12%.[7] Patients who received curative treatment for the recurrent NPC, however, have an improved survival than those who had not received curative treatment.[8] Curative treatment for local failure of NPC after radiotherapy can be in the form of reirradiation or salvage surgery. Significant morbidities can occur in patients receiving reirradiation, including osteonecrosis, cranial nerve palsies and tissue fibrosis. The efficacy of reirradiation has also been questioned, as there may be radio-resistant clones of tumor cells in the recurrent tumor.[9]

Open nasopharyngectomy has been shown to be an efficacious treatment for recurrent NPC. From the largest case series in the literature, the 5-year actuarial local control rate was 74% and 5-year disease free survival was 56%. The factors affecting local control and survival were negative resection margin and tumor size smaller than 1.5 cm.[10] Another smaller study also showed superior results in 5-year survival in patients with clear margins compared to those patients with close margins or positive margins.[11] Therefore, for open nasopharyngectomy, the goal is to achieve an en bloc complete resection of the tumor with an adequate margin and thus a similar goal should be attained in robotic nasopharyngectomy. Piecemeal excision or a debulking type of surgery would risk incomplete excision and latter recurrence.

Nasopharyngeal carcinoma frequently arises from the fossa of Rosenmüller, which is located in the posterolateral part of the nasopharynx, posterior to the Eustachian tube cushion.[12] Tumors in the fossa of Rosenmüller have been shown to frequently invade the Eustachian tube cartilage.[13] Therefore, for tumors that involve the fossa of Rosenmüller, the ipsilateral Eustachian tube cartilage should be removed. An anterolateral approach such as the maxillary swing operation offers better access to the lateral nasopharyngeal wall, Eustachian tube cartilage and parapharyngeal space than an anterior approach. One retrospective nonrandomized study showed that the maxillary swing approach had a superior survival rate and local control rate compared to the midfacial degloving approach in recurrent T1 and T2 tumors.[14] Therefore, in robotic nasopharyngectomy, the resection technique of the tumor in the nasopharynx should emulate open nasopharyngectomy by the maxillary swing approach in order to achieve similar oncological results. This robot-assisted operation provides exposure and instrumentation without the need for retracting the midface and maxillary sinus laterally.

APPLIED ANATOMY

The nasopharynx is a box-shaped cavity situated behind the nasal cavity approximately 10 cm posterior to the nostril. The lateral and posterior walls are composed of an outer fibrous layer, a middle muscular layer and an inner mucosal layer. The roof of the nasopharynx is the basisphenoid bone anteriorly and the clivus bone posteriorly. The anterior part of the nasopharynx communicates with the nasal cavity via the posterior choana and the inferior wall of the nasopharynx is absent and freely communicates with the oropharynx. The lower limit of the nasopharynx is defined as the level of the soft palate.

The outer fascial wall of the nasopharynx is formed by the pharyngobasilar fascia. This fascia attaches to the medial pterygoid plate anteriorly. The superior constrictor muscles form the muscular layer of the lateral and posterior nasopharyngeal wall.

The Eustachian tube openings pierce the lateral wall of the nasopharynx on both sides. A recess is formed by the posterior crus of the Eustachian tube and the posterior wall of the nasopharynx. This recess is called the fossa of Rosenmüller or lateral pharyngeal recess. Nasopharyngeal carcinoma frequently arises from the mucosa of the fossa of Rosenmüller and can invade the cartilage of the Eustachian tube. This causes dysfunction of the Eustachian tube and ipsilateral otitis media with effusion. Visualization of the extent of the tumor in the fossa of the Rosenmüller can be difficult during operation and the ipsilateral cartilaginous Eustachian tube should be resected en bloc with the tumor unless the tumor is distant from the fossa of the Rosenmüller.

The parapharyngeal space abuts the lateral wall of the nasopharynx and tumors frequently spread into this space. Anterior to the parapharyngeal space, the medial pterygoid muscle abuts the anterior part of the lateral wall of the nasopharynx. A venous plexus, the pharyngeal plexus, drains through the medial pterygoid muscle and the parapharyngeal space. Significant venous bleeding can occur during dissection in this area.

The internal carotid artery (ICA) is situated posterolateral to the fossa of Rosenmüller. A separate fascia, the carotid sheath, wraps the ICA. The distance of the fossa of Rosenmüller and the ICA can be variable. In cases of an ectatic ICA, this vessel can abut the fossa of Rosenmüller. These patients may not be suitable candidates for robotic nasopharyngectomy as there is a risk of accidental exposure and injury to this vessel.

The pterygoid plates form the anterior boundary of the parapharyngeal space in the nasopharynx. This bony structure limits the lateral reach of robotic instruments. Unfortunately, current robotic instruments lack the tools for bone removal. Unless an alternative method is employed to remove the pterygoid plates, it is difficult to resect tissues lateral to the lateral pterygoid plates.

INDICATIONS AND CONTRAINDICATIONS

Indications

- Local recurrence of NPC after radiotherapy
- Primary surgery for malignant salivary gland tumors in the nasopharynx
- Other benign tumors within the nasopharynx.

Characteristics of the Tumor

- Small centrally located tumors. Invasion to the sphenoid floor is not a contraindication
- Tumors with minimal parapharyngeal space invasion
- The lateral extent of the tumor should not be more lateral than the lateral pterygoid plate
- Tumor should be at least 1 cm away from the ICA

- Minimal clivus invasion
- Tumors with invasion of cartilaginous part of the Eustachian tube or prevertebral muscles are not contraindicated.

Contraindications

- Large tumor with skull base or gross clivus invasion
- Tumor abutting or close to the ICA
- Presence of retropharyngeal lymph node metastasis
  - The retropharyngeal lymph nodes are usually situated proximal to the internal carotid artery. In cases of recurrence after radiotherapy, it can be difficult to locate the lymph nodes within the fibrous tissue risking injury to the ICA.
- Tumor involvement of the pterygomaxillary fissure or ethmoid sinuses
  - Current robotic instruments cannot remove bone
- Patients with trismus
  - Unable to open mouth for transoral procedure
- Patients with a narrow velopharyngeal airway with the hard palate close to the posterior wall of the nasopharynx
  - Inadequate room for robotic arm movement.

PREOPERATIVE WORKUP

The extent of the local tumor needs to be determined with cross-sectional imaging to assess the suitability for robotic nasopharyngectomy. A contrast enhanced magnetic resonance imaging (MRI) is preferred as MRI provides superior soft tissue contrast at the skull base. A contrast computed tomography (CT) scan is helpful to delineate the extent of bony invasion in cases where invasion into the sphenoid or clivus are suspected. A positron emission tomography-computed tomography (PET-CT) scan is also helpful to differentiate post-treatment changes with recurrent tumor.

An endoscopy of the nasal cavities and the nasopharynx is complementary to imaging for assessment as the mucosal extent of the tumor is better determined by endoscopy. Involvement of the Eustachian tube opening is also better identified on endoscopy. Patients with tumors extending into the nasal cavity, sphenoethmoidal recess or sphenoid sinus would need additional transnasal endoscopic procedures for complete removal of the tumors.

For malignant disease, the patient should also be evaluated for the presence of nodal metastasis. We prefer an ultrasound of the neck with or without fine needle aspiration to assess for nodal metastasis. Cross-sectional imaging such as CT or MRI and functional imaging such as PET-CT scans are also helpful in determining the presence of nodal metastasis. If nodal metastases are present, a neck dissection is required, either at the same time as the robotic nasopharyngectomy or at another separate session.

The patient requires clinical assessment of the upper aerodigestive tract with special attention to the presence of trismus or if the patient has a large tongue as both conditions could impede the transoral approach to the nasopharynx. The patient should have a dental gap of more than 3 cm for successful transoral robotic surgery. The distance of the hard palate to the posterior wall of the nasopharynx should also be assessed. If the distance is too narrow, it may not provide enough room for the movements of the robotic arm. The elevation of the soft palate and the presence of velopharyngeal incompetence should also be assessed. Patients with impaired elevation of the soft palate should be warned that the velopharyngeal incompetence could increase after robotic nasopharyngectomy.

Many patients after nasopharyngectomy suffer from otitis media with effusion. Preoperative otoscopic assessment of the ears and audiological assessment of hearing will be beneficial for counseling and planning of postoperative treatment of hearing dysfunction.

INSTRUMENTATION

Robotic nasopharyngectomy is performed transorally and usually soft tissue dissection including splitting the soft palate is required to facilitate exposure of the nasopharynx. A mouth gag is required to open the mouth and depress the tongue. A Boyle Davis gag or Dingman mouth retractor can be used. The mouth gag needs to be supported with a Mayo table or a Unitrac (Aesculap, Braun, Center Valley, PA) retractor holder secured to the operating table.

Robotic nasopharyngectomy is performed with two robotic arms and one camera arm for operation. All models of the da Vinci surgical robot (Intuitive Surgical, Inc., Sunnyvale, CA) can be used for robotic nasopharyngectomy although the da Vinci Si HD with the high definition camera provides better visualization of the surgical site.

Either the 8-mm or 12-mm binocular telescope can be used. A 12-mm telescope is preferable as it offers a better illumination and brighter images. Both 0° and 30° telescopes can be used depending on the surgeon's preference. The 0° telescope offers a view more in line with the robotic instruments. Alternatively, after turning the scope towards one side, the 30° telescope allows better visualization of the lateral wall of the nasopharynx and the parapharyngeal space. The surgeon can alternate the telescopes during the operation depending on the part of the dissection that is being performed.

Dissection instruments include a 5-mm Maryland retractor mounted on one robotic arm for tissue retraction. For dissection, either a 5-mm monopolar cautery or an 8-mm bipolar scissors can be used. For patients with a very narrow nasopharynx, one will need to use 5-mm instruments for dissection with an 8-mm telescope. Alternative energy sources for hemostasis and dissection such as ultrasonic dissectors are too bulky to be used within the nasopharynx so cautery remains the choice for hemostasis and dissection.

The bedside surgeon will need additional suction devices, bipolar diathermy and endoscopic clip applicator for smoke evacuation and assistance in hemostasis, respectively. Occasionally, the bedside surgeon may need to assist in retraction of the specimen by passing an endoscopic ethmoidal biopsy forcep transnasally to lift the specimen.

OPERATIVE SETUP AND OPERATIVE TECHNIQUE

Patient Placement

The operation is performed under general anesthesia with the patient lying supine intubated with an oral Rae endotracheal tube or a nonkinking endotracheal tube. The endotracheal tube should be taped to the lower lip at the midline with the blade of the mouth gag placed over it. The patient can be tilted head up 10° to decrease the venous pressure and allow more room for the camera arm to move. A plastic suction catheter connected to suction can be placed in the posterior choana of contralateral side of the tumor for smoke evacuation.

Palatal Split and Exposure of the Nasopharynx

The surgeon can now apply the mouth gag to depress the tongue and open the mouth. Care must be taken not to compress the endotracheal tube and prevent ventilation. The next step is to perform splitting of the soft palate to facilitate exposure of the nasopharynx. The soft palate can be split in the midline or on the side of the tumor. For a midline palatal split, an incision is placed from the uvula to the hard palate in the midline, ending just posterior to the incisor foramen. The medial part of the soft palate is detached from the hard palate on both sides. Stay sutures are then placed over the incised edge of the soft palate to retract the soft palate laterally.[15] If the posterior edge of the hard palate is blocking the view to the roof of the nasopharynx, a 1 cm area of bone can be removed with a rongeur. Care must be taken not to remove too much bone in the posterior edge of the hard palate as this may increase the risk of palatal fistula formation. Figures 12.1A and B show the incision of the midline palate split and Figure 12.2 shows the view of the nasopharynx with the tumor from the telescope after the midline palatal split (12.1).

For the lateral palatal flap approach, an incision is made from the incisive foramen towards the ipsilateral medial upper alveolus mucosa, passing through the greater palatine foramen, splitting the soft palate laterally and ending in the upper pole of the tonsil.[16] The greater palatine vessels are ligated and divided. The hard palate mucosa with the periosteum is elevated from the underlying bone just beyond midline. The soft palate is detached from the hard palate with cautery just beyond midline. Care must be taken not to damage the contralateral greater palatine vessels as they are the sole blood supply to the palatal mucosa flap. The palatal flap is then retracted to the contralateral side with stay sutures. The benefit of the lateral palatal flap approach is that it offers better exposure and instrument reach of the ipsilateral lateral nasopharyngeal wall and parapharyngeal space. The disadvantage is that the ipsilateral blood supply to the palate is sacrificed with slightly increased difficulty in closure of the palatal incision. Figures 12.1A and B show the incision of the lateral palatal flap approach and Figure 12.2 shows the view of the nasopharynx from the telescope (12.1).

Hemostasis to the palatal wound edge should be achieved at the conclusion of the palate split procedure. The operative field is then irrigated with normal saline and is ready for the robotic part of the operation.

Docking of the Patient Cart

After draping the surgical robot, the patient cart is docked from the head end of the patient. The robot should not be too close to the head end of the operating table to allow more room for the robot arms to move. The bedside surgeon sits on the side of the patient, facing the head. A video monitor is placed next to the robot for the bedside surgeon to observe and assist in the procedure. The scrub nurse sits next to the bedside surgeon facing the bedside surgeon and hands the instruments to the bedside surgeon. Another monitor at the foot end of the operating table allows the scrub nurse to observe the operation. Figure 12.2 shows the setup.

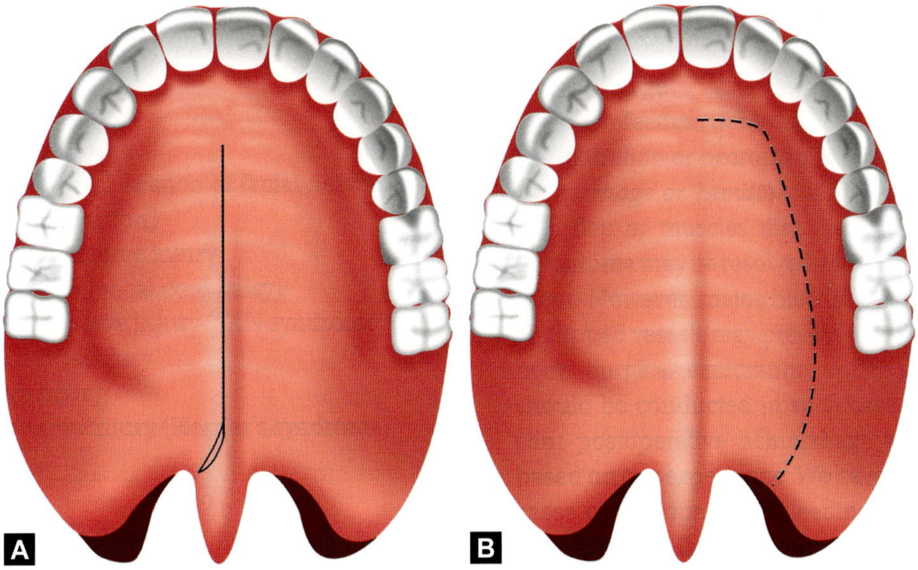

Figs. 12.1A and B: (A) Diagram illustrating the incision for midline palatal split. (B) Diagram illustrating the incision for a left side lateral palatal flap.

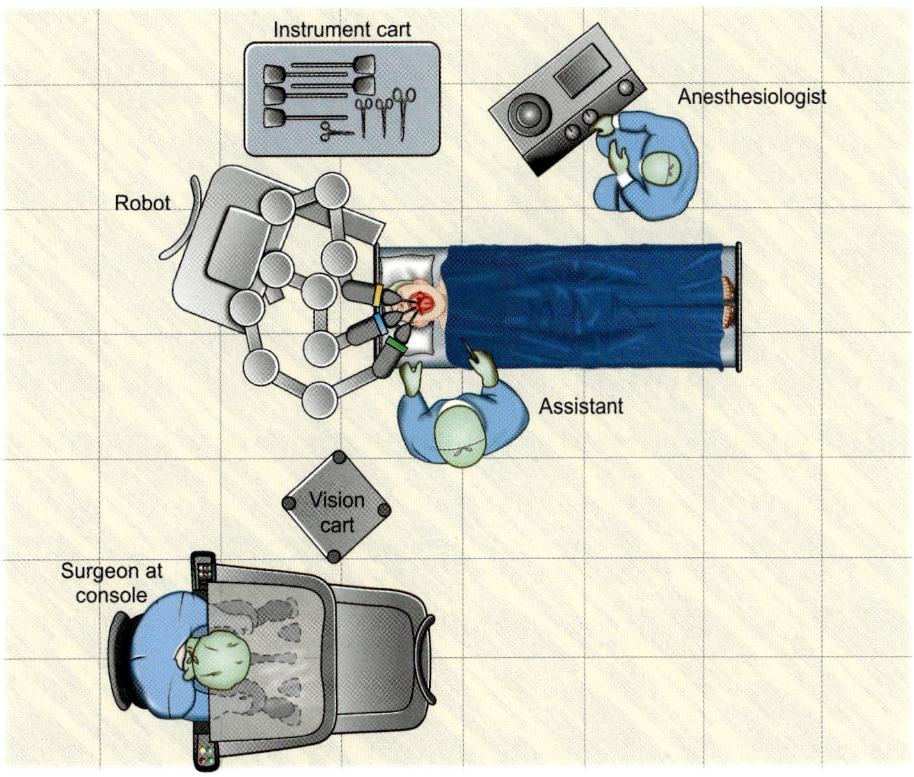

Fig. 12.2: Operating room layout for transoral robotic surgery nasopharyngectomy.

Operative Techniques at the Console

The console surgeon identifies the pathology and then marks the resection limits with a margin of 1.5 cm around the periphery of the tumor with index cuts using cautery (🎥 12.1). For lesions not involving the ipsilateral fossa of Rosenmüller, the medial crus of the Eustachian tube should be included in the resection. For lesions epicentered at the fossa of Rosenmüller, the whole ipsilateral Eustachian tube cartilage should be removed.

For the midline palatal split approach, the dissection starts inferiorly. The inferior resection margin is incised down to the prevertebral muscles. Depending on the depth of the tumor from imaging, the incision can be carried down through the prevertebral muscles to the clivus bone. The bedside surgeon can confirm that the bone is reached by sticking a metal suction catheter into the incision and palpating for bone. For lesions that have not invaded the prevertebral muscles, a small cuff of prevertebral muscle can be left to protect the clivus from exposure and subsequent osteonecrosis. The Maryland forceps are used to grasp the tumor and the surrounding tissue to provide countertraction for the dissection to proceed from an inferior to superior direction, reaching the middle part of the tumor. On the lateral aspect of the lesion, the Maryland forceps grasp the Eustachian tube cushion and the cautery spatula or cautery scissor are used to incise the Eustachian tube cartilage. The dissection then proceeds from lateral to medial on both sides. For the superior part of the dissection, the prevertebral muscles are absent. The incision is carried down to bone and then the mucosa and soft tissue of the nasopharynx is dissected away from the bone. The dissection converges towards the center of the resection specimen and the whole specimen can be delivered from the oral cavity. Soft tissue resection margins should be assessed by frozen section. The resection wound should then be irrigated and inspected for any bleeding, which then be controlled by the robotic cautery or the bipolar cautery of the bedside surgeon. 🎥 12.1 is an edited video showing the robotic assisted nasopharyngectomy performed via a transoral midline palatal split approach.

For the lateral palatal flap approach, the first part of the dissection is the detachment of the pharyngobasilar fascia and the lateral Eustachian tube cartilage from the medial pterygoid plate, in an inferior to superior direction. Following detachment of the pharyngobasilar fascia, the parapharyngeal fat and the medial part of the medial pterygoid muscle will be exposed. Depending on the lateral extent of the tumor, a decision is required whether or not to resect part of the medial pterygoid muscles. By grasping the medial pterygoid muscle with the Maryland forceps, the medial part of the muscle can be resected en bloc with the nasopharynx. Visualization of the parapharyngeal space during this part of the dissection can be improved by employing an upward facing 30° telescope turned towards the side of the dissection. The pharyngeal venous plexus runs through the medial pterygoid muscle and significant bleeding can be expected during the dissection of the medial pterygoid muscle. The bedside surgeon can assist hemostasis by introducing a bipolar cautery forceps through the mouth to cauterize these bleeders. Care must be taken during the dissection of the medial pterygoid muscles as the ICA lies posterior laterally and overzealous resection of the medial pterygoid muscle can expose or injure the ICA. The inferior incision is then performed, carried laterally to cut the inferior part of the medial pterygoid muscle. The specimen is then retracted superiorly and dissected out in an inferior to superior fashion similar to the midline palatal split approach. Care must be taken when dividing the Eustachian tube cartilage in the lateral aspect of the resection. The lateral palatal flap approach allows further lateral reach of the robotic instruments. The ICA turns medially towards midline and enters the foramen lacerum just lateral to the cartilaginous Eustachian tube at the skull base. Dividing the cartilaginous Eustachian tube too lateral and too close to the skull base can inadvertently injure the ICA. The rest of the resection is similar to the midline palatal split approach.

Incorporation of Transnasal Endoscopic Resection

One of the disadvantages of using the da Vinci surgical robot is the lack of instruments for bone removal. For tumors epicentered at the roof the nasopharynx, the floor of the sphenoid sinus may need to be removed to achieve an adequate resection margin. In other cases, tissue in the posterior choana or posterior nasal septum may need to be removed. Using robotic resection alone, disease in the posterior nasal cavities cannot be adequately visualized and resected from a transoral approach. In these situations, the operation can be assisted by transnasal endoscopic resection.[17] The inferior part of the resection is first performed with the da Vinci surgical robot but leaving the superior part of the dissection, namely the floor of the sphenoid or the posterior nasal cavities untouched. The patient cart of the robot is then undocked and the procedure is switched to a transnasal endoscopic resection with conventional transnasal endoscopic instruments. The superior mucosal resection margins are then marked and the mucosa dissected with dissectors. The bones in the floor of the sphenoid and posterior nasal cavities can then be removed with endoscopic drills or a Kerrison type of rongeur. The dissection is completed when the whole resection specimen is freed from the superior attachment and is removed inferiorly via the oral cavity.

Coverage of the Nasopharynx after Resection

After robotic nasopharyngectomy, the bone of the clivus is exposed. The area of exposed bone can increase depending on the extent of prevertebral muscle resection. Exposure of radiated clivus bone can lead to osteoradionecrosis (ORN). Osteoradionecrosis of the bone of the skull base is a significant long-term complication of nasopharyngectomy in the irradiated nasopharynx and has been shown to significantly affect the quality of life of the patients.[18] Covering the exposed raw bone in the clivus can decrease the chance of ORN. The best method of coverage is provided by vascularized tissue of the nasoseptal flap. The use of the nasoseptal flap has been popularized by the Pittsburg group and they have described the use of this flap in their transpterygoid endoscopic resection of the nasopharynx.[6] The nasoseptal flap can be used when one side of the sphenopalatine artery and nasal septum have not been disturbed. The flap is usually harvested at the end of the robotic resection using the endoscopic techniques described by the Pittsburg group.[19] The flap is rotated down to line the nasopharynx after applying fibrin glue to the raw area. The flap is kept in place by posterior nasal packs.

If utilization of the nasoseptal flap is not possible, an alternative method of coverage is to use a free mucosal graft harvested from the inferior turbinate or the posterior wall of the oropharynx. We have no experience in using allograft dermal matrix materials such as AlloDerm, for coverage of the nasopharynx.

Closure of the Palatal Wound

The closure of the palatal wound is extremely important to prevent the occurrence of palatal fistula and long-term velopharyngeal insufficiency. After confirming hemostasis, a nasogastric tube is inserted for feeding. Care must be taken not to dislodge the nasoseptal flap or graft in the posterior nasopharynx. A posterior nasal pack is used to bolster the nasoseptal flap or graft to the nasopharynx and prevent postoperative bleeding. The posterior nasal packing can be an inflated balloon of a Foley catheter or a long Merocel (Medtronics, Inc., Jacksonville, FL) nasal tampon (🎥 12.1).

The hard palate mucosa is closed in a single layer with interrupted absorbable sutures. Two or three holes are drilled in the posterior hard palate near the incision for attachment of the soft palate to the hard palate with absorbable sutures. Finally, the soft palate should be closed with absorbable sutures in three layers, one layer applied to the nasopharynx side of the soft palate, one layer to the tensor veli palatini muscle and finally the oral cavity side of the soft palate. The closure of tensor veli palatini muscle is especially important to restore the soft palate elevation motion.

Finally, the mouth gag is removed and the upper airway is checked for patency before extubation. If the soft tissue in the upper airway is swollen so that extubation may fail, the patient can either be kept intubated for 24 or 48 hours or a temporary tracheostomy is performed to protect the airway.

POSTOPERATIVE CARE

The patient is advised not to eat orally and avoid excessive talking to allow the palatal wound to heal. Nutritional support is given in the form of nasogastric tube feeding. The period of tube feeding usually lasts from 7 to 10 days. The patient is maintained on a soft diet until the palatal wound has healed. While the patient is not eating solids, he/she needs to perform regular mouth opening exercises with or without assistive devices such as Therabite (Amos, Sweden) to prevent fibrosis of the pterygoid muscles that can lead to trismus.

Antibiotics should be given until the nasal packs are removed. The posterior nasal packing should be removed after 5–7 days to allow time for the nasoseptal flap or graft to firmly adhere to the posterior nasopharynx wall.

After removal of the nasal packs, the patient should be instructed to irrigate the nasal cavities with normal saline to remove blood clots or dried secretions 3–5 times per day. The surgeon can clean the nasopharynx with gentle suction using nasoendoscopy weekly or fortnightly until the whole area is epithelialized. The patient should also be assessed for the presence of middle ear effusion and treated accordingly.

COMPLICATIONS

Major complications after robotic nasopharyngectomy are rare. The most fearsome complication is ICA injury. This can be prevented by careful case selection. In open nasopharyngectomy, the pulse of ICA can be palpated lateral to the parapharyngeal space and the course of the vessel can be traced from the oropharyngeal level up to the skull base without exposure of the artery. Tactile sensation is absent in robotic surgery and currently there is no reliable way to locate the ICA in robotic nasopharyngectomy. The best way to prevent ICA injury is by staying away from the artery.

All patients should have cross-sectional imaging to determine the relationship of the tumor to the ICA. Tumors closely abutting the ICA are not ideal candidates for robotic nasopharyngectomy. The whole course of the ICA should be traced from the neck up to the foramen lacerum on the cross-sectional imaging. Patients with ectatic ICAs that run medially abutting the fossa of Rosenmüller should also be excluded from robotic nasopharyngectomy.

Venous bleeding from the venous plexus in the pterygoid muscles can be troublesome. Control of the venous bleeding can be done with bipolar cautery applied by the bedside surgeon, or by using hemostatic agents such as Floseal (Baxter, Deerfield, IL) and packing.

Other intraoperative complications include inadvertent damage to the teeth and structures of the face and edema of the upper airway. Inadvertent damage to the teeth and oral cavity can be avoided by careful application of the mouth gag. A plastic lip retractor placed around the lip can prevent injury to the soft tissue of the lips and oral cavity by the shaft of the robotic instruments. The bedside surgeon needs to be vigilant of the robotic arms and shafts to prevent injury to the soft tissue of the face by the robotic arms. After the conclusion of the procedure, the mouth gag is released and removed. The patient should not be extubated immediately but instead left intubated for a period of 15–30 minutes to observe for any edema of the tongue, floor of mouth or larynx. If there is any edema or risk of airway obstruction, the patient should be kept intubated and send to the intensive care unit for 24-48 hours to allow the edema to subside before extubation. Alternatively, a tracheostomy can be performed.

Long-term complications of robotic nasopharyngectomy include dehiscence of the palatal wound leading to palatal fistula, trismus from fibrosis of the pterygoid muscles and ORN of the clivus and skull base. Palatal fistula is best prevented by good surgical techniques. The tissues of the palatal wound should be well approximated. The soft palate should be accurately reattached to the hard palate by stitches passing through holes drilled in the hard palate. The muscles of the soft palate, especially the tensor veli palatine muscles should be closed in a separate layer to restore the function of the muscle. The patient should avoid eating for 7–10 days to allow the soft palate wound to heal. A small dehiscence of the soft palate wound could be repaired primarily provided that there is no tension in the repair. Larger defects require a rotational palatal flap to close the defect. Alternatively, an obturator can prevent nasal regurgitation during speech and swallowing.

Following robotic nasopharyngectomy, patients typically experience trismus in the early postoperative period. The medial pterygoid muscle has received surgical trauma and stretching the muscle will cause pain, which in turn, produces trismus. However, long-term immobility of the medial pterygoid muscle will result in fibrosis and permanent trismus. It is imperative that the patient practice mouth opening exercises in the early postoperative period with under adequate pain control. A nonsteroidal anti-inflammatory drug and mouth opening assistive devices such as Therabite (Atos Medical AB, Sweden) can facilitate the mouth opening exercises.

Osteoradionecrosis of the skull base occurs after robotic nasopharyngectomy due to the exposure of the radiated skull bone to nasal secretions and microbes. Risks of ORN increase with increasing radiation and area of exposed bone. As mentioned before, coverage of the raw exposed bone after robotic nasopharyngectomy decreases the occurrence of ORN. For established ORN, conservative treatment includes a combination of long-term antibiotics and regular endoscopic debridement of necrotic tissue and crusts and pain control. Severe ORN may require surgical debridement and coverage of the debrided area with vascularized tissue such as a free flap.

FOLLOW-UP

In the early postoperative period, the patient should be advised to come for monthly or twice monthly follow-up for endoscopic cleaning of the nasopharynx. When the nasopharynx is completely epithelialized in 3 or 4 months, the patient can then be followed up less frequently. As the nasopharynx may be covered with mucosal flaps, regular cross-sectional imaging using MRI scan or PET-CT scan may be helpful in addition to nasoendoscopy in detecting early recurrences.

RESULTS

An early case series of 12 cases showed promising results using robotic nasopharyngectomy. Mean operative time was 240 minutes with a mean hospital stay of 7 days. Clear margins were achieved in nine patients and two patients had close margins. Only one patient had positive margin within the clivus bone. The 2-year local control rate was 87%. Patients were able to return to a normal oral diet with minimal morbidity. Long-term oncological results are still pending.[20]

FUTURE DIRECTIONS

The surgical robot is a relatively new tool in performing minimally invasive surgery. At the time of writing, the line-up of robotic instruments is not intentionally designed for surgery in the head and neck region. The instruments are comparatively bulky to be used intraorally. Alternative energy sources for dissection and hemostasis such as ultrasonic dissectors are available but they are not small and flexible enough to be used in the nasopharynx. Robotic instruments for bone removal have not yet been developed. In the near future, we hope to see the miniaturization of the current robotic instruments, which will be better adapted for use in the head and neck region.

The complexity of the anatomy in the head and neck region makes endoscopic dissection of the head and neck and skull base challenging. Computer-aided surgery in the form of navigation has greatly assisted the endoscopic surgeon to identify the anatomy and pathology during operation. There are still several obstacles that need to be overcome to integrate the computer navigation system with the surgical robot. For optical navigation systems, the placement of the optical cameras of the navigation system and the reference landmarks may need to be redesigned to prevent the robotic arms blocking the line of sight. The robotic arms may also affect magnetic fields and accuracy of the electromagnetic navigation systems. In the future, we hope the navigation system and robotic system can be integrated in one machine and the imaging scans can be overlaid on the 3D view from the telescope. This would greatly facilitate operations within the head and neck.

VIDEO LEGEND

Video 12.1: Robotic-Assisted Surgery for recurrent Nasopharyngeal cancer.

REFERENCES

1. Fee WE, Jr, Gilmer PA, Goffinet DR. Surgical management of recurrent nasopharyngeal carcinoma after radiation failure at the primary site. Laryngoscope. 1988;98(11):1220-6.
2. Morton RP, Liavaag PG, McLean M, et al. Transcervico-mandibulo-palatal approach for surgical salvage of recurrent nasopharyngeal cancer. Head Neck. 1996;18(4):352-8.
3. Wei WI, Lam KH, Sham JS. New approach to the nasopharynx: the maxillary swing approach. Head Neck. 1991; 13(3):200-7.
4. Fisch U. The infratemporal fossa approach for nasopharyngeal tumors. Laryngoscope. 1983;93(1):36-44.
5. Chen MK, Lai JC, Chang CC, et al. Minimally invasive endoscopic nasopharyngectomy in the treatment of recurrent T1-2a nasopharyngeal carcinoma. Laryngoscope. 2007;117(5): 894-6.
6. Al-Sheibani S, Zanation AM, Carrau RL, et al. Endoscopic endonasal transpterygoid nasopharyngectomy. Laryngoscope. 2011;121(10):2081-9.
7. Lee AW, Sze WM, Au JS, et al. Treatment results for nasopharyngeal carcinoma in the modern era: the Hong Kong experience. Int J Radiat Oncol Biol Phys. 2005;61(4):1107-16.
8. Yu KH, Leung SF, Tung SY, et al. Survival outcome of patients with nasopharyngeal carcinoma with first local failure: a study by the Hong Kong Nasopharyngeal Carcinoma Study Group. Head Neck. 2005;27(5):397-405.
9. Teo PM, Kwan WH, Chan AT, et al. How successful is high-dose (> or = 60 Gy) reirradiation using mainly external beams in salvaging local failures of nasopharyngeal carcinoma? Int J Radiat Oncol Biol Phys. 1998;40(4):897-913.
10. Wei WI, Chan JY, Ng RW, et al. Surgical salvage of persistent or recurrent nasopharyngeal carcinoma with maxillary swing approach—Critical appraisal after 2 decades. Head Neck. 2011;33(7):969-75.
11. Vlantis AC, Tsang RK, Yu BK, et al. Nasopharyngectomy and surgical margin status: a survival analysis. Arch Otolaryngol Head Neck Surg. 2007;133(12):1296-301.
12. Woo JKS. Clinical diagnosis. In: Van Hasselt CA, Gibb AG (Eds). Nasopharyngeal Carcinoma. Hong Kong: The Chinese University Press; 1999. p. 337.
13. Wei WI. Carcinoma of the nasopharynx. In: Myers EN, Bluestone CD, Brackmann DE, Krause CJ (Eds). Advances in Otolaryngology—Head and Neck Surgery. St. Louis: Mosby; 1998. p. 320.
14. Vlantis AC, Yu BK, Kam MK, et al. Nasopharyngectomy: does the approach to the nasopharynx influence survival? Otolaryngol Head Neck Surg. 2008;139(1):40-6.
15. Wei WI, Ho WK. Transoral robotic resection of recurrent nasopharyngeal carcinoma. Laryngoscope. 2010;120(10): 2011-4.
16. Tsang RK, Ho WK, Wei WI, et al. Transoral robotic assisted nasopharyngectomy via a lateral palatal flap approach. Laryngoscope. 2013;123(9):2180-3.
17. Yin Tsang RK, Ho WK, Wei WI. Combined transnasal endoscopic and transoral robotic resection of recurrent nasopharyngeal carcinoma. Head Neck. 2012;34(8):1190-3.
18. Chan YW, Chow VL, Wei WI. Quality of life of patients after salvage nasopharyngectomy for recurrent nasopharyngeal carcinoma. Cancer. 2012;118(15):3710-8.
19. Hadad G, Bassagasteguy L, Carrau RL, et al. A novel reconstructive technique after endoscopic expanded endonasal approaches: vascular pedicle nasoseptal flap. Laryngoscope. 2006;116(10):1882-6.
20. Tsang RK, To VS, Ho AC, et al. Early results of robotic assisted nasopharyngectomy for recurrent nasopharyngeal carcinoma. Head Neck. 2014. Epup ahead of print. doi:10.1002/hed.23672.

Chapter 13 Robot-Assisted Otologic and Neurotologic Surgery

Betty S Tsai Do

INTRODUCTION

The fields of otology and neurotology saw significant growth throughout the 20th century as new technologies were introduced, which then permitted a deeper understanding of the anatomy, promoting the development of better surgical techniques to address hearing and vestibular disorders, which required improved instrumentation and tools, thereby creating a continuous cycle of advancement. This included the introduction of the surgical microscope in the 1920s, the application of a drill for aural surgery, surgery for otosclerosis, the birth of skull base surgery in the 1960s, and more recently, the development of cochlear implants.[1-4] New technologies continue to shape these fields in the 21st century.

Robotic surgery, "the use of surgical robots in the performance of a surgery procedure", has been present since the mid-1980s.[5] Initially used for orthopedic and neurosurgical applications, robots are now used in various surgical subspecialties since the development of the Da Vinci surgical system.[6] While the use of the Da Vinci system is primarily limited to oral cavity, oropharyngeal and thyroid surgery, the first robots designed for otolaryngologic surgery targeted otologic applications.[7-9] Despite this, the use of robots in otologic and neurotologic surgery has yet to gain popularity.

This chapter will review the development of robotic surgery in the temporal bone and describe potential applications in otologic and neurotologic surgery.

RATIONALE FOR THE USE OF ROBOTICS IN SURGERY OF THE TEMPORAL BONE

A cortical mastoidectomy is a basic procedure that is performed in many otologic and neurotologic surgeries. The drilling of this cavity is a prerequisite for cochlear implants. Additionally, this procedure is commonly done as part of the translabyrinthine approach to the skull base. This portion of the procedure can sometimes be time consuming leaving the surgeon fatigued for the microscopic fine-motor work later in the case. Proponents of robotic-assisted surgery have suggested that the robot be employed for the early macroscopic drilling to leave the surgeon for the finer details, thereby improving surgical outcomes. However, as robotic technology continues to advance, human limitations on tactile sensitivity and dexterity may eventually be overcome in microsurgical procedures.[8,10] With that in mind, the finer microsurgical dissections also may benefit from the use of robotics in the future.

POTENTIAL APPLICATIONS IN OTOLOGIC AND NEUROTOLOGIC SURGERY

To date, a few prototype robotic systems have been described. Robots can be classified as surgical assist devices or as autonomous robots.[10] Because otologic and neurotologic surgery involves manipulation around bony landmarks, the use of image-guidance for autonomous robots is a possibility. This is significantly different from many other subspecialty surgeries in which soft tissue deformation will make it difficult for an autonomous robot to complete the planned task.

Robots that function as a surgical extender can eliminate hand tremor or allow a surgeon to perform more dexterous operations. One of the first robots described has been described to assist with the stapedotomy procedure.[7] The challenges typically presented to surgeons include the variable thickness of the stapes footplate, which can vary between 0.1–2.5 mm as well as the limited access to the stapes from the external auditory canal, which often requires removal of a small amount of bone from the scutum as shown in Figure 13.1. Robotic systems that automatically drill the footplate have been shown to have better force control on the footplate and minimize the protrusion of the instrument tip beyond the medial surface of the footplate in the micropick fenestration technique.[7,8] These robotic systems have also been shown to significantly

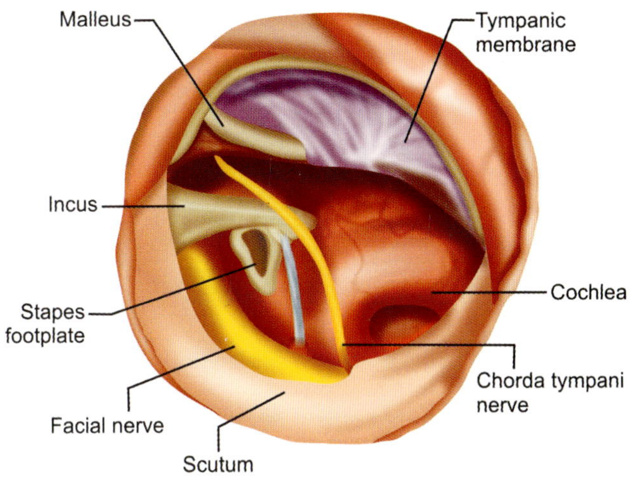

Fig. 13.1: Surgery in the middle ear space requires precise manipulation around some key structures as documented in the figure. Specifically, the close proximity of the facial nerve, stapes, and cochlea necessitates a great degree of accuracy in targeting the correct structure to minimize complications.

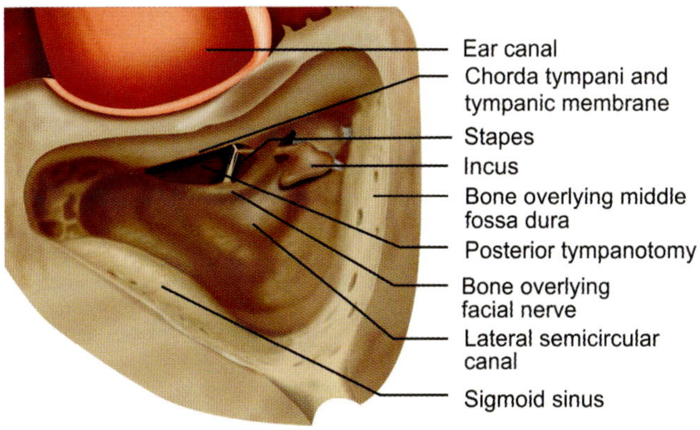

Fig. 13.2: Ideal result after drilling a cortical mastoidectomy and facial recess (posterior tympanotomy). These are common steps to otologic and neurotologic procedures such as a cochlear implant and removal of tumors from the temporal bone. Structures that are typically identified during the procedure include the tegmen mastoideum (bone overlying the middle fossa dura), sigmoid sinus, horizontal semicircular canal (horizontal canal), incus, chorda tympani nerve and facial nerve.

reduce the cumulative force applied to the stapes footplate.[8] While these results are promising, to date, both of these systems have only been tested in cadaveric bones.

Two of the first systems were designed for milling through the temporal bone.[9,11] Federspil et al. demonstrated that an industrial robot could be used to drill a well to house a cochlear implant.[9] Danilchenko et al. more recently showed that mastoid milling could be safely performed in a cadaveric model by integrating an image guidance system with an industrial robot without injury to any critical structures. Figure 13.2 demonstrates the typical landmarks that are identified during a cortical mastoidectomy. Because these landmarks are osseous, robots have been shown to reliably drill around these structures.

However, in order to accurately remove 96–99% of the target mastoid in their study, multiple additional steps need to be taken into account, including the ability to accurately register the mastoid with the image guidance system and to sterilize the robot. Additionally, the extra time taken for registration needs to be considered before a robot such as this can be made commercially available. Nevertheless, it is one of the first steps in creating a robot for otologic and neurotologic surgery. A different type of robot relying on ultrasound technology had also been proposed. Instead of relying on an intraoperative or preoperative computed tomography (CT) scan, the robot relies on live three-dimensional (3D) ultrasound scanning to generate intraoperative images thereby decreasing the planning time.[12] The authors demonstrated that bone thickness could be measured with an accuracy of about 0.5 mm and a maximum estimated imprecision of about 0.35 mm. Further research would be needed to determine potential applications of such a robot.

More recent research has been focused on developing a robot for cochlear implantation. The steps are fairly consistent from patient to patient, especially in those with normal anatomy. While a cortical mastoidectomy is fairly straightforward, the degree of precision and accuracy required for the creation of the facial recess and subsequent cochleostomy increases significantly as the room for error decreases. Additionally, studies have correlated better cochlear implant outcomes with decreased trauma during insertion making it more critical to be able to control the insertion force. Studies of the width of the extended facial recess have shown a maximum distance from 3.01 ± 0.40 to 4.11± 0.67 at the level of the facial nerve.[13,14] The actual space at the level of the round window during cochlear implantation is even less as sacrifice of the chorda tympani nerve is not routine for such surgeries. An average facial recess measurement is about 2.65 ± 0.63 mm in the plane of the round window.[15] Nevertheless, Labadie et al. have proven that using image-guidance, temporal bone drilling of the facial recess can be performed to an accuracy within 0.76 ± 0.23 mm as a precursor study to percutaneous cochlear implantation.[16] This study also demonstrated the ability to access the facial recess in a minimally invasive approach from the lateral mastoid cortex without drilling a mastoidectomy. Such an approach could potentially decrease operative time as well as postoperative recovery time.

Much of the focus on robotic surgery in otology has been its development for use in cochlear implantation. There are multiple factors that may affect patient outcomes including duration of deafness, duration of cochlear implant use, choice of processing algorithm, and method and quality of fitting.[17-20] However, there are also surgical factors that vary across patients that may affect their outcomes. One that has been well-studied is the electrode placement. Electrode insertions through the scala vestibuli have an increased risk of insertion-induced trauma to intracochlear structures with a negative impact to outcome.[21-23] Greater insertion depth has also been associated with lower outcome scores.[22] In the study by Finley et al., they hypothesized that these two variables may be improved by careful selection of cochleostomy sites with control of insertion depth.[22]

However, one of the most variable aspects of cochlear implantation is the cochleostomy. In a survey conducted in 2007 of 55 cochlear implant surgeons, there was significant variability in cochleostomy locations between surgeons with the majority selecting an anterior or inferior cochleostomy.[24] One of the benefits of robotic surgery is the more precise selection of the cochleostomy site using image guidance in order to optimize placement of the electrode into the scala tympani. Using bone-implanted fiducial markers for navigation, Klenzer et al., built a force-controlled robot to reliably create a cochleostomy at a predefined point on the cochlear promontory.[25] They demonstrated that using a 64 multi slice CT, middle and inner ear structures could be identified and properly segmented with the appropriate software, providing an excellent planning tool. Additionally, the target registration error using bone fiducials were 0.13–.37 mm (mean 0.25 mm), an acceptable level of accuracy for performing a precise cochleostomy.

One of the key features in drilling the cochleostomy is to avoid violation of the endosteal membrane especially in hearing preservation surgery. However, "blue-lining" the endosteal membrane with subsequent sharp opening with a knife or needle has been proven to be difficult.[26] The ideal robot should start drilling at point A as demonstrated in Figure 13.3 and stop at point B, just prior to entry through the endosteum (breakthrough point) as demonstrated in point C. Additionally, there have been suggestions that contamination of the inner ear by bone dust may result in early postoperative meningitis.[27] Fortunately, robotic technology has proven that this can be possible. Brett et al. described the first autonomous robot that relies on force and torque feedback during drilling to create a bony cochleostomy without entering the endosteal layer.[28] They subsequently proved this concept in a porcine trial by demonstrating the relative increase in the force to torque ratio during the drilling of the bony cochleostomy up unto the breakthrough point, after which the force feedback decreases significantly whereas the torque continues to increase as the endosteal membrane is penetrated.[29] Because the cochleostomy is accessed through a limited opening through the facial recess, Du et al. created a smart micro-drill that permitted alignment of the drill several millimeters away from the target site that could still penetrate through a narrow aperture such as a the facial recess. Using a chuck, they were able to stabilize the drill bits and align them to the desired trajectory.[30]

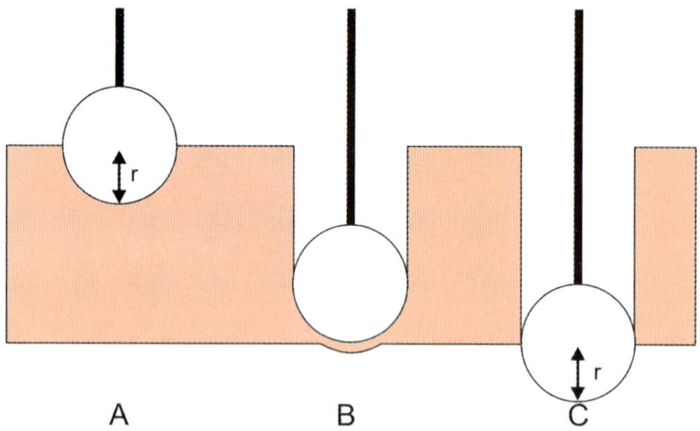

Figs. 13.3A to C: Drill positions at different stages of the cochleostomy drilling. Initially as the drill advances through the bone (A), the surface area of the drill on the bone increases, increasing the force by the drill on the surrounding bone. It continues to increase until the bone adjacent to the endosteum is thinned out (B). However, there needs to be a quick drop in force prior to breaking through the bone (C) in order to minimize trauma into the cochlea. Force feedback from the drill during this process has been shown to protect autonomous drills from breaking through the endosteum.

More recently, the technique is being applied to the pediatric population. Unlike the adult patients in which the inner ear and mastoid have already developed, pediatric temporal bones are developing in the early years of life. Specifically, as the mastoids develop in the first few years of life, imaging characteristics may change significantly between preoperative and intraoperative imaging.[31] This requires modification of the preoperative registration technique. However, an excellent understanding of the anatomy can make this possible.

In addition to the cochleostomy, another factor involved in cochlear implant outcomes is the amount of trauma sustained by the cochlea during the insertion of the electrodes. This is especially important in preserving cochlear structures to accommodate for concurrent electro-acoustic stimulation (EAS). Manufacturers have designed a variety of electrode arrays such as perimodiolar arrays, thin electrodes and shorter electrodes to minimize the trauma. Additionally, surgeons have modified their techniques such as the soft surgery approach to insertion or the advance off-stylet approach to limit cochlear damage. One of the benefits of robot-assisted surgery is the ability to measure and limit the force applied during the insertion of the implant electrode compared to the variability from that of a human hand. Studies have shown that robotic insertion forces regardless of insertion technique (traditional insertion versus advance off-stylet) average approximately 0.006 N up to an insertion depth of 7 mm. On the other hand, for deeper insertions beyond 9.74 mm, located at the end of the basal turn, the advance off-stylet insertion force averaged 0.008 ± 0.006 N with a peak of 0.034 N compared to the traditional insertion force which averaged 0.046 ± 0.027 N with a peak force of 0.093 N.[32] Compared to manual insertions by experienced surgeons, the forces across the entire insertion depth are similar (0.005 ± 0.014 N for the robot, 0.004 ± 0.001 N for the surgeon in advance off-stylet technique) with surgeons out-performing the robot.[32] However, the peak insertion forces between 120° and 200° are much higher by the surgeons, which the authors attributed to an increased insertion speed by the surgeons compared to the automated robotic insertion. The authors concluded that the difference between the average insertion forces are not significant enough clinically but that the decreased force peaks may be more significant for minimizing trauma-induced damage.[32]

While electrode and insertion modifications seek to limit the amount of trauma generated within the cochlea, straight electrodes inevitably come into contact with the external wall while perimodialar electrodes have the potential to injure the modiolus or turn on themselves as they curl. To address this, Zhang et al. have developed a robot-assisted steerable electrode prototype.[33] They designed a robot that not only could sense forces but also has four degrees of freedom to steer the electrode through the scala tympani with a maximum insertion force reduction by 59.6%. While conceptually this robot-assisted steerable array allows for more precise placement with less trauma, the ability to limit traumatic forces still is dependent on the characteristics of the electrode when it is fabricated.

Surgical access to the petrous apex has also been proven to be challenging whether it be through an infralabyrinthine, infracochlear, subarcuate, or retrolabyrinthine approaches. For surgical drainage of lesions such as the cholesterol granuloma, only a small surgical opening is needed and robots can create such tracts with submillimeter accuracy. Recently, a case report described success with an approach using an image-guided automated approach with the stereotactic microframes.[34] In using robot-assisted guidance, limited mastoid exposure was required to create an infralabyrinthine tract to the petrous apex. Additionally, critical structures such as the posterior semicircular canal, facial nerve, carotid artery and sigmoid sinus were not exposed or violated. The subarcuate path, which requires the creation of the tract through the center of the superior semicircular canal, about 4.7 mm in diameter, would have been extremely difficult without robotic assistance. In this case report, the use of the image-guidance permitted the creation of such a tract with considerable accuracy. Furthermore, the total intraoperative time was significantly less than what would traditionally have been expected. Images demonstrating such a trajectory are shown in Figures 13.4A and B.

Future applications of robotic surgery include the development of an automated system to mill the bone up until the opening of the internal auditory canal during a translabyrinthine approach for skull base surgeries. Oftentimes, a significant amount of time is spent on drilling out the mastoid, facial recess and labyrinth prior to exposing the tumor in the internal auditory canal. With similar principles to the drilling of the cochlear implant and mastoidectomy, using image guidance, one could design robotic surgery techniques to mill the bone adjacent to the sigmoid sinus, middle fossa and facial nerve in addition to the internal auditory canal as each of these structures are embedded within or serve as borders for the temporal bone. With a robot performing much of the tedious task to drilling, the surgeon can then focus on decompressing the sigmoid sinus, middle fossa and internal auditory canal in addition to the finer task of dissecting tumors, such as peeling the acoustic neuroma off the facial nerve.

Another potential application of robotic surgery is using the automated system to drill the temporal bone via a middle fossa approach. Unlike the retrosigmoid and translabyrinthine approaches where landmarks are easily visualized, identification of structures in the middle fossa is more nebulous. Even the relationship between the arcuate eminence and the superior semicircular canal has

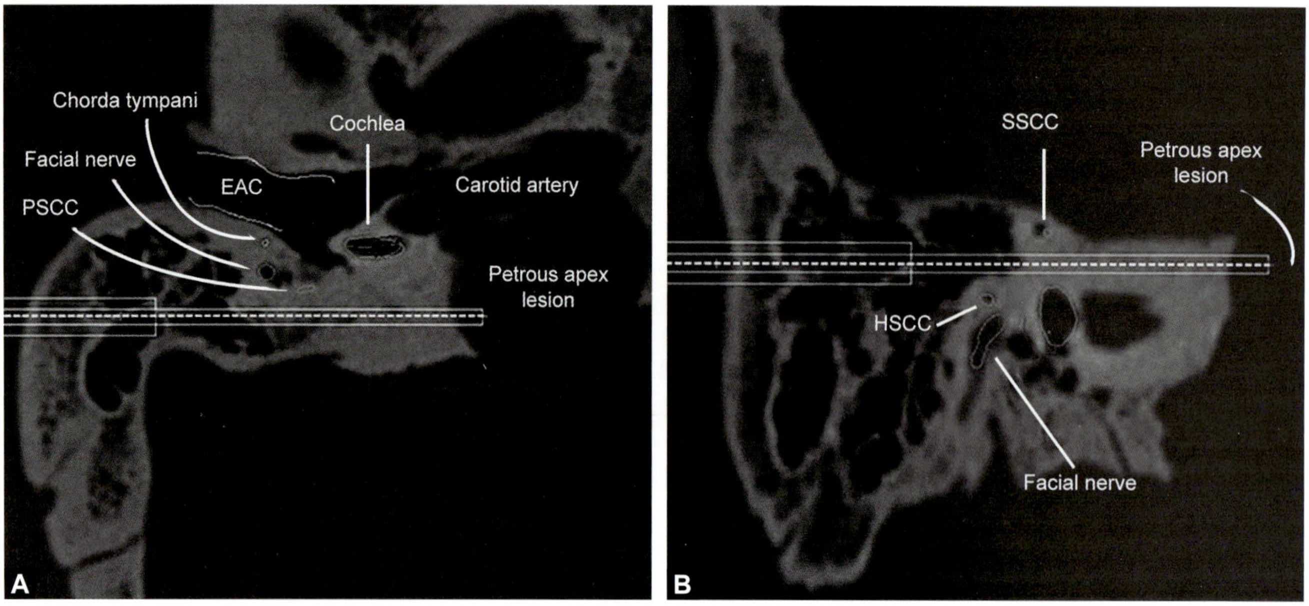

Figs. 13.4 A and B: During the preoperative imaging evaluation, a pathway that does not violate important key structures to the target needs to be identified. In the figure here, it is important to ensure that the facial nerve, external auditory canal, sigmoid sinus, and semicircular canals are safe from the anticipated trajectory of the drill with some margin of safety. If such a path does not exist, robotic surgery is not recommended. (PSCC: Posterior semicircular canal; HSCC: Horizontal semicircular canal; SSCC: Superior semicircular canal; EAC: External auditory canal).
Source: Taken from Balachandran et al.[34] with permission.

been described to be variable.[35] In otologic surgery, the middle fossa approach is often used to achieve hearing preservation for the resection of intracanalicular acoustic neuromas. Not only does this require careful dissection within the internal auditory canal protecting both the facial and cochlear nerves, it also requires that the surgeon avoid drilling the cochlea, which lies in close proximity to the lateral internal auditory canal. While image-guided surgery would be useful for such an approach, the accuracy of a robot would be beneficial in minimizing injury to critical structures.

INDICATIONS AND CONTRAINDICATIONS

While difficult to access anatomy may be considered an indication for image-guided robotic otology surgery, it could also be considered a contraindication. With most robots with limited degrees of freedom (DOF), if the following structures on imaging studies reveal abnormalities, i.e. congenital, then a traditional approach may be recommended:

- Facial nerve
- External auditory canal
- Cochlear anatomy

Imaging obtained during the preoperative workup may be the deciding factor as to whether or not to proceed with robot-assisted otologic surgery. The lack of a safe drilling path for the robot, such as obstruction by the facial nerve or external auditory canal would be considered a contraindication to robotic surgery. On the other hand, a difficult to visualize anatomic location such as an ossified cochlea may be considered an indication if there exists a path for the robot to drill and open up.

PREOPERATIVE WORKUP

Before any patients are considered candidates for robotic surgery, they must be surgical candidates first. The standard otologic and neurotologic workup including history, physical exam, audiogram, and relevant imaging should have already been completed. During this time, the preoperative imaging can be used to determine if there exists an accessible pathway from the lateral head to the area of interest whether it be the cochlea, petrous apex, or middle ear. In the rare circumstance in which this pathway does not exist, the robotic approach cannot be used.

In order for a robot to accurately drill in the targeted area, a high-resolution CT scan for image-guidance is required. Current commonly used image guidance

Table 13.1: Image guidance systems used in otolaryngologic surgery

Image-guidance system	*Manufacturer*	*TRE (mm)*	*Fiducial*	*Reference*
BrainLAB™	BrainLAB, Heimstetten, Germany	1.31 ± 0.87 2.77 ± 1.64 2.28 ± 0.91	Skin affixed markers Laser skin contour Proprietary headset	Schlaier, et al. 2002[41]
InstaTrak™	GE Medical Systems, Lawrence, MA	1.97	Skin affixed markers	Fried, et al. 1997[42]
StealthStation™	Medtronic Surgical Navigation Technologies, Louisville, CO	1.14 2.3 0.96	Skin affixed markers Anatomic landmarks Surface-merged	Pfisterer, et al. 2008[43]
Stryker Image Guidance System™	Stryker Instruments, Kalamazoo, MI	0.48 ± 0.21	Bone-implanted fiducials	Pillai. et al. 2008[44]

Listed in this table are the target registration errors (TRE) for various navigation systems that have been used in otolaryngologic surgery. Because data for the Medtronic Fusion system was not available from the manufacturer at the time of publication, data from the Medtronic Stealth Station, which is commonly used for combined skull base procedures was listed.

systems have been reported to accuracies of 2 mm or less as shown in Table 13.1.[36] However, studies have shown that the most accurate systems rely on bone-implanted fiducial markers.[37,38] Given that the error margin most of these systems that do not rely on bone-implanted fiducial markers overlap with the maximum distance of the facial recess, to minimize injury to the facial nerve, imaging with bone-implanted fiducials is required. The fiducials may be placed the day before as part of the preoperative imaging or on the day of surgery with intraoperative imaging. From this imaging, software can be used to design a stereotactic microframe secured to these bone fiducial markers in order to maintain the accuracy during the robotic drilling. Benefits of placing the fiducials the day before allow for preoperative surgical planning that can cut down intraoperative surgical time, such as the fabrication of a custom microtable. However, this requires that the patient undergo two procedures, one to implant the fiducials, the other for the actual otologic surgery itself. Alternatively, the fiducials and the surgery could be performed on the same day with a slight extension in the intraoperative surgical time instead.

Another consideration is prior surgery in a patient, especially prior craniotomies, whether it be middle fossa or suboccipital. The presence of a bony defect may limit the ability to place fiducials close to the intended target area thereby increasing the margin of error. This must be taken into account when deciding whether or not an image-guidance approach is possible.

COMPLICATIONS

Much of the mastoidectomy drillout in otologic and neurotologic procedures allows for identification of key structures in order to minimize complications while accessing a very specific portion of the ear. In cochlear implantation, a cortical mastoidectomy with facial recess drillout requires that the tegmen, horizontal semicircular canal and incus be identified in order to safely drill out the facial recess which requires more precise identification of the facial and chorda tympani nerves. Once that is done, only can the search for the cochlear round window begin. In robotic surgery, these landmarks are not necessarily searched in a sequential pattern, but rather, advance planning with navigational technologies help to limit the error in obtaining a direct path to the target. As demonstrated in Figures 13.4A and B and previously described, a direct trajectory avoiding key structures needs to be identified. Structures at risk for most otologic and neurotologic surgeries include the facial nerve, chorda tympani nerve, sigmoid sinus, carotid artery and labyrinth. Specifically, higher priorities are given to the facial nerve which innervates the muscles of facial expression and the carotid artery, the main blood supply to the brain. However, injury to the sigmoid sinus can also result in significant blood loss, and injury to the labyrinth can result in complete hearing loss and vertigo.

Simulations on temporal bones using image-guidance with bone-implanted fiducials, which have been demonstrated to have the highest degree of accuracy (*see* Table 13.1), have been imperfect. In a study with 10 temporal bones in an attempt to drill a cochleostomy in preparation for a cochlear implant, 3/10 bones resulted in violation of nearby structures (2 stapes, 1 chorda tympani).[39] On the other hand, there was no injury to the facial nerve in any of the temporal bones. When the authors of the study reviewed the preoperative imaging, it was noted that in those specimens, the facial recess was more narrow and that these structures were already at risk. While sacrifice of the chorda tympani nerve occurs in 20% of pediatric cochlear implant cases, injury to the stapes in the era of hearing preservation is not considered acceptable.[40] The authors therefore concluded that a narrow facial recess may be considered a contraindication to robotic surgery given the higher rate of potential complications.

CONCLUSION

While robotic surgery is commonly being used in many aspects of otolaryngology, and significant advances have been made for use in otologic and neurotologic surgery, additional modifications are required to make them safe for routine otologic surgery. While preliminary temporal bone studies are promising, the close proximity of key structures requiring a high degree of accuracy with currently available commercial image-guidance systems may limit the use of automated systems at this time. However, as technology continues to advance, the greater precision of robots may eventually improve surgical outcomes in select situations in the future.

REFERENCES

1. Holmgren G. Operations on the temporal bone carried out with the help of the lens and the microscope. Acta Otolaryngol 1922;4:383-93.
2. Holmgren G. Some experiences in the surgery of otosclerosis. Acta Otolaryngol 1923;5:460-6.
3. Shambaugh GE, Jr. Julius Lempert and the fenestration operation. Am J Otol 1955;16:247-52.
4. Glasscock ME, 3rd. The history of neuro-otology. A personal perspective. Otolaryngol Clin North Am 2002;35:227-38.
5. Gourin CG, Terris DJ. Surgical robotics in otolaryngology: expanding the technology envelope. Current opinion in otolaryngology & head and neck surgery 2004;12:204-8.
6. Nguyen Y, Miroir M, Kazmitcheff G, et al. From conception to application of a tele-operated assistance robot for middle ear surgery. Surgical innovation 2012;19:241-51.
7. Brett PN, Baker DA, Reyes L, et al. An automatic technique for micro-drilling a stapedotomy in the flexible stapes footplate. Proceedings of the Institution of Mechanical Engineers Part H, Journal of engineering in medicine 1995; 209:255-62.
8. Rothbaum DL, Roy J, Stoianovici D, et al. Robot-assisted stapedotomy: micropick fenestration of the stapes footplate. Otolaryngol Head Neck Surg 2002;127:417-26.
9. Federspil PA, Geisthoff UW, Henrich D, et al. Development of the first force-controlled robot for otoneurosurgery. Laryngoscope 2003;113:465-71.
10. Taylor RH. A perspective on medical robotics. P Ieee 2006;94:1652-64.
11. Danilchenko A, Balachandran R, Toennies JL, et al. Robotic mastoidectomy. Otol Neurotol 2011;32:11-6.
12. Stolka PJ, Henrich D, Tretbar SH, et al. First 3D ultrasound scanning, planning, and execution of CT-free milling interventions with a surgical robot. Conference proceedings: Annual International Conference of the IEEE Engineering in Medicine and Biology Society IEEE Engineering in Medicine and Biology Society Conference 2008;2008:5605-10.
13. Young YS, Nadol JB, Jr. Dimensions of the extended facial recess. The Annals of otology, rhinology, and laryngology 1989;98:336-8.
14. Teszler CB, Ruimi D, Bar-Meir E, Luntz M. Width of the extended facial recess: a numerical study of ultrahigh-resolution computed tomography and its implications in minimally invasive otologic surgery. Otol Neurotol 2005;26:782-9.
15. Bielamowicz SA, Coker NJ, Jenkins HA, et al. Surgical dimensions of the facial recess in adults and children. Arch Otolaryngol Head Neck Surg 1988;114:534-7.
16. Labadie RF, Chodhury P, Cetinkaya E, et al. Minimally invasive, image-guided, facial-recess approach to the middle ear: demonstration of the concept of percutaneous cochlear access in vitro. Otol Neurotol 2005;26:557-62.
17. Blamey P, Arndt P, Bergeron F, et al. Factors affecting auditory performance of postlinguistically deaf adults using cochlear implants. Audiol Neurootol 1996;1:293-306.
18. Friedland DR, Venick HS, Niparko JK. Choice of ear for cochlear implantation: the effect of history and residual hearing on predicted postoperative performance. Otol Neurotol 2003;24:582-9.
19. Skinner MW. Optimizing cochlear implant speech performance. Ann Otol Rhinol Laryngol Suppl 2003;191:4-13.
20. Wilson BS, Finley CC, Farmer JC, Jr., et al. Comparative studies of speech processing strategies for cochlear implants. Laryngoscope 1988;98:1069-77.
21. Briggs RJ, Tykocinski M, Stidham K, et al. Cochleostomy site: implications for electrode placement and hearing preservation. Acta Otolaryngol 2005;125:870-6.
22. Finley CC, Holden TA, Holden LK, et al. Role of electrode placement as a contributor to variability in cochlear implant outcomes. Otol Neurotol 2008;29:920-8.
23. Aschendorff A, Kubalek R, Turowski B, et al. Quality control after cochlear implant surgery by means of rotational tomography. Otol Neurotol 2005;26:34-7.
24. Adunka OF, Buchman CA. Scala tympani cochleostomy I: results of a survey. Laryngoscope 2007;117:2187-94.
25. Klenzner T, Ngan CC, Knapp FB, et al. New strategies for high precision surgery of the temporal bone using a robotic approach for cochlear implantation. Eur Arch Otorhinolaryngol 2009;266:955-60.
26. James C, Albegger K, Battmer R, et al. Preservation of residual hearing with cochlear implantation: how and why. Acta Otolaryngol 2005;125:481-91.
27. Nadol JB, Jr., Eddington DK. Histologic evaluation of the tissue seal and biologic response around cochlear implant electrodes in the human. Otol Neurotol 2004;25:257-62.
28. Brett PN, Taylor RP, Proops D, et al. A surgical robot for cochleostomy. Conference proceedings: Annual International Conference of the IEEE Engineering in Medicine and Biology Society IEEE Engineering in Medicine and Biology Society Conference 2007;2007:1229-32.

29. Coulson CJ, Taylor RP, Reid AP, et al. An autonomous surgical robot for drilling a cochleostomy: preliminary porcine trial. Clinical otolaryngology : official journal of ENT-UK; official journal of Netherlands Society for Oto-Rhino-Laryngology & Cervico-Facial Surgery 2008;33:343–7.
30. Du X, Assadi MZ, Jowitt F, et al. Robustness analysis of a smart surgical drill for cochleostomy. The international journal of medical robotics + computer assisted surgery : MRCAS 2013;9:119–26.
31. Balachandran R, Reda FA, Noble JH, et al. Minimally invasive image-guided cochlear implantation for pediatric patients: clinical feasibility study. Otolaryngol Head Neck Surg 2014;150:631–7.
32. Schurzig D, Webster RJ, 3rd, Dietrich MS, et al. Force of cochlear implant electrode insertion performed by a robotic insertion tool: comparison of traditional versus Advance Off-Stylet techniques. Otol Neurotol 2010;31:1207–10.
33. Zhang J, Wei W, Ding J, et al. Inroads toward robot-assisted cochlear implant surgery using steerable electrode arrays. Otol Neurotol 2010;31:1199–206.
34. Balachandran R, Tsai BS, Ramachandra T, et al. Minimally invasive image-guided access for drainage of petrous apex lesions: a case report. Otol Neurotol 2014;35:649–55.
35. Kartush JM, Kemink JL, Graham MD. The arcuate eminence. Topographic orientation in middle cranial fossa surgery. The Annals of otology, rhinology, and laryngology 1985;94:25–8.
36. Labadie RF, Davis BM, Fitzpatrick JM. Image-guided surgery: what is the accuracy? Current opinion in otolaryngology & head and neck surgery 2005;13:27–31.
37. Labadie RF, Shah RJ, Harris SS, et al. In vitro assessment of image-guided otologic surgery: submillimeter accuracy within the region of the temporal bone. Otolaryngol Head Neck Surg 2005;132:435–42.
38. Grauvogel TD, Soteriou E, Metzger MC, et al. Influence of different registration modalities on navigation accuracy in ear, nose, and throat surgery depending on the surgical field. Laryngoscope 2010;120:881–8.
39. Majdani O, Rau TS, Baron S, et al. A robot-guided minimally invasive approach for cochlear implant surgery: preliminary results of a temporal bone study. International journal of computer assisted radiology and surgery 2009; 4:475–86.
40. Bhatia K, Gibbin KP, Nikolopoulos TP, et al. Surgical complications and their management in a series of 300 consecutive pediatric cochlear implantations. Otol Neurotol 2004;25: 730–9.
41. Schlaier J, Warnat J, Brawanski A. Registration accuracy and practicability of laser-directed surface matching. Computer aided surgery : official journal of the International Society for Computer Aided Surgery 2002;7:284-90.
42. Fried MP, Kleefield J, Gopal H, et al. Image-guided endoscopic surgery: results of accuracy and performance in a multicenter clinical study using an electromagnetic tracking system. Laryngoscope 1997;107:594–601.
43. Pfisterer WK, Papadopoulos S, Drumm DA, et al. Fiducial versus nonfiducial neuronavigation registration assessment and considerations of accuracy. Neurosurgery 2008;62: 201–7; discussion 7–8.
44. Pillai P, Sammet S, Ammirati M. Application accuracy of computed tomography-based, image-guided navigation of temporal bone. Neurosurgery 2008;63:326-32; discussion 32–3.

Index

Note: Page numbers followed by *f* and *t* refer to figure and table, respectively.

U

V

W

Z